D0425617

PERSONALITY AND PSYCHOPATHOLOGY

PERSONALITY
AND
PSYCHOPATHOLOGY

Edited by
ROBERT F. KRUEGER
JENNIFER L. TACKETT

THE GUILFORD PRESS
New York   London

© 2006 The Guilford Press
A Division of Guilford Publications, Inc.
72 Spring Street, New York, NY 10012
www.guilford.com

Printed in the United States of America

This book is printed on acid-free paper.

Last digit is print number: 9 8 7 6 5 4 3 2 1

Library of Congress Cataloging-in-Publication Data

Personality and psychopathology / edited by Robert F. Krueger
and Jennifer L. Tackett.
       p. cm.
Includes bibliographical references and index.
ISBN-13: 978-1-59385-288-7
ISBN-10: 1-59385-288-6
1. Personality disorders. 2. Personality. 3. Psychology, Pathological.
I. Krueger, Robert F. II. Tackett, Jennifer L.
RC554.P452 2006
616.85'81—dc22
                                           2006002863

For our families

About the Editors

Robert F. Krueger, PhD, is Associate Professor of Clinical Psychology and Individual Differences, Personality, and Behavior Genetics in the Department of Psychology, and Adjunct Associate Professor of Child Psychology in the Institute of Child Development, at the University of Minnesota, Twin Cities. He received the American Psychological Association's 2006 Theodore Millon Mid-Career Award in Personality and Psychology, the American Psychological Association's 2005 Distinguished Scientific Award for Early Career Contribution to Psychology, a 2003 Early Career Award from the International Society for the Study of Individual Differences. He also holds a McKnight Presidential Fellowship from the University of Minnesota. Dr. Krueger obtained his doctorate from the University of Wisconsin at Madison and completed his clinical internship at Brown University. He is currently an associate editor of the *Journal of Abnormal Psychology* and the *Journal of Personality*, and has served on the editorial boards of a variety of other journals.

Jennifer L. Tackett, MA, is a doctoral candidate in the Clinical Science and Psychopathology Training Program at the University of Minnesota, Twin Cities. She has published work on childhood antisocial behavior, personality–psychopathology relationships, and childhood personality in the *Journal of Abnormal Child Psychology*, the *Journal of Abnormal Psychology*, and the *Journal of Personality Disorders*. She was a recipient of a 2-year (2001–2003) National Institute of Mental Health fellowship from a training grant titled "Neurobehavioral Aspects of Personality and Psychopathology." Currently, Ms. Tackett is completing her clinical internship at the Veterans Affairs Medical Center in Minneapolis. In the fall of 2006, she will begin an appointment as Assistant Professor of Psychology at the University of Toronto.

Contributors

Susan M. Andersen, PhD, Department of Psychology, New York University, New York, New York

Edward M. Bernat, PhD, Department of Psychology, University of Minnesota, Twin Cities, Minneapolis, Minnesota

Pavel Blagov, MA, Department of Psychology, Emory University, Atlanta, Georgia

Richard A. Depue, PhD, Laboratory of Neurobiology of Personality, Cornell University, Ithaca, New York

Glen O. Gabbard, MD, Department of Psychiatry, Baylor College of Medicine, Houston, Texas

Wakiza Gamez, MA, Department of Psychology, University of Iowa, Iowa City, Iowa

Kerry L. Jang, PhD, Department of Psychiatry, University of British Columbia, Vancouver, British Columbia, Canada

Roman Kotov, MA, Department of Psychology, University of Iowa, Iowa City, Iowa

Robert F. Krueger, PhD, Department of Psychology, University of Minnesota, Twin Cities, Minneapolis, Minnesota

Benjamin B. Lahey, PhD, Department of Health Studies, University of Chicago, Chicago, Illinois

Roseann Larstone, PhD, Department of Psychiatry, University of British Columbia, Vancouver, British Columbia, Canada

Mark F. Lenzenweger, PhD, Department of Psychology, State University of New York at Binghamton, Binghamton, New York; Department of Psychiatry, Weill Medical College of Cornell University, New York, New York

Björn Meyer, PhD, Department of Psychology, City University, London, United Kingdom

Regina Miranda, PhD, Department of Psychology, Hunter College, City University of New York, New York, New York

Stephanie N. Mullins-Sweatt, MA, Department of Psychology, University of Kentucky, Lexington, Kentucky

Thomas F. Oltmanns, PhD, Department of Psychology, Washington University, St. Louis, Missouri

Christopher J. Patrick, PhD, Department of Psychology, University of Minnesota, Twin Cities, Minneapolis, Minnesota

Paul A. Pilkonis, PhD, Department of Psychiatry, University of Pittsburgh Medical Center, Western Psychiatric Institute and Clinic, Pittsburgh, Pennsylvania

Amber L. Singh, MS, Department of Psychology, Emory University, Atlanta, Georgia

Jennifer L. Tackett, MA, Clinical Science and Psychopathology Training Program, University of Minnesota, Twin Cities, Minneapolis, Minnesota

Eric Turkheimer, PhD, Department of Psychology, University of Virginia, Charlottesville, Virginia

Irwin D. Waldman, PhD, Department of Psychology, Emory University, Atlanta, Georgia

David Watson, PhD, Department of Psychology, University of Iowa, Iowa City, Iowa

Drew Westen, PhD, Department of Psychology and Department of Psychiatry and Behavioral Sciences, Emory University, Atlanta, Georgia

Thomas A. Widiger, PhD, Department of Psychology, University of Kentucky, Lexington, Kentucky

Heike Wolf, PhD, Differential Psychology and Psychological Diagnostics, University of the Saarland, Saarbrücken, Germany

Contents

1   Introduction   1
Robert F. Krueger and Jennifer L. Tackett

2   Basic Dimensions of Temperament in Relation to Personality   7
and Psychopathology
David Watson, Roman Kotov, and Wakiza Gamez

3   The Five-Factor Model of Personality Disorder: A Translation across Science   39
and Practice
Stephanie N. Mullins-Sweatt and Thomas A. Widiger

4   Perceptions of Self and Others Regarding Pathological Personality Traits   71
Thomas F. Oltmanns and Eric Turkheimer

5   Dispositional Dimensions and the Causal Structure of Child and Adolescent   112
Conduct Problems
Irwin D. Waldman, Amber L. Singh, and Benjamin B. Lahey

6   What Is the Role of Personality in Psychopathology?:   153
A View from Behavior Genetics
Kerry L. Jang, Heike Wolf, and Roseann Larstone

7   The Construct of Emotion as a Bridge between Personality   174
and Psychopathology
Christopher J. Patrick and Edward M. Bernat

8   A Multidimensional Neurobehavioral Model of Personality Disturbance   210
    Richard A. Depue and Mark F. Lenzenweger

9   Developing Treatments That Bridge Personality and Psychopathology   262
    Björn Meyer and Paul A. Pilkonis

10 Through the Lens of the Relational Self: Triggering Emotional Suffering   292
    in the Social-Cognitive Process of Transference
    Susan M. Andersen and Regina Miranda

11 Back to the Future: Personality Structure as a Context for Psychopathology 335
    Drew Westen, Glen O. Gabbard, and Pavel Blagov

    Index   385

Chapter 1

Introduction

ROBERT F. KRUEGER
JENNIFER L. TACKETT

Historically, personality and psychopathology have been relatively distinct areas of inquiry. There are numerous instantiations of this split. In academic departments of psychology, the study of personality is often represented in social psychology area groups rather than clinical psychology area groups, and clinical psychologists are more likely to study psychopathology than are social psychologists. In the *Diagnostic and Statistical Manuals* of the American Psychiatric Association, from DSM-III to the current DSM-IV-TR, personality is described separately from current psychopathology, on a distinct descriptive "axis"; personality disorders are recorded on Axis II, and current psychopathological syndromes are recorded on Axis I. Moreover, distinct journals exist to serve the study of personality and psychopathology. For example, among journals published by the American Psychological Association, personality research tends to appear in the *Journal of Personality and Social Psychology*, whereas basic research on psychopathology tends to appear in the *Journal of Abnormal Psychology*.

In spite of this historical separation in both psychology and psychiatry, a number of influential programs of research and theorizing have emerged at the intersection of these areas. These programs are diverse in their inspiration and focus. For example, some programs begin with the notion of basic temperaments and extrapolate to the idea that the normal ranges of those temperaments manifest as personality, whereas abnormal range temperament confers risk to psychopathology. Some programs begin with the classic psychodynamic observation that psychopathology is best under-

stood in the context of the patient's character structure. Some begin with
the observation that fundamental neurobehavioral and genetic systems underlie manifest personality traits and that these systems might serve as underlying bases (or "endophenotypes") for psychopathology. Although these
perspectives have distinct historical and intellectual origins, they share the
common premise that psychopathology is better understood when viewed
in the context of personality, and that personality theorizing and research is
enriched by considering how personality can be manifested in psychopathology. The aim of *Personality and Psychopathology* is to bring together the most eminent scholars driving these integrative programs of research and theorizing in one volume.

The volume begins with a pair of chapters focused on the relationship
between temperament, personality and psychopathology. Watson, Kotov,
and Gamez (Chapter 2) address relationships between personality and
psychopathology within the context of a hierarchical model of temperament constructs. Specifically, they focus on the Big Two dimensions of temperament: Neuroticism or Negative Emotionality (N/NE) and Extraversion
or Positive Emotionality (E/PE). The authors utilize these two superfactors
as well as associated lower-order factors as a framework for understanding
psychopathology. Broad connections between the Big Two and mental disorders are reviewed, with an emphasis on the mood and anxiety disorders.
Data are presented to illustrate specific relationships between disorders and
lower-order facets of the temperament dimensions, highlighting the importance of utilizing multiple levels of the hierarchical structure of personality.
In addition, the authors seek to integrate "clinical traits" related to the
mood and anxiety disorders, such as anxiety sensitivity and self-criticism,
into our understanding of the connections between personality and psychopathology. Throughout the chapter, the authors present compelling evidence for an organizing framework of personality and psychopathology
that captures these diverse constructs in an integrative hierarchical structure.

The five-factor model (FFM) is proposed as a bridge between personality and personality pathology by Mullins-Sweatt and Widiger (Chapter 3).
Their chapter provides a review of support for the FFM as a model of personality structure, including the lexical basis of the FFM, validity of the
model, temporal stability, heritability, cross-cultural replications and robustness of the FFM across various constructs and areas of study. The authors argue that there is strong evidence for the FFM as a comprehensive
model of personality traits, which makes the FFM an ideal springboard for
understanding maladaptive expressions of personality traits. They go on to
discuss research speaking to the connection between the FFM traits and
DSM-defined personality disorders. Specifically, they note high reliabilities
for clinicians utilizing the FFM to describe personality disorders, more

comprehensive descriptions of personality disorders when using the FFM (as opposed to the DSM), FFM traits accounting for the temporal stability of personality disorder symptoms, and use of the FFM to account for comorbidity between personality disorders. An underlying theme of this chapter is that conceptualizing personality pathology from an FFM perspective is a viable and desirable alternative to the Axis II categories in the DSM.

Oltmanns and Turkheimer (Chapter 4) tackle a variety of issues related to the perception of individuals with personality pathology. In their chapter, they deal with such important questions as: How well do informants report others' personality pathology? Are there systematic biases found in informant reports for specific types of pathology? Do discrepancies between self- and informant reports of personality pathology reflect disagreement or lack of self-insight? The authors present data from a variety of studies, focusing on nonclinical samples such as military recruits and undergraduates. The results indicate that symptoms of personality pathology are associated with distress and impairment, even in these nonclinical samples. In addition, self–informant agreement was higher for positive traits and differed in systematic ways for negative traits (e.g., people described by others as paranoid are more likely to describe themselves as angry but not suspicious). Furthermore, discrepancies between self- and other reports are smaller when individuals are asked how others would rate them on certain characteristics, as opposed to how they would rate themselves. This suggests that discrepancies between self- and other reports may often reflect a lack of actual agreement, as opposed to a lack of self-insight. The work of Oltmanns and Turkheimer has important implications for how we assess and conceptualize personality pathology, and provides a much needed guide to understanding how specific data may be gleaned from specific informants about specific varieties of personality pathology.

Waldman, Singh, and Lahey (Chapter 5) bridge personality and psychopathology by presenting a developmental model of childhood and adolescent antisocial behavior that incorporates personality traits, or "dispositions." Specifically, personality characteristics labeled Negative Emotionality, Prosociality, and Daring were selected as particularly relevant to the pathological domain of antisocial behavior in children. These dispositions, along with differences in cognitive ability, are defined as the major components of antisocial propensity. The authors propose that these dispositions are mediators between direct causal effects from genetic and environmental influences and later manifestations of antisocial behavior. They also review literature on genetic contributions to the relevant personality dispositions and psychopathology and specify mediational models to investigate processes linking these dispositions to antisocial behavior.

Jang, Wolf, and Larstone (Chapter 6) continue with this theme of genetic contributions to personality and psychopathology. Traditionally, behavior-genetic inquiry has focused on the study of genetic and environmental influences on specific psychological constructs. Having demonstrated non-negligible genetic influence on diverse constructs, behavior geneticists have recently turned their attention more toward elucidating the interplay of genetic and environmental factors across constructs. Jang, Wolf, and Larstone provide an excellent introduction to this "new look" in behavior genetics and how it can inform our understanding of models of the personality–psychopathology interface. In particular, they show how traditional models of personality–psychopathology relations (e.g., does personality act as a risk factor for psychopathology?) can be elaborated and refined in a behavior-genetic context (e.g., does personality confer genetic risk, environmental risk, or some combination?)

Patrick and Bernat (Chapter 7) pursue a strategy similar to Depue and Lenzenweger (Chapter 8), in the sense that their chapter focuses on the development of a neurobehavioral model to bridge personality and psychopathology. However, Patrick and Bernat's approach is focused more specifically on the constructs of emotion and emotion regulation, and on the ability of those constructs to bridge not only personality and psychopathology but also neurobiology and the classification of psychopathology. Specifically, Patrick and Bernat propose connections between neurobiological systems influencing emotion and its regulation, on the one hand, and spectrum concepts emerging from quantitative research on the organization of psychopathology, on the other. They focus in particular on the internalizing (mood and anxiety) and externalizing (substance problems and antisocial behavior) spectra and propose testable hypotheses about brain systems underlying the observed coherence of these spectra and their links to emotional phenomena. They thereby provide a fundamental road map for linking a number of heretofore distinct literatures in a more unified model, bringing together ideas from neurobiology, emotion science, personality, and quantitative research on the classification of psychopathology.

Continuing with the theme of biological bases of the personality–psychopathology interface, Depue and Lenzenweger (Chapter 8) outline a highly comprehensive model of personality disturbance based in neurobiology. As a starting point, Depue and Lenzenweger delineate specific neurobehavioral systems underlying major personality domains. Nevertheless, they go beyond these correspondence maps by suggesting that personality disturbance can be understood in terms of interactions among neurobehavioral systems underlying major personality traits. In Depue and Lenzenweger's model, personality disturbance is not simply the extremity along a single neurobehavioral dimension but, rather, can be better understood as a function of the confluence of multiple systems. This sophisticated interactive model goes a long way toward capturing the complexity of personality disturbance in the real world while anchoring it to generative ideas about the relevant underlying neurobiology.

Meyer and Pilkonis (Chapter 9) agreed to undertake one of the most challenging topics for this volume: approaches to conceptualizing personality and psychopathology in an integrated way, in order to frame clinical intervention more suitably. As noted by these authors, in clinical settings, straightforward presentations are rare; the vast majority of patients who present with "personality pathology" (an "Axis II disorder") also present with "acute pathology" (an "Axis I disorder"). Various strategies for dealing with such complex presentations can be articulated, but these are often piecemeal in nature. Meyer and Pilkonis argue against this piecemeal approach and for a shift toward conceptual models and constructs that transcend personality and psychopathology. In particular, they discuss how constructs such as temperament, early adversity, cognitive-emotional dysfunction, and failure to engage with valued and need-fulfilling life tasks bridge personality and psychopathology. They then argue that each of these areas can form a focus for intervention, and that effective approaches focusing on these areas can be implemented even in the time-limited framework imposed by current managed care conditions.

A focus on constructs transcending personality and psychopathology in the clinic is a hallmark of a psychodynamic approach. We were fortunate to be able to include two chapters that draw inspiration from this approach, yet broaden it considerably. Andersen and her colleagues have been pioneers in studying the process of transference—the ways in which representations of key figures from a person's past influence his or her current behavior. In their contribution to this volume, Andersen and Miranda (Chapter 10) review a systematic program of research documenting the transference phenomenon and discuss the implications of this phenomenon for understanding emotional distress. They show how the personality process of transference can be linked to mood and anxiety pathology. Their work deepens our understanding of the interpersonal aspects of mood and anxiety disorders by showing how transference processes influence the likelihood of emotional suffering versus resilience in an interpersonal context.

Our volume concludes with an unusually rich and thoughtful contribution from Westen, Gabbard, and Blagov (Chapter 11). Their chapter focuses on the construct of personality structure and its link to psychopathology. From a measurement perspective, personality structure typically refers to the organization of individual differences in personality traits across people, such as the distinction between the traits of neuroticism and extraversion discussed by Watson, Kotov, and Gamez (in Chapter 2) and by Mullins-Sweatt and Widiger (in Chapter 3). From a psychodynamic perspective, however, personality structure refers to the intraindividual organization of psychological constructs, such as motives, goals, cognitive strategies, and the like. Westen, Gabbard, and Blagov provide a bridge between these two conceptions of personality structure. They argue that a key consideration in working to integrate trait constructs with intraindividual personality structures will be the extent to which these constructs can be brought together in a system that proves useful in the clinic. The work of Westen, Gabbard, and Blagov thereby goes a long way toward bridging not only different conceptions of personality structure but also science and practice.

As we noted earlier, our aim in assembling these diverse chapters for *Personality and Psychopathology* was to make the case that a rich variety of bridges were being built to link personality and psychopathology. Hopefully, readers of this volume will come to agree with us that this is an exciting and productive area for both basic and applied research and theorizing. Moreover, in looking toward the future, we also hope that these chapters can point to ways to link the various bridges to one another. From our editorial perch and our work in assembling this volume, we have come to feel that the next major challenge in this area will entail bringing together work coming from distinct perspectives to yield novel insights and integrative models. For example, how would one link psychological processes inspired by psychodynamic theory to broad traits such as those of the five-factor model and then to underlying neurobiological systems? We hope the chapters in this volume can inspire this kind of integrative inquiry and thereby further strengthen and broaden the bridge between personality and psychopathology.

Chapter 2

Basic Dimensions of Temperament in Relation to Personality and Psychopathology

DAVID WATSON
ROMAN KOTOV
WAKIZA GAMEZ

Beginning in the 1980s, a remarkable series of developments has led to the emergence of temperament-based models of personality (see L. A. Clark & Watson, 1999; McCrae et al., 2000). With the emergence of these temperament-based approaches, traits now provide plausible causal explanations of behavior rather than mere descriptions of it. The primary goal of this chapter is to explicate the nature of two basic dimensions of temperament and then to use them as an organizing framework for studying the links between personality and psychopathology.

THE BIG TWO DIMENSIONS OF TEMPERAMENT

The Hierarchical Structure of Personality

After several decades of frustratingly slow progress, trait researchers finally began to converge on a consensual taxonomy during the 1990s (L. A. Clark & Watson, 1999; Watson, Clark, & Harkness, 1994). This development enabled investigators to focus more intensively on a relatively small number of consensually recognized traits, thereby helping them to articulate more complex and sophisticated theoretical models. This consensus was facilitated by the recognition that personality traits are ordered hierarchically, so that there is no inherent incompatibility between structural schemes emphasizing a few general "superfactors" and those that model a much larger number of narrower traits (Digman, 1997; Markon, Krueger, & Watson, 2005; Watson et al., 1994). At the apex of this hierarchy are the "big" traits that constitute the superfactor models. At the next lower level of the hierarchy, these traits can be decomposed into several distinct yet correlated subtraits, or "facets." For instance, the broad trait of Extraversion can be subdivided into narrower facets such as assertiveness, gregariousness, energy, and adventurousness (Watson & Clark, 1997a). These facets, in turn, can be further decomposed into even narrower traits (e.g., talkativeness) and behavioral habits (Digman, 1997). In this chapter, we will focus initially on the superfactors that form the highest level of this hierarchy, and then consider facet-level relations between personality and psychopathology.

Superfactor Models of Personality

What are the superfactors that constitute the apex of this structural hierarchy? Here, consensus is less than complete, because the contemporary field is divided between two prominent models. Fortunately, these models are closely related and can easily be integrated with each other (see L. A. Clark & Watson, 1999; Markon et al., 2005; Watson et al., 1994).

The Big Five

First, the five-factor, or Big Five, model developed out of a series of attempts to understand the natural language of trait descriptors (John & Srivastava, 1999; McCrae et al., 2000). Structural analyses of these descriptors consistently revealed five broad factors: Extraversion, Agreeableness, Conscientiousness, Neuroticism, and Openness to Experience (or Imagination, Intellect, or Culture). This structure has proven to be remarkably robust, with the same five factors emerging in both self- and peer-ratings (McCrae & Costa, 1987), in analyses of both children and adults (Digman, 1997) and across a wide variety of languages and cultures (McCrae & Costa, 1997).

The Big Three

Second, the Big Three structure is based on a reduced set of superfactors: Neuroticism/Negative Emotionality (N/NE), Extraversion/Positive Emotionality (E/PE), and Disinhibition versus Constraint (DvC) (see L. A. Clark & Watson, 1999; Markon et al., 2005). This structural scheme arose from the pioneering work of Eysenck and his colleagues (see Eysenck, 1997). Eysenck originally created a widely influential two-factor model consisting of Neuroticism (vs. Emotional Stability) and Extraversion (vs. Introversion). Subsequent analyses led to the identification of a third broad dimension, labeled Psychoticism; despite its name, however, this dimension is better viewed as assessing individual differences in disinhibition versus constraint (see L. A. Clark & Watson, 1999; Watson & Clark, 1993).

Other theorists subsequently posited very similar three-factor models. Tellegen (1985) proposed a structure consisting of Negative Emotionality (paralleling Neuroticism), Positive Emotionality (cf. Extraversion), and Constraint (which is strongly negatively correlated with Psychoticism). Watson and Clark (1993) articulated a very similar model, with factors named Negative Temperament, Positive Temperament, and Disinhibition (vs. Constraint), respectively. Finally, in his reformulation of the California Psychological Inventory, Gough (1987) introduced the higher-order "vectors" of Self-Realization, Internality, and Norm-Favoring, which represent the low ends of Neuroticism, Extraversion, and Psychoticism, respectively. L. A. Clark and Watson (1999) established that these three-factor models all converged well and defined a single common structure.

Relating the Big Three and Big Five

The accumulating data establish that the Big Five model essentially represents an expanded and more differentiated version of the Big Three (L. A. Clark & Watson, 1999; Markon et al., 2005). Most notably, the Neuroticism and Extraversion dimensions of the Big Five essentially are equivalent to the N/NE and E/PE factors, respectively, of the Big Three (L. A. Clark & Watson, 1999; Markon et al., 2005; Watson et al., 1994). Thus, N/NE and E/PE are common to both schemes and constitute a basic Big Two of personality. Accordingly, these dimensions are the primary focus of this chapter.

Furthermore, the DvC dimension of the Big Three is an amalgam of (low) Conscientiousness and Agreeableness; that is, disinhibited individuals tend to be impulsive, reckless, and irresponsible (i.e., low Conscientiousness), as well as uncooperative, unsympathetic, and manipulative (i.e., low Agreeableness). Finally, Openness is less strongly related to the Big Three, although it does show a moderate positive association with E/PE (Digman, 1997; Markon et al., 2005). Putting these data together, one can transform the Big Three into the Big Five by (1) decomposing DvC into Agreeableness and Conscientiousness and (2) incorporating the additional dimension of Openness (L. A. Clark & Watson, 1999; Markon et al., 2005; Watson et al., 1994).

THE TEMPERAMENTAL BASIS OF N/NE AND E/PE

Definition of a Temperament

As noted, we focus primarily on the Big Two dimensions of N/NE and E/PE in this chapter. As we document in the following sections, it now is clear that these traits represent basic dimensions of temperament (L. A. Clark & Watson, 1999). Three key features of temperaments are that they (1) are at least partly attributable to innate biological factors and are present at some form at birth, (2) are substantially stable over time, and (3) have emotional processes as core defining features (L. A. Clark & Watson, 1999; Digman, 1994).

The Genetic Bases of the Dimensions

N/NE and E/PE clearly show all three of these characteristics. First, L. A. Clark and Watson (1999) review extensive evidence establishing that both traits have a substantial genetic component. Heritability estimates based on twin studies typically fall in the .40 to .60 range, with a median value of approximately .50. Adoption studies yield lower—yet still substantial—heritability estimates, but this may be due largely to their inability to model nonadditive genetic variance (Plomin, Corley, Caspi, Fulker, & DeFries, 1998). It is noteworthy, however, that several studies have reported lower heritability estimates for both N/NE and E/PE in older participants (e.g., McGue, Bacon, & Lykken, 1993; Viken, Rose, Kaprio, & Koskenvuo, 1994). The causes of these age-related declines are not yet clear. However, McGue et al. (1993) found that, whereas the reduced estimate for N/NE was due to a true decline in heritability, that for E/PE was attributable to the increased influence of the unshared environment (coupled with a stable genetic component).

The Temporal Stability of the Dimensions

Second, scores on these dimensions are strongly stable over time; in fact, impressive levels of stability can be observed as early as late adolescence (L. A. Clark & Watson, 1999; Roberts & DelVecchio, 2000). For instance, McGue et al. (1993) retested twins between the ages of 20 and 30 (i.e., a 10-year interval) and obtained stability correlations of .60 (N/NE) and .59 (E/PE). Even higher stability coefficients are obtained after the age of 30; across retest intervals ranging from 6 to 12 years, stability correlations for the traits generally fall in the .70–.80 range (Costa & McCrae, 1992b). Helson and Klohnen (1998) report particularly impressive evidence of long-term stability. They assessed a sample of women at ages 27 and 52 (i.e., a span of 25 years) and obtained stability coefficients of .65 (N/NE) and .62 (E/PE).

The Affective Basis of the Dimensions

Finally, as their labels suggest, both traits have strong and systematic links to emotional experience. Specifically, neuroticism is strongly and broadly correlated with individual differences in negative affectivity, whereas extraversion is strongly associated with positive affectivity (Watson, 2000; Watson & Clark, 1992). For example, in an analysis using combined samples (with an overall N of 4,457), Watson, Wiese, Vaidya, and Tellegen (1999) obtained a correlation of .58 between neuroticism and the trait form of the Negative Affect scale from the Positive and Negative Affect Schedule (PANAS; Watson, Clark, & Tellegen, 1988). Extraversion had a parallel correlation of .51 with the PANAS Positive Affect scale.

To explicate these relations further, we will examine the associations between the Big Five and measures of specific lower-order affective traits. These data are based on several college student samples. The Big Five were assessed using various instruments, including the NEO Five-Factor Inventory (Costa & McCrae, 1992a) and the Big Five Inventory (BFI; John & Srivastava, 1999); to eliminate differences in metrics across measures, we standardized the scores on a within-sample basis and then combined them into a single analysis with an overall N of 5,028. Trait affectivity was assessed using the Expanded Form of the Positive and Negative Affect Schedule (PANAS-X; Watson & Clark, 1999). The trait version of this instrument asks respondents to indicate on a 5-point scale (1 = *very slightly or not at all*, 5 = *extremely*) "to what extent you generally feel this way, that is, how you feel on average." The PANAS-X includes four scales measuring specific negative emotions (Watson & Clark, 1997b, 1999): Fear (6 items; e.g., *scared, nervous*), Sadness (5 items; e.g., *blue, lonely*), Guilt (6 items; e.g., *ashamed, angry at self*), and Hostility (6 items; e.g., *angry, scornful*). In addition, three scales assess discrete positive affects: Joviality (8 items; e.g., *happy, enthusiastic*), Self-Assurance (6 items; e.g., *proud, confident*), and Attentiveness (4 items; e.g., *alert, concentrating*).

Table 2.1 presents correlations between these PANAS-X scales and the Big Five. For our purposes, the most noteworthy aspect of this table is that it clearly establishes the affective basis of both neuroticism and extraversion. Consistent with previous research (Watson, 2000; Watson & Clark, 1992), neuroticism is strongly and broadly associated with individual differences in negative emotionality (r's ranged from .41 to .55). Thus, individuals who are high on this dimension experience frequent and intense episodes of fear, sadness, anger, and guilt; they also report relatively low levels of self-confidence. Furthermore, a multiple regression analysis revealed that the seven lower-order PANAS-X scales jointly accounted for 45.1% of the variance in neuroticism (see also Watson, 2000).

In contrast, extraversion displays somewhat greater specificity in its links to positive emotionality. Specifically, extraversion correlated very

TABLE 2.1. Correlations between Negative and Positive Emotionality and the Big Five Personality Traits

	Neur	Extra	Open	Agree	Con
Specific Negative Affects					
Fear	.51	−.22	−.11	−.19	−.20
Sadness	.55	−.35	−.04	−.25	−.22
Guilt	.50	−.25	−.08	−.26	−.28
Hostility	.41	−.20	−.10	−.52	−.24
Specific Positive Affects					
Joviality	−.38	.58	.17	.33	.22
Self-Assurance	−.40	.47	.24	.00	.17
Attentiveness	−.26	.26	.22	.23	.52

Note: $N = 5,028$. Correlations of |.40| are highlighted. Correlations of |.04| and greater are significant at $p < .01$, two-tailed. Neur, Neuroticism; Extra, Extraversion; Open, Openness; Agree, Agreeableness; Con, Conscientiousness.

strongly (.58) with Joviality, more moderately (.47) with Self-Assurance, and rather modestly (.26) with Attentiveness. Thus, extraverts tend to be cheerful, energetic, enthusiastic, confident, and bold individuals. Moreover, paralleling our results for neuroticism, a multiple regression analysis indicated that the seven lower-order PANAS-X scales jointly predicted 39.8% of the variance in extraversion.

THE BIG TWO AND PSYCHOPATHOLOGY

Etiology of the Relations between Personality and Psychopathology

As noted earlier, we will use the Big Two dimensions of N/NE and E/PE as an organizing framework for studying the associations between personality and psychopathology. We initially summarize evidence related to the two general higher-order dimensions and then examine data regarding the lower-order facets within these domains.

Before reviewing this evidence, we first must briefly address the issue of *etiology*—that is, what factor or factors are causally responsible for the observed relations between personality and psychopathology? Four basic explanatory models have been proposed in this literature (see L. A. Clark, Watson, & Mineka, 1994; Watson & Clark, 1995; Widiger, Verheul, & van den Brink, 1999). Two models assume that trait/temperament dimensions exert a causal influence on psychopathology. First, the *vulnerability* model postulates that maladaptive personality traits increase the likelihood that a person eventually will develop clinically significant psychopathology. In a related vein, the *pathoplasty* model posits that once a disorder has developed, trait factors will interact with psychopathology to influence its severity, course, or response to treatment. A third basic model reverses the direction of causality, arguing that psychopathology influences personality, either transiently (what is often called a *complication* model) or permanently (a *scar* model). The final model asserts that personality and psychopathology reflect the same underlying processes; for instance, a *common cause* model posits that a shared etiological factor (e.g., a common genetic diathesis) gives rise to individual differences in both personality and psychopathology, whereas a *spectrum* model argues that normal and abnormal processes fall on the same underlying continua, such that individual differences in temperament essentially represent subclinical manifestations of psychopathology.

The relations between personality and psychopathology are extraordinarily complex. Indeed, the available evidence provides at least some support for all of these models (L. A. Clark et al., 1994; Watson & Clark, 1995; Widiger et al., 1999). In this chapter, we will emphasize the importance of data that are consistent with spectrum/common cause models and that affirm Widiger et al.'s (1999) conclusion that "personality and psychopathology at times fail to be distinct conditions" (p. 351). Specifically, we argue that these basic dimensions of temperament reflect individual differences across a very broad range of functioning, subsuming both normal (i.e., personality) and abnormal (i.e., psychopathology) processes. Thus, we echo L. A. Clark and Watson's (1999) assertion that it is necessary "to recognize that what we call personality in one context shares a common origin (not only a genetic diathesis but perhaps environmental or learning-based etiologies as well) with what we call psychopathology in another" (p. 418).

Relations between N/NE and Psychopathology

N/NE as a General Predictor of Psychopathology

Among the general dimensions of personality, N/NE is the strongest, broadest predictor of psychopathology. In fact, elevated levels of the trait have been linked to virtually all Axis I and Axis II disorders. Thus, significant elevations in N/NE have been reported in a diverse array of syndromes, including mood disorders, anxiety disorders, substance use disorders, somatoform disorders, eating disorders, personality and conduct disorders, and schizophrenia (L. A. Clark et al., 1994; Krueger, Caspi, Moffitt, Silva, & McGee, 1996; Mineka, Watson, & Clark, 1998). Indeed, Widiger and Costa (1994) concluded that N/NE "is an almost ubiquitously elevated trait within clinical populations" (p. 81). To a considerable extent, therefore, N/NE can be viewed as a general predictor of the overall level of psychological functioning rather than a specific predictor of particular syndromes. In support of this conclusion, Gamez, Watson, and Doebbeling

(2005) reported that a marker of N/NE correlated –.51 with Global Assessment of Functioning (GAF) ratings in a sample of Gulf War veterans (this sample is described in greater detail shortly).

N/NE and the Mood and Anxiety Disorders

Although N/NE is a broad and general predictor of psychopathology, it is more strongly linked to some syndromes than to others. More specifically, in light of the temperamental basis of this dimension, it makes good sense that it is more strongly related to disorders with a substantial component of subjective distress than to syndromes that primarily are characterized by thought disturbance, social/occupational dysfunction, behavioral avoidance, or other types of psychopathology. Subjective distress is a core element in most of the mood and anxiety disorders. Thus, it is hardly surprising that N/NE shows particularly strong links to these disorders. For example, Watson, Gamez, and Simms (2005) report correlations between basic personality traits—including both N/NE and E/PE—and lifetime DSM-III-R (American Psychiatric Association, 1987) diagnoses in the National Comorbidity Survey (NCS; Kessler et al., 1994). They found that N/NE had a significantly stronger association with a lifetime diagnosis of any mood disorder ($r = .30$) and any anxiety disorder ($r = .29$) than with any substance use disorder ($r = .11$) (see Watson et al., 2005, Table 1). Consequently, we focus on the mood and anxiety disorders in this chapter.

Differential Relations within the Mood and Anxiety Disorders

This systematic association with distress/dysphoria also can be used to understand and model differential relations between N/NE and individual mood and anxiety disorders. In this regard, Mineka et al. (1998) summarize evidence indicating that some of these disorders have much stronger subjective distress components than others. Specifically, major depression and generalized anxiety disorder (GAD) both are characterized by the pervasive experience of distress. In contrast, many of the anxiety disorders are associated with a more limited expression of negative affectivity. Individuals with these disorders do experience marked subjective distress, but this distress tends to be concentrated in either (1) specific classes of situations (e.g., social phobia) or (2) temporally discrete episodes (e.g., panic disorder). Finally, some disorders (e.g., subtypes of specific phobia) primarily are characterized by behavioral avoidance and have relatively modest components of distress/negative affectivity.

This analysis, in turn, suggests that N/NE should correlate more strongly with distress-based disorders such as major depression and GAD than with anxiety disorders containing a more modest distress component.

Gamez et al. (2005) provide evidence supporting this idea in a large (N = 563) sample of military veterans who served during the 1991 Gulf War. The participants in this follow-up study were selected from a larger initial sample (Doebbeling et al., 2002; Simms, Watson, & Doebbeling, 2002) to investigate three common problems among Gulf War veterans: cognitive dysfunction, chronic widespread pain, and depression. Current diagnoses were obtained from all participants, using the Structured Clinical Interview for DSM-IV (SCID; First, Spitzer, Gibbon, & Williams, 1997). N/NE scores were assessed using the Negative Temperament scale from the Schedule for Nonadaptive and Adaptive Personality (SNAP; L. A. Clark, 1993). As expected, N/NE had significantly stronger correlations with major depression (r = .38), GAD (r = .31), and posttraumatic stress disorder (r = .35) than with social phobia, panic disorder, agoraphobia, and specific phobia (r's ranged from .12 to .20).

Symptom-Based Analyses

We can further illustrate the basic points that N/NE (1) relates more strongly to some types of dysfunction than to others and (2) is a particularly strong predictor of subjective distress and dysphoria by examining how it relates to specific types of anxiety and depression symptoms. In this regard, Watson et al. (2005) examined symptom-level relations in the sample of Gulf War veterans that was described earlier. They examined nine anxiety and depression symptoms that were taken either from the SCID screening module or from the SCID current depressive episode module. Replicating results obtained at the syndromal level, Watson et al. found that N/NE was significantly related to every symptom. In addition, however, they reported that N/NE had significantly stronger correlations with the distress-based symptoms of depressed mood (r = .41), loss of interest or pleasure (r = .40), and nervousness/anxiety (r = .39) than with panic attacks, social anxiety, agoraphobic fears, specific phobias, obsessive intrusions and compulsions (r's ranged from .12 to .31).

Analyses of Heterogeneous Syndromes

Symptom heterogeneity is a prominent feature of many of the current DSM-IV (American Psychiatric Association, 1994) mood and anxiety disorders, including obsessive–compulsive disorder (OCD; Watson & Wu, 2005), posttraumatic stress disorder (PTSD; Simms et al., 2002; Watson, 2005), specific phobia (Cutshall & Watson, 2004), and major depression (see Watson et al., 2005). These symptom dimensions can be expected to correlate differently with other variables, including basic traits such as N/NE.

Accordingly, Watson et al. (2005) examined relations between N/NE and the specific symptom dimensions that constitute these heterogeneous disorders. These analyses revealed the same basic pattern as in other types of data: once again, N/NE clearly was a stronger predictor of distress/dysphoria than of other types of symptoms. For instance, Watson et al. report relevant data based on five-factor analytically derived scales assessing specific symptoms of depression (see Watson et al., 2005, Table 7). They found that two markers of N/NE had significantly stronger correlations with a measure of depressed affect (r's = .62 and .69) than with scales assessing lassitude/anergia, suicidal ideation, insomnia/sleep problems, and loss of appetite (r's ranged from .27 to .50).

As another example, Watson et al. (2005) examined relations between N/NE and four factor analytically derived PTSD symptom scales in the Gulf War sample described previously. As would be expected, N/NE had a significantly stronger correlation with Dysphoria (r = .45) than with Intrusions (r = .32), Hyperarousal (r = .30), and Avoidance (r = .28). It is especially noteworthy that there was a time lag of approximately 6 years between the administration of the trait and symptom scales; consequently, these differential relations were maintained across a substantial time interval.

Taxonomic Implications of the Data

These data all lead to the same general conclusion: N/NE correlates more strongly and consistently with subjective distress and dysphoria than with other types of dysfunction. Thus, among the mood and anxiety disorders, it is most strongly related to disorders characterized by chronic, pervasive distress (e.g., depression and GAD), moderately related to syndromes characterized by more specific and limited forms of distress (e.g., panic disorder, social phobia), and weakly related to syndromes characterized primarily by behavioral avoidance (e.g., specific phobia) (Mineka et al., 1998; Watson et al., 2005). Symptom-level results reveal the same basic pattern: once again, N/NE is a significantly better predictor of subjective distress (e.g., depressed affect) than of other types of symptoms (e.g., lassitude, insomnia)

These data have important structural/taxonomic implications for the mood and anxiety disorders. In this regard, structural analyses of DSM-III-R and DSM-IV diagnoses consistently have found evidence for a three-factor model consisting of Externalizing (alcohol dependence, drug dependence, antisocial personality disorder), Anxious–Misery (major depression, dysthymia, GAD, PTSD), and Fear (panic disorder, agoraphobia, social phobia, simple phobia); the latter two factors are strongly correlated and so define a higher-order "Internalizing" dimension (Krueger, 1999; Vollebergh et al., 2001; see Watson, 2005, for a review). It is noteworthy, furthermore, that this alternative model fits the data significantly better than a structure based on the current DSM classification, in which all of the anxiety disorders mark one factor, and depression and dysthymia define the other.

These consistent structural findings lead to a very striking conclusion: the traditional distinction between sad/depressed mood and anxious/fearful mood does not provide a suitable basis for organizing these syndromes into diagnostic classes (see also Watson, 2005). Rather, the syndromes can be classified more accurately based on the magnitude of their subjective distress component. That is, one recurrent factor (Anxious–Misery) is defined by disorders that are characterized by pervasive distress (major depression, dysthymic disorder, GAD, PTSD), whereas the other dimension (Fear) is marked by syndromes involving more limited forms of distress and more prominent behavioral avoidance (panic disorder, agoraphobia, social phobia, specific phobia).

This further suggests that N/NE should be more strongly related to the Anxious–Misery factor than to Fear. We can test this idea using the SCID symptom data in the Gulf War veteran sample that was described previously. Earlier, we noted that nine anxiety and depression symptoms had been culled from the SCID screening module and the SCID current depressive episode module. In addition, two externalizing symptoms (excessive drinking, drug use) were taken from the SCID screening module. We subjected these 11 symptoms to a principal components analysis; we extracted three factors, which then were rotated to oblique simple structure using promax. These rotated loadings are presented in Table 2.2. It is noteworthy that the resulting structure closely replicates the three-factor structure that has been reported in previous disorder-based analyses (Krueger, 1999; Vollebergh et al., 2001). That is, the three factors in Table 2.2 clearly can be identified as Anxious–Misery (defined by both depressed mood and nervousness/anxiety), Fear (marked by symptoms of panic/agoraphobia, specific phobia, social phobia, and OCD), and Externalizing, respectively.

Next, we computed regression-based factor scores on these three dimensions and then correlated these scores with the three higher-order factor scales from the SNAP—Negative Temperament (a marker of N/NE), Positive Temperament (a measure of E/PE), and Disinhibition (which assesses the final Big Three dimension of Disinhibition vs. Constraint). These correlations are presented in Table 2.3. As expected, N/NE had a significantly stronger correlation with the Anxious–Misery factor ($r = .49$) than with the Fear ($r = .38$; $z = 2.59$, $p < .05$, two-tailed) and Externalizing ($r = .04$; $z = 8.21$, $p < .01$, two-tailed) factors.

These data illustrate how a distress-based approach helps to explicate our understanding of both personality and psychopathology. As we have seen, the existing DSM-IV syndromes empirically cluster according to the magnitude of their subjective distress component. Indeed, Watson (2005)

TABLE 2.2. Promax-Rotated Factor Loadings of SCID-Based Symptoms in the Gulf War Sample

Symptom	Factor 1	Factor 2	Factor 3
Depressed mood	.94	−.14	−.05
Loss of interest or pleasure	.85	.01	−.03
Nervousness/anxiety	.64	.06	.14
Panic attacks	.13	.62	.05
Obsessive intrusions	−.08	.60	.06
Specific phobias	−.10	.55	−.09
Compulsions	−.08	.53	.02
Agoraphobic fears	.24	.48	.10
Social anxiety	.21	.46	−.22
Excessive drinking	−.11	−.04	.78
Drug use	.16	.03	.71

Note. N = 559. Loadings of |.40| and greater are highlighted. SCID, Structured Clinical Interview for DSM-IV.

has proposed that the existing diagnostic classes be eliminated, arguing that the current anxiety and unipolar mood disorders should be reorganized into the "distress disorders" (which would include major depression, dysthymia, GAD, and PTSD) and the "fear disorders" (which would include panic disorder/agoraphobia, social phobia, and specific phobia). Because of its strong association with subjective distress and dysphoria, N/NE shows a particularly strong affinity to the distress disorders and, in fact, helps to explain the comorbidity among them (see Mineka et al., 1998; Watson, 2005).

Etiology of the Relations

Finally, we briefly consider the etiological basis of these relations between N/NE and psychopathology. As noted previously, these associations are extraordinarily complex, such that there is at least some evidence sup-

TABLE 2.3. Correlations between the Higher Order SNAP Scales and SCID Symptom Factors in the Gulf War Data

Symptom factor	NT	PT	DIS
Factor 1 (Anxious–Misery)	.49**	−.34**	.20**
Factor 2 (Fear)	.38**	−.17**	.09*
Factor 3 (Externalizing)	.04	.03	.18**

Note. N = 526. SNAP, Schedule for Nonadaptive and Adaptive Personality; SCID, Structured Clinical Interview for DSM-IV; NT, Negative Temperament; PT, Positive Temperament; DIS, Disinhibition.
*p < .05, two-tailed. **p < .01, two-tailed.

porting both vulnerability/pathoplasty and scar/complication models (see L. A. Clark et al., 1994; Watson & Clark, 1995). Thus, to some extent, individual differences in N/NE are both a cause and an effect of psychopathology.

Furthermore, twin studies indicate that temperament and psychopathology also reflect a shared genetic diathesis (Mineka et al., 1998; Watson & Clark, 1995). In an analysis of nearly 4,000 pairs of Australian twins, Jardine, Martin, and Henderson (1984) found that a single genetic factor was responsible for most of the observed overlap between N/NE and symptoms of depression and anxiety. Kendler, Neale, Kessler, Heath, and Eaves (1993) and Hettema, Prescott, and Kendler (2004) subsequently replicated these findings at the diagnostic level, reporting that major depression, GAD, and N/NE all were strongly linked to a common genetic diathesis. Kendler et al. (1993) argued that this shared genetic factor represents a general tendency to cope poorly with stress and, therefore, to experience frequent and intense episodes of distress and negative affect. These data support our earlier assertion that these basic dimensions of temperament reflect individual differences across a very broad range of functioning, subsuming both normal (i.e., personality) and abnormal (i.e., psychopathology) processes.

Relations between E/PE and Psychopathology

E/PE and Depression

In contrast to N/NE, E/PE shows relatively specific links to particular types of dysfunction. Early reviews of this topic especially emphasized the association between low levels of E/PE and depression. Most notably, Watson, Clark, and Carey (1988)—based on the seminal work of Tellegen (1985)— argued that low E/PE is a specific feature of depression that distinguishes it from anxiety. In support of this view, Watson, Clark, and Carey showed that a measure of E/PE was consistently negatively correlated with indicators of depression but was largely unrelated to manifestations of anxiety. For instance, E/PE had significant associations with 11 of 20 depressive symptoms (median $r = -.25$), and correlated $-.40$ with the total number of depressive complaints. In sharp contrast, E/PE was significantly related to only 3 of 33 anxiety-related complaints (median $r = -.10$), and had correlations ranging from only $-.11$ to $-.15$ with composite indexes of panic, phobia, and OCD symptoms. Furthermore, E/PE was substantially related to lifetime DSM-III (American Psychiatric Association, 1980) diagnoses of major depression ($r = -.41$) and dysthymic disorder ($r = -.37$), but had corresponding correlations ranging from only $-.01$ to $-.23$ with various anxiety disorders.

Several subsequent studies have replicated this negative association between E/PE and depression (L. A. Clark & Watson, 1991; Jolly, Dyck, Kramer, & Wherry, 1994). For instance, Watson et al. (2005) examined relations between the SNAP Positive Temperament scale and symptoms derived from the SCID current depressive episode module. They found that this E/PE marker correlated –.30 with depressed mood and –.28 with loss of interest or pleasure. Similarly, Brown, Chorpita, and Barlow (1998) obtained a correlation of –.53 between E/PE and a latent depression factor that was composed of both self-report and interview-based indicators. Thus, the available evidence clearly establishes that E/PE is a significant predictor of anhedonia (i.e., the loss of pleasure) and depressed affect.

E/PE and Other Disorders

At the same time, however, the accumulating data have revealed that low levels of E/PE are not unique to depression but also characterize other types of psychopathology. In fact, after reviewing the literature, Mineka et al. (1998) concluded that low levels of E/PE "are not confined solely to depression but also characterize—to a lesser degree, perhaps—schizophrenia, social phobia, and other disorders" (p. 398). Berenbaum and Fujita (1994), for instance, conducted a meta-analysis of seven studies that compared the E/PE scores of schizophrenics with those of normal controls. Their results indicated that E/PE levels were approximately 1 SD lower ($d = -.98$) in the schizophrenics across these samples. It is noteworthy, moreover, that a parallel analysis of eight studies revealed that E/PE scores also were substantially lower in schizophrenics than in general samples of neurotic patients ($d = -.61$).

Of course, anhedonia is a prominent feature of schizophrenia and schizotypy (Blanchard, Gangestad, Brown, & Horan, 2000; Herbener & Harrow, 2002; Joiner, Brown, & Metalsky, 2003). Accordingly, these results might simply reaffirm the substantial link between E/PE and anhedonia. However, it now is clear that E/PE is associated with problems beyond anhedonia. The most consistent evidence concerns its link to social anxiety and social phobia. Amies, Gelder, and Shaw (1983) initially identified low levels of E/PE in a sample of 87 social phobics. Watson, Clark, and Carey (1988) subsequently reported significant negative correlations between various symptoms of social phobia and E/PE; they also found a significant negative association ($r = -.23$) with DSM-III diagnoses of social phobia. Similarly, Brown et al. (1998) found that E/PE correlated –.39 with their latent social phobia factor. Furthermore, this association was significantly stronger than those between E/PE and GAD, panic/agoraphobia, and OCD (r's ranged between –.16 and –.27). Finally, Watson et al. (2005)

reported a significant ($r = -.18$) link between E/PE and lifetime DSM-III-R diagnoses of social phobia in the NCS data.

Specificity of Relations across Different E/PE Measures

Watson et al. (2005) also obtained clear evidence indicating that the magnitude of these relations varied as a function of the type of E/PE measure that was used. For instance, they found that self-rated social anxiety had significantly stronger associations with extraversion/sociability (r's ranged from $-.50$ to $-.54$) than with trait positive affectivity (r's ranged from $-.29$ to $-.35$). Thus (and not surprisingly), scales that contain explicit interpersonally oriented content are better predictors of social anxiety/social phobia than are specific measures of positive emotionality. Conversely, trait positive affectivity tended to correlate more highly with various kinds of depression symptoms than did extraversion/sociability. These results illustrate the importance of moving beyond the broad superfactors and examining specific facets within these domains. We return to this issue shortly.

Etiology of These Relations

Thus, markers of E/PE are most strongly and consistently correlated with indicators of (1) anhedonia/depressed affect [which are especially prominent features of major depression and also characterize other syndromes, such as schizophrenia and schizotypy) and (2) social/interpersonal anxiety (the core symptom of social phobia). As was the case with N/NE, the causal bases of these relations are quite complex. L. A. Clark et al. (1994) summarize findings consistent with virtually all of the models described earlier (see also Watson & Clark, 1995). For instance, low premorbid E/PE scores predicted subsequent depression in a 4-year follow-up study, thereby supporting a vulnerability model (Holohan & Moos, 1991). Consistent with a pathoplasty model, high E/PE scores are associated with a quicker return to normal functioning and better overall outcome following an episode of depression (L. A. Clark et al., 1994). Conversely, other data indicate that E/PE scores are significantly influenced by episodes of depression, either temporarily (Roy, 1991) or permanently (Hirschfield et al., 1989). Thus, as with N/NE, E/PE appears to be both a cause and an effect of psychopathology.

In addition, it seems reasonable to argue that these trait-disorder relations partly reflect common underlying processes, thereby supporting spectrum/common cause models. This seems particularly likely with regard to the well-replicated link between E/PE and social phobia. To a considerable extent, showing that low levels of extraversion/sociability can be linked to social phobia is tantamount to demonstrating that "Introversion contributes to the development of extreme Introversion" (Widiger et al., 1999, p. 351).

LOWER-ORDER RELATIONS BETWEEN PERSONALITY AND PSYCHOPATHOLOGY

Overview

Analyses of the Big Two dimensions of N/NE and E/PE have led to important insights into the nature and organization of the mood and anxiety disorders. Nevertheless, as research in this area progresses, it will be important to move beyond these superfactors and examine the specific types of content that are subsumed within these domains. We already have presented evidence demonstrating that sociability and positive emotionality measures are differentially related to psychopathology. We now consider these lower-order relations in greater detail.

Incremental Validity Analyses of the MASQ Symptom Scales

Outline of the Regression Analyses

To establish the importance of examining relations at the lower-order level, it is necessary to demonstrate that these specific traits have incremental validity and provide explanatory power above and beyond the effects of the higher-order dimensions. We present two series of hierarchical regression analyses that address this issue in the large sample of Gulf War veterans that was described earlier. In both sets of analyses, the 15 SNAP scales were entered in a series of four steps. First, as noted previously, the SNAP includes higher-order scales assessing the Big Three dimensions of temperament; these were entered in Step 1 to control for these general traits. Next, structural analyses of the SNAP (L. A. Clark, 1993; Markon et al., 2005) indicate that six of its lower-order scales—Mistrust, Manipulativeness, Self-Harm, Eccentric Perceptions, Aggression, and Dependency—load primarily on the higher-order N/NE factor; these scales were entered in a block in Step 2. In Step 3, we entered the three lower-order scales that define the E/PE dimension (Exhibitionism, Entitlement, Detachment). Finally, the three remaining scales that load primarily on the Disinhibition versus Constraint factor—Impulsivity, Propriety, and Workaholism—were entered as a block in Step 4.

In the first series of analyses, we used the symptom scales from the 62-item short form of the Mood and Anxiety Symptom Questionnaire (MASQ; Watson & Clark, 1991) as criteria. The MASQ was constructed to test key aspects of the tripartite model of depression and anxiety (L. A. Clark &

Watson, 1991). The MASQ short form contains two anxiety and depression scales. The General Distress: Anxious Symptoms Scale (GD: Anxiety; 11 items) includes several indicators of anxious mood, whereas Anxious Arousal (17 items) assesses various manifestations of somatic arousal (e.g., feeling dizzy, shortness of breath). The General Distress: Depressive Symptoms Scale (GD: Depression; 12 items) contains several items tapping depressed mood along with other nonspecific symptoms of mood disorder (e.g., feelings of disappointment, self-blame); in contrast, Anhedonic Depression contains 8 items reflecting anhedonia, disinterest, and low energy (e.g., felt nothing was interesting or enjoyable) and 14 reverse-keyed items assessing positive emotional experiences (e.g., had a lot of energy).

Regression Results

The results of these hierarchical regression analyses are summarized in Table 2.4, which shows the cumulative R^2 (as well as the significance of the R^2 change) associated with each step. These findings clearly demonstrate that the Big Three dimensions contribute the bulk of the predictive power. Indeed, across the four analyses, they account for 24.5% (Anxious Arousal) to 55.8% (Anhedonic Depression) of the criterion variance. Even so, the lower-order traits contribute significantly in every analysis, accounting for an additional 3.5% (GD: Anxiety) to 12.5% (GD: Depression) of the variance. It is noteworthy that this incremental variance is attributable primarily to the six lower-order N/NE markers, which added a significant contribution (ranging from 2.1% to 12.1% incremental variance) in every analysis. In contrast, the lower-order E/PE and Disinhibition markers contributed less than 2% incremental variance in every case.

Which lower-order scales provided this incremental predictive power? The Self-Harm scale—which contains content reflecting low self-esteem, parasuicidal behaviors, and suicidal ideation—was the strongest predictor of depressive symptoms, contributing 10.9% and 2.8% incremental variance to the prediction of GD: Depression and Anhedonic Depression, respectively. Self-Harm also was the strongest predictor of GD: Anxiety, contributing an additional 1.9% of the variance. These results establish that this lower-order trait contains important, clinically relevant variance not tapped by the higher-order dimensions; it therefore merits closer scrutiny in future research. In addition, Mistrust (which assesses a pervasive suspiciousness and cynical attitudes toward others) and Workaholism (which taps a tendency toward perfectionism and self-imposed demands for excellence) made lesser contributions to the prediction of GD: Depression and Anhedonic Depression, respectively. Finally, Eccentric Perceptions (4.4% incremental variance) and Impulsivity (1.1%) contributed significantly to the prediction of Anxious Arousal.

TABLE 2.4. Hierarchical Regression Analyses Using the MASQ Symptom Scales as Criteria

	Cumulative R^2 at:			
	Step 1 Big Three Scales	Step 2 N/NE Scales	Step 3 E/PE Scales	Step 4 Disinhibition Scales
GD: Anxiety	.405**	.426**	.428	.440**
GD: Depression	.446**	.567**	.569	.571
Anxious Arousal	.245**	.292**	.297	.309*
Anhedonic Depression	.558**	.616**	.624*	.633**

Note. N = 555. MASQ, Mood and Anxiety Symptom Questionnaire; N/NE, Neuroticism/Negative Emotionality; E/PE, Extraversion/Positive Emotionality; GD: Anxiety, General Distress: Anxious Symptoms; GD: Depression, General Distress: Depressive Symptoms.
*R^2 change is significant at $p < .05$, two-tailed; **R^2 change is significant at $p < .01$, two-tailed.

Incremental Validity Analyses of the SCID Symptoms

The second series of hierarchical regressions was identical, except that the nine anxiety and depression symptoms derived from the SCID (described earlier in connection with the analyses reported in Tables 2.2 and 2.3) were used as the criteria. The results of these analyses are summarized in Table 2.5, which again shows the cumulative R^2 (as well as the significance of the R^2 change) associated with each step. Once again, the Big Three dimensions clearly contribute the bulk of the predictive power. Across the nine analyses, they account for 1.8% (compulsions) to 20.9% (depressed mood) of the variance, with a median value of 9.6%. In contrast, the lower-order scales contributed from 2.4% (compulsions) to 7.4% (loss of interest or pleasure) of the variance, with a median value of 4.7%. Still, the lower-order scales made significant incremental contributions in seven of the nine analyses. Replicating the MASQ results, the lower-order N/NE traits generally showed the strongest predictive power, contributing significantly in six analyses (with values ranging from 2.3% to 6.4%). In addition, the specific E/PE scales contributed significantly to both social anxiety (an additional 3.3%) and agoraphobic fears (an additional 1.5%). Finally, the lower-order Disinhibition scales contributed less than 1% of the variance in every case.

As in the MASQ analyses, Self-Harm emerged as the strongest and broadest predictor among the lower-order traits. It was the strongest single predictor of four symptoms: depressed mood (5.4% incremental variance), loss of interest or pleasure (4.4%), nervousness/anxiety (2.5%), and panic attacks (2.7%). It also contributed significantly to the prediction of obsessions (1.4%) and agoraphobic fears (1.3%). Detachment—which assesses a tendency toward aloofness and emotional reserve, as well as a preference for being alone—was the strongest predictor of both social anxiety (1.9%)

TABLE 2.5. Hierarchical Regression Analyses Using the SCID Symptoms as Criteria

	Cumulative R^2 at:			
	Step 1 Big Three Scales	Step 2 N/NE Scales	Step 3 E/PE Scales	Step 4 Disinhibition Scales
Depressed mood	.209**	.273**	.276	.279
Loss of interest or pleasure	.195**	.254**	.264	.269
Nervousness/anxiety	.174**	.201**	.206	.208
Social anxiety	.128**	.151*	.184**	.185
Panic attacks	.096**	.135**	.138	.143
Obsessive intrusions	.077**	.133**	.138	.143
Agoraphobic fears	.053**	.075	.090*	.098
Specific phobias	.020*	.036	.045	.048
Compulsions	.018*	.033	.035	.042

Note. N = 555. SCID, Structured Clinical Interview for DSM-IV; N/NE, Neuroticism/Negative Emotionality; E/PE, Extraversion/Positive Emotionality.
*R^2 change is significant at $p < .05$, two-tailed; **R^2 change is significant at $p < .01$, two-tailed.

and agoraphobic fears (1.9%), suggesting that it shows a specific link to social/interpersonal dysfunction; Detachment also contributed significantly to the prediction of loss of interest or pleasure (1.6%). In addition, Dependency made a lesser contribution to the prediction of social anxiety (1.1%). Finally, Eccentric Perceptions—which assesses unusual perceptions, cognitions, and beliefs—was the strongest predictor of obsessive intrusions (2.5%). This finding is consistent with other evidence establishing systematic links between OCD symptoms and unusual cognitions and perceptions (Watson, Wu, & Cutshall, 2004). Mistrust also contributed significantly (1.0%) to the prediction of obsessions.

Incremental Validity Analyses of DSM-IV Anxiety and Mood Disorders

Finally, it is important to examine incremental validity at the diagnostic level. Gamez et al. (2005) report partial correlations (controlling for Negative Temperament) between the lower-order SNAP scales and current DSM-IV diagnoses for major depression, GAD, PTSD, social phobia, specific phobia, panic disorder, and agoraphobia. We reran these partial correlation analyses, controlling for all three higher-order SNAP scales. Consistent with our symptom-level analyses, Self-Harm made the strongest incremental contribution to the prediction of psychopathology. Specifically, Self-Harm was significantly related to current diagnoses of major depression (partial $r = .26$), GAD (partial $r = .14$), and social phobia (partial $r = .11$). Two other lower-order N/NE scales also displayed incremental validity:

Mistrust was related to major depression (partial $r = .11$) and PTSD (partial $r = .12$), whereas Eccentric Perceptions had links to both PTSD (partial $r = .18$) and social phobia (partial $r = .11$). Finally, Workaholism had a significant association with major depression (partial $r = .12$).

Summary

Our results consistently indicate that the higher-order dimensions—especially N/NE—contribute the bulk of the variance to the prediction of psychopathology. Nevertheless, the lower-order SNAP traits also contributed significantly in the large majority of our analyses. Among these specific traits, the SNAP Self-Harm scale shows the strongest and broadest links to psychopathology; it displays particularly strong associations with indicators of depression. In addition, Detachment shows a specific affinity to social/interpersonal dysfunction. Finally, Eccentric Perceptions displayed incremental validity in relation to OCD and PTSD symptoms. Lower-order analyses of this type provide a useful complement to those focusing at the broad superfactor level and can play an important role in explicating the links between personality and psychopathology. We therefore encourage future researchers to examine these relations at both levels of the personality hierarchy.

INTEGRATING CLINICAL TRAITS INTO THE BIG TWO FRAMEWORK

Additional Traits from the Clinical Literature

Overview

Throughout this chapter, we have emphasized the heuristic and practical value of a structural framework based on two general dimensions of temperament—N/NE and E/PE. Of course, clinical researchers have examined the connections between many other dispositional constructs and the mood and anxiety disorders. In this final section, we demonstrate how several of these clinical measures can be integrated into our Big Two framework.

Psychopathology researchers have identified a number of trait-like constructs that are believed to contribute to the development of mental disorders. These constructs were developed outside of the mainstream personality field, usually in the context of a particular model of psychopathology. They tend to be rather narrow in scope and are hypothesized to have relatively specific links to psychopathology. It is noteworthy that the researchers who study these concepts often do not consider them to be classic personality traits. On the other hand, these phenomena are conceptualized as dispositional characteristics (e.g., Blatt, 1974; Reiss & McNally, 1985), and the empirical evidence shows that their stability is comparable to that of typical personality dimensions (e.g., Kasch, Klein, & Lara, 2001; Taylor, 1999). Accordingly, these clinical constructs may not differ substantially from traditional personality traits. In this final section, we discuss some of the most important of these clinical measures. The literature is too large and diverse to be fully reviewed here, so we will focus on four of the most studied clinical traits: ruminative response style, anxiety sensitivity, self-criticism, and perfectionism.

Ruminative Response Style

Ruminative response style is a tendency to dwell on the negative thoughts and feelings associated with depression. The trait was originally proposed as a moderator that influenced the course of depression (Nolen-Hoeksema & Morrow, 1991), but it eventually became evident that it also plays a role in the development of depression. The Response Styles Questionnaire (RSQ; Nolen-Hoeksema & Morrow, 1991) is the best-established measure of this dimension. It includes 22 items describing a variety of responses to depressed mood (e.g., "listen to sad music"). Research has established that the RSQ predicts the severity of depressed mood (e.g., Nolen-Hoeksema & Morrow, 1993; Nolen-Hoeksema, Morrow, & Fredrickson, 1993), and that instructions to ruminate following a negative mood induction prolong dysphoric mood (e.g., Morrow & Nolen-Hoeksema, 1990). Finally, RSQ scores were found to predict depression over an 18-month period (Just & Alloy, 1997).

Anxiety Sensitivity

Anxiety sensitivity reflects the extent to which one fears anxiety and anxiety-related sensations (Reiss & McNally, 1985). For example, individuals with high anxiety sensitivity may perceive that heart palpitations are symptoms of a heart attack. This trait is an established risk factor for panic attacks and panic disorder, as is evident from both prospective and laboratory studies (McNally, 2002; Taylor, 1999). Anxiety sensitivity is most frequently assessed using the Anxiety Sensitivity Index (ASI; Peterson & Reiss, 1992), which contains 16 items (e.g., "It scares me when I become short of breath").

Self-Criticism

Blatt's (1974) theory of depression posits two key trait vulnerability factors: dependency and self-criticism. These traits are most often operationalized using the Depressive Experiences Questionnaire (DEQ; Blatt, D'Afflitti, &

Quinlan, 1976). The DEQ is a well-established risk factor for depression (for reviews, see Nietzel & Harris, 1990; Enns & Cox, 1997). However, findings for the DEQ Dependency scale have shown that it lacks specificity to depression (D. A. Clark, Steer, & Beck, 1994; Enns & Cox, 1997). Thus, we only consider DEQ Self-Criticism here.

Self-criticism can be defined as a tendency to experience feelings of failure, inadequacy, and guilt stemming from unrealistically high expectations for oneself. The DEQ Self-Criticism scale has been found to predict physiological and affective responses to an induced-failure task, and to interact with negative life events to predict depressed mood (D. A. Clark et al., 1994; Enns & Cox, 1997). There have been several revisions of the original DEQ Self-Criticism scale; the most recent version (Bagby, Parker, Joffe, & Buis, 1994) consists of nine items (e.g., "I often find that I don't live up to my own standards or ideals").

Perfectionism

Perfectionism is defined by the setting of excessively high standards. However, recent research has revealed that it is a multifaceted phenomenon (e.g., Frost, Marten, Lahart, & Rosenblate, 1990). Frost's model posits that perfectionism consists of five dimensions, which are operationalized by the Frost Multidimensional Perfectionism Scale (FMPS; Frost et al., 1990). The FMPS is becoming widely accepted as a useful measure of the construct, and there is growing evidence that perfectionism is associated with both anxiety and depression (Enns & Cox, 1999; Frost & Steketee, 1997). Of the five subscales, Concern over Mistakes (FMPS-COM) shows the strongest associations with psychopathology (Kawamura, Hunt, Frost, & DiBartolo, 2001; Lynd-Stevenson & Hearne, 1999). Thus, only this subscale will be considered here; it contains 9 items and reflects an overconcern with mistakes (e.g., "I should be upset if I make a mistake").

Relations among the Constructs

These four traits arose independently out of very distinct theoretical models. Nevertheless, the empirical evidence indicates that the constructs are more strongly related than one might initially expect. For instance, Enns and Cox (1999) reported a correlation of .61 between DEQ Self-Criticism and FMPS-COM in a sample of 145 depressed patients. Similarly, the RSQ and DEQ Self-Criticism correlated .57 in a sample of 88 depressed undergraduates (Kasch et al., 2001). Furthermore, correlations between the RSQ, the ASI, and DEQ Self-Criticism ranged from .45 to .75 in a mixed sample of 76 patients with major depression or panic disorder (Cox, Enns, Walker, Kjernisted, & Pidlubny, 2001).

To augment these scattered findings, we administered these four measures to 232 undergraduate psychology students at the University of Iowa. Correlations between the measures ranged from .43 to .66 in this sample. These moderate to strong correlations suggest that the four clinical traits can be viewed as facets of an overarching general construct. Analyses of the relations between these clinical traits and the general dimensions of temperament can help us evaluate this possibility; we examine these associations in the following section.

Associations between the Clinical Traits and the Big Two

Prior Evidence

The available evidence indicates that all of these traits are substantially related to N/NE. DEQ Self-Criticism shows a particularly strong link to N/NE, with correlations ranging from .56 to .78 across various studies (Cox, Enns, Walker, et al., 2001; Dunkley, Blankstein, & Flett, 1997; Enns & Cox, 1999). Similarly, correlations between N/NE and the RSQ have ranged from .46 to .79 (Cox, Enns, & Taylor, 2001; Cox, Enns, Walker, et al., 2001; Kasch et al., 2001). Associations with the FMPS-COM are slightly lower, with coefficients ranging from .48 to .55 across studies (e.g., Enns & Cox, 1999; Rosser, Issakidis, & Peters, 2003). Finally, correlations between N/NE and the ASI tend to be moderate, generally falling in the .40 to .50 range (Cox, Borger, Taylor, Fuentes, & Ross, 1999; Cox, Enns, & Taylor, 2001; Cox, Enns, Walker, et al., 2001; Taylor, Koch, & Crockett, 1991).

The data regarding E/PE are less extensive, but generally suggest more modest negative associations. Enns and Cox (1999) reported a −.28 correlation between E/PE and the FMPS-COM. Correlations with the other traits have ranged from −.18 to −.49 for the RSQ (Kasch et al., 2001; Cox, Enns, Walker, et al., 2001), from −.26 to −.36 for the ASI (Cox et al., 1999; Cox, Enns, Walker, et al., 2001) and from −.25 to −.52 for DEQ Self-Criticism (Cox, Enns, Walker, et al., 2001; Dunkley et al., 1997; Enns & Cox, 1999).

Factor Analytic Evidence

These correlational results broadly support our suggestion that these traits can be integrated into a Big Two framework. Of course, factor analyses offer more direct and compelling structural evidence. To date, however, only one study has examined this issue. Lilienfeld (1997) performed a joint factor analysis of the 11 lower-order scales of the Multidimensional Personality Questionnaire (Tellegen, in press), together with four measures of anxiety sensitivity, including the ASI. Lilienfeld extracted three factors, which were clearly interpretable as the Big Three. For our purposes, it is noteworthy that all of the anxiety sensitivity scales had high loadings on the N/NE dimension (ranging from .65 to .78) and very low loadings on the other two factors (ranging from only −.09 to .14). Thus, these data establish that anxiety sensitivity falls within the domain of N/NE.

To explore this issue further, we conducted a principal factor analysis in the sample of 232 undergraduates described earlier. The analyzed variables included all four clinical traits, two markers of N/NE (the SNAP Negative Temperament and BFI Neuroticism scales), and two indicators of E/PE (SNAP Positive Temperament and BFI Extraversion). We extracted two factors and rotated them to oblique simple structure using promax. The resulting loadings are presented in Table 2.6. All four clinical traits were strong, clear markers of the N/NE dimension: they had loadings ranging from .62 (ASI) to .77 (DEQ Self-Criticism) on this factor, and loadings ranging from only .07 to −.08 on the E/PE dimension. Together with the data reviewed earlier, these results suggest that these clinical traits can be considered facets of N/NE.

Incremental Validity of the Clinical Traits

A number of studies have shown that these clinical traits contribute incremental predictive power beyond that attributable to the Big Two. For instance, the RSQ predicts self-reported symptoms of depression even after controlling for N/NE (Cox, Enns, & Taylor, 2001), and for both N/NE and E/PE (Enns, Cox, & Borger, 2001). Moreover, RSQ scores differentiated patients with major depressive disorder from patients with panic disorder even after both N/NE and E/PE were controlled (Cox, Enns, Walker, et al., 2001).

Similarly, the ASI predicted the development of spontaneous panic attacks after controlling for N/NE (Schmidt, Lerew, & Jackson, 1997, 1999). Furthermore, it predicted fearful responses to biological challenges—such as CO_2 inhalation—better than N/NE (McNally, 2002). Lilienfeld (1997) found that a composite of four anxiety sensitivity measures predicted anxiety symptoms after controlling for the Big Two. Finally, the ASI differentiated patients with panic from patients with depression even after both N/NE and E/PE were controlled (Cox, Enns, Walker, et al., 2001).

The DEQ Self-Criticism scale predicted self-reported symptoms of depression above and beyond N/NE in samples of 276 depressed patients (Clara, Cox, & Enns, 2003) and 233 undergraduates (Dunkley et al., 1997). Moreover, it predicted depression severity—assessed using both an interview and a self-report measure—after controlling for both N/NE and E/PE (Enns & Cox, 1999). In the same study, FMPS-COM also showed incremental predictive validity in relation to the Big Two.

TABLE 2.6. Promax-Rotated Factor Loadings of the Big Two and Clinical Trait Scales

Scale	Factor 1	Factor 2
SNAP Negative Temperament	.85	.01
DEQ Self-Criticism	.77	-.08
BFI Neuroticism	.77	-.08
FMPS Concern over Mistakes	.73	.07
Response Styles Questionnaire	.67	-.01
Anxiety Sensitivity Index	.62	.06
SNAP Positive Temperament	.05	.89
BFI Extraversion	-.03	.68

Note. N = 232. Loadings of |.40| and greater are highlighted. SNAP, Schedule for Nonadaptive and Adaptive Personality; DEQ, Depressive Experiences Questionnaire; BFI, Big Five Inventory; FMPS, Frost Multidimensional Perfectionism Scale.

Summary

The reviewed evidence indicates that these four clinical traits—ruminative response style, anxiety sensitivity, self-criticism, and perfectionism—are moderately to strongly related to the higher-order N/NE factor. Nevertheless, these dimensions also contain unique, clinically interesting variance beyond that attributable to the Big Two. Overall, these data suggest that these clinical traits basically can be viewed as lower-order facets of N/NE.

It seems likely that many other clinical traits can be incorporated into this structural framework as well. Unfortunately, the field has been slow to recognize the commonality between clinical traits and more traditional personality traits. We strongly encourage psychopathology researchers to recognize this commonality and to integrate their clinical trait measures into established personality structures, such as the Big Two. One important implication of these hierarchical structures is that observed associations between clinical traits and psychopathology simply may be due to the variance that these lower-order traits share with the higher-order temperament dimensions (i.e., the classic third-variable problem). Accordingly, studies investigating clinical traits routinely should include measures of general temperament and control for their contributions.

CONCLUSION

We explicated the nature of two basic dimensions of temperament—N/NE and E/PE—and then used them as an organizing framework for studying the links between personality and psychopathology. Our review of the literature established that N/NE is a broad and general predictor of psychopathology, but that it correlates more strongly and consistently with subjective distress and dysphoria than with other types of dysfunction. In contrast, E/PE is most strongly and consistently correlated with indicators of depression (including anhedonia and depressed affect) and social anxiety/social phobia.

These Big Two dimensions are substantial predictors of dysfunction, and they should be routinely included in studies investigating the links between personality and psychopathology. By themselves, however, they provide an incomplete picture of these relations. Of course, any comprehensive analysis also would include the other major superfactors of personality, such as Disinhibition (versus Constraint) and the dimensions included in the popular Big Five model. In addition, throughout this chapter we have emphasized that these models all are *hierarchical* in nature. Accordingly, a complete analysis also must assess and model the narrower traits that constitute the lower-order level of the personality hierarchy.

Our analyses of the SNAP scales consistently indicated that the higher-order traits—especially N/NE—contribute the bulk of the variance to the prediction of psychopathology. Nevertheless, the specific lower-order scales also contributed significantly in the large majority of our analyses. Most notably, Self-Harm showed the broadest links to psychopathology and was a particularly strong predictor of depression. The Detachment and Eccentric Perceptions scales also showed incremental power and merit further attention. In a related vein, we established that four widely studied clinical traits—ruminative response style, anxiety sensitivity, self-criticism, and perfectionism—(1) essentially can be viewed as facets of N/NE and (2) show incremental predictive validity beyond the Big Two.

Based on the data we have reviewed in this chapter, we believe that hierarchical structural models should play a more prominent and comprehensive role in research examining the links between personality and psychopathology. We therefore encourage future researchers to examine these relations at both levels of the structural hierarchy.

REFERENCES

American Psychiatric Association. (1980). *Diagnostic and statistical manual of mental disorders* (3rd ed.). Washington, DC: Author.

American Psychiatric Association. (1987). *Diagnostic and statistical manual of mental disorders* (3rd ed., rev.). Washington, DC: Author.

American Psychiatric Association. (1994). *Diagnostic and statistical manual of mental disorders* (4th ed.). Washington, DC: Author.

Amies, P. L., Gelder, M. G., & Shaw, P. M. (1983). Social phobia: A comparative clinical study. *British Journal of Psychiatry, 142,* 174–179.

Bagby, R. M., Parker, J. D. A., Joffe, R. T., & Buis, T. (1994). Reconstruction and validation of the Depressive Experiences Questionnaire. *Assessment, 1*, 59–68.

Berenbaum, H., & Fujita, F. (1994). Schizophrenia and personality: Exploring the boundaries and connections between vulnerability and outcome. *Journal of Abnormal Psychology, 103*, 148–158.

Blanchard, J. J., Gangestad, S. W., Brown, S. A., & Horan, W. P. (2000). Hedonic capacity and schizotypy revisited: A taxometric analysis of social anhedonia. *Journal of Abnormal Psychology, 109*, 87–95.

Blatt, S. J. (1974). Levels of object representation in anaclitic and introjective depression. *Psychonalytic Study of the Child, 29*, 107–157.

Blatt, S. J., D'Afflitti, J. P., & Quinlan, D. M. (1976). *Depressive Experiences Questionnaire*. New Haven, CT: Yale University Press.

Brown, T. A., Chorpita, B. F., & Barlow, D. H. (1998). Structured relationships among dimensions of the DSM-IV anxiety and mood disorders and dimensions of negative affect, positive affect, and autonomic arousal. *Journal of Abnormal Psychology, 107*, 179–192.

Clara, I. P., Cox, B. J., & Enns, M. W. (2003). Hierarchical models of personality and psychopathology: The case of self-criticism, neuroticism, and depression. *Personality and Individual Differences, 35*, 91–99.

Clark, D. A., Steer, R. A., & Beck, A. T. (1994). Common and specific dimensions of self-reported anxiety and depression: Implications for the cognitive and tripartite models. *Journal of Abnormal Psychology, 103*, 645–654.

Clark, L. A. (1993). *Schedule for Nonadaptive and Adaptive Personality: Manual for Administration, Scoring, and Interpretation*. Minneapolis, MN: University of Minnesota Press.

Clark, L. A., & Watson, D. (1991). Tripartite model of anxiety and depression: Psychometric evidence and taxonomic implications. *Journal of Abnormal Psychology, 100*, 316–336.

Clark, L. A., & Watson, D. (1999). Temperament: A new paradigm for trait psychology. In L. A. Pervin & O. P. John (Eds.), *Handbook of personality* (2nd ed., pp. 399–423). New York: Guilford Press.

Clark, L. A., Watson, D., & Mineka, S. (1994). Temperament, personality, and the mood and anxiety disorders. *Journal of Abnormal Psychology, 103*, 103–116.

Costa, P. T., Jr., & McCrae, R. R. (1992a). *Revised NEO Personality Inventory (NEO-PI-R) and NEO Five-Factor Inventory (NEO-FFI) professional manual*. Odessa, FL: Psychological Assessment Resources.

Costa, P. T., Jr., & McCrae, R. R. (1992b). Trait psychology comes of age. In T. B. Sonderegger (Ed.), *Nebraska Symposium on Motivation: Psychology and aging* (pp. 169–204). Lincoln: University of Nebraska Press.

Cox, B. J., Borger, S. C., Taylor, S., Fuentes, K., & Ross, L. M. (1999). Anxiety sensitivity and the five-factor model of personality. *Behaviour Research and Therapy, 37*, 633–641.

Cox, B. J., Enns, M. W., & Taylor, S. (2001). The effect of rumination as a mediator of elevated anxiety sensitivity in major depression. *Cognitive Therapy and Research, 25*, 525–534.

Cox, B. J., Enns, M. W., Walker, J. R., Kjernisted, K., & Pidlubny, S. R. (2001). Psychological vulnerabilities in patients with major depression vs. panic disorder. *Behaviour Research and Therapy, 39,* 567–573.

Cutshall, C., & Watson, D. (2004). The Phobic Stimuli Response Scales: A new self-report measure of fear. *Behaviour Research and Therapy, 42,* 1193–1201.

Digman, J. M. (1994). Child personality and temperament: Does the five-factor model embrace both domains? In C. F. Halverson, G. A. Kohnstamm, & R. P. Martin (Eds.), *The developing structure of temperament and personality from infancy to adulthood* (pp. 323–338). Hillsdale, NJ: Erlbaum.

Digman, J. M. (1997). Higher-order factors of the Big Five. *Journal of Personality and Social Psychology, 73,* 1246–1256.

Doebbeling, B. N., Jones, M. F., Hall, D. B., Woolson, R. F., Clarke, W. R., Crumley, T., et al. (2002). Methodological issues in a population-based health survey of Gulf War veterans. *Journal of Clinical Epidemiology, 55,* 477–487.

Dunkley, D. M., Blankstein, K. R., & Flett, G. L. (1997). Specific cognitive–personality vulnerability styles in depression and the five-factor model of personality. *Personality and Individual Differences, 23,* 1041–1053.

Enns, M. W., & Cox, B. J. (1997). Personality dimensions and depression: Review and commentary. *The Canadian Journal of Psychiatry, 42,* 274–284.

Enns, M. W., & Cox, B. J. (1999). Perfectionism and depression symptom severity in major depressive disorder. *Behaviour Research and Therapy, 37,* 783–794.

Enns, M. W., Cox, B. J., & Borger, S. C. (2001). Correlates of analogue and clinical depression: A further test of the phenomenological continuity hypothesis. *Journal of Affective Disorders, 66,* 175–183.

Eysenck, H. J. (1997). Personality and experimental psychology: The unification of psychology and the possibility of a paradigm. *Journal of Personality and Social Psychology, 73,* 1224–1237.

First, M. B., Spitzer, R. L., Gibbon, M., & Williams, J. B. W. (1997). *Structured Clinical Interview for DSM-IV Axis I Disorders— Patient Edition (SCID- I/P).* New York: Biometrics Research, New York State Psychiatric Institute.

Frost, R. O., & Steketee, G. (1997). Perfectionism in obsessive–compulsive disorder patients. *Behaviour Research and Therapy, 35,* 291–296.

Frost, R. O., Marten, P., Lahart, C., & Rosenblate, R. (1990). The dimensions of perfectionism. *Cognitive Therapy and Research, 14,* 449–468.

Gamez, W., Watson, D., & Doebbeling, B. N. (2005). *Abnormal personality and the mood and anxiety disorders: Implications for structural models of anxiety and depression.* Manuscript submitted for publication.

Gough, H. G. (1987). *California Psychological Inventory* [administrator's guide]. Palo Alto, CA: Consulting Psychologists Press.

Helson, R., & Klohnen, E. C. (1998). Affective coloring of personality from young adulthood to midlife. *Personality and Social Psychology Bulletin, 24,* 241–252.

Herbener, E. S., & Harrow, M. (2002). The course of anhedonia during 10 years of schizophrenic illness. *Journal of Abnormal Psychology, 111,* 237–248.

Hettema, J. M., Prescott, C. A., & Kendler, K. S. (2004). Genetic and environmental sources of covariation between generalized anxiety disorder and neuroticism. *American Journal of Psychiatry, 161,* 1581–1587.

Hirschfeld, R. M. A., Klerman, G. L., Lavori, P., Keller, M., Griffith, P., & Coryell, W.

(1989). Premorbid personality assessments of first onset of major depression. *Archives of General Psychiatry, 46,* 345–350.

Holohan, C. J., & Moos, R. H. (1991). Life stressors, personal and social resources, and depression: A 4–year structural model. *Journal of Abnormal Psychology, 100,* 31–38.

Jardine, R., Martin, N. G., & Henderson, A. S. (1984). Genetic covariation between neuroticism and symptoms of anxiety and depression. *Genetic Epidemiology, 1,* 89–107.

John, O. P., & Srivastava, S. (1999). The Big Five trait taxonomy: History, measurement, and theoretical perspectives. In L. A. Pervin & O. P. John (Eds.), *Handbook of personality* (2nd ed., pp. 102–138). New York: Guilford Press.

Joiner, T. E., Brown, J. S., & Metalsky, G. I. (2003). A test of the tripartite model's prediction of anhedonia's specificity to depression: Patients with major depression versus patients with schizophrenia. *Psychiatry Research, 119,* 243–250.

Jolly, J. B., Dyck, M. J., Kramer, T. A., & Wherry, J. N. (1994). Integration of positive and negative affectivity and cognitive content-specificity: Improved discrimination of anxious and depressive symptoms. *Journal of Abnormal Psychology, 103,* 544–552.

Just, N., & Alloy, L. B. (1997). The response styles theory of depression: Tests and an extension of the theory. *Journal of Abnormal Psychology, 106,* 221–229.

Kasch, K. L., Klein, D. N., & Lara, M. E. (2001). A construct validation study of the Response Styles Questionnaire Rumination scale in participants with a recent-onset major depressive episode. *Psychological Assessment, 13,* 375–383.

Kawamura, K. Y., Hunt, S. L., Frost, R. O., & DiBartolo, P. M. (2001). Perfectionism, anxiety, and depression: Are the relationships independent? *Cognitive Therapy and Research, 25,* 291–301.

Kendler, K. S., Neale, M. C., Kessler, R. C., Heath, A. C., & Eaves, L. J. (1993). A longitudinal twin study of personality and major depression in women. *Archives of General Psychiatry, 50,* 853–862.

Kessler, R. C., McGonagle, K. A., Zhao, S., Nelson, C. B., Hughes, M., Eshleman, S., et al. (1994). Lifetime and 12–month prevalence of DSM-III-R psychiatric disorders in the United States: Results from the National Comorbidity Survey. *Archives of General Psychiatry, 51,* 8–19.

Krueger, R. F. (1999). The structure of common mental disorders. *Archives of General Psychiatry, 56,* 921–926.

Krueger, R. F., Caspi, A., Moffitt, T. E., Silva, P. A., & McGee, R. (1996). Personality traits are differentially linked to mental disorders: A multitrait–multidiagnosis study of an adolescent birth cohort. *Journal of Abnormal Psychology, 105,* 299–312.

Lilienfeld, S. O. (1997). The relation of anxiety sensitivity to higher and lower order personality dimensions: Implications for the etiology of panic attacks. *Journal of Abnormal Psychology, 106,* 539–544.

Lynd-Stevenson, R. M., & Hearne, C. M. (1999). Perfectionism and depressive affect: The pros and cons of being a perfectionist. *Personality and Individual Differences, 26,* 549–562.

Markon, K. E., Krueger, R. F., & Watson, D. (2005). Delineating the structure of normal and abnormal personality: An integrative hierarchical approach. *Journal of Personality and Social Psychology, 88,* 139–157.

McCrae, R. R., & Costa, P. T., Jr. (1987). Validation of a five-factor model of personality across instruments and observers. *Journal of Personality and Social Psychology, 52,* 81–90.

McCrae, R. R., & Costa, P. T., Jr. (1997). Personality trait structure as a human universal. *American Psychologist, 52,* 509–516.

McCrae, R. R., Costa, P. T., Jr., Ostendorf, F., Angleitner, A., Hrebíčková, M., Avia, M. D., et al. (2000). Nature over nurture: Temperament, personality, and life span development. *Journal of Personality and Social Psychology, 78,* 173–186.

McGue, M., Bacon, S., & Lykken, D. T. (1993). Personality stability and change in early adulthood: A behavioral genetic analysis. *Developmental Psychology, 29,* 96–109.

McNally, R. J. (2002). Anxiety sensitivity and panic disorder. *Biological Psychiatry, 52,* 938–946.

Mineka, S., Watson, D., & Clark, L. A. (1998). Comorbidity of anxiety and unipolar mood disorders. *Annual Review of Psychology, 49,* 377–412.

Morrow, J., & Nolen-Hoeksema, S. (1990). Effects of responses to depression on the remediation of depressed affect. *Journal of Personality and Social Psychology, 58,* 519–527.

Nietzel, M. T., & Harris, M. J. (1990). Relationship of dependency and achievement/autonomy to depression. *Clinical Psychology Review, 10,* 279–297.

Nolen-Hoeksema, S., & Morrow, J. (1991). *Responses to Depression questionnaire.* Unpublished manuscript, Department of Psychology, Stanford University.

Nolen-Hoeksema, S., & Morrow, J. (1993). Effects of rumination and distraction on naturally occurring depressed mood. *Cognition and Emotion, 7,* 561–570.

Nolen-Hoeksema, S., Morrow, J., & Fredrickson, B. L. (1993). Response styles and the duration of episodes of depressed mood. *Journal of Abnormal Psychology, 102,* 20–28.

Peterson, R. A., & Reiss, S. (1992). *Test manual for the Anxiety Sensitivity Index* (2nd ed.). Orland Park, IL: International Diagnostic Systems.

Plomin, R., Corley, R., Caspi, A., Fulker, D. W., & DeFries, J. (1998). Adoption results for self-reported personality: Evidence for nonadditive genetic effects? *Journal of Personality and Social Psychology, 75,* 211–218.

Reiss, S., & McNally, R. J. (1985). Expectancy model of fear. In S. Reiss & R. R. Bootzin (Eds.), *Theoretical issues in behavior therapy* (pp. 107–121). San Diego: Academic Press.

Roberts, B. W., & DelVecchio, W. F. (2000). The rank-order consistency of personality traits from childhood to old age: A quantitative review of longitudinal studies. *Psychological Bulletin, 126,* 3–25.

Rosser, S., Issakidis, C., & Peters, L. (2003). Perfectionism and social phobia: Relationship between the constructs and impact on cognitive behavior therapy. *Cognitive Therapy and Research, 27,* 143–151.

Roy, A. (1991). Personality variables in depressed patients and normal controls. *Neuropsychobiology, 23,* 119–123.

Schmidt, N. B., Lerew, D. R., & Jackson, R. J. (1997). The role of anxiety sensitivity in the pathogenesis of panic: Prospective evaluation of spontaneous panic attacks during acute stress. *Journal of Abnormal Psychology, 106*, 355–364.

Schmidt, N. B., Lerew, D. R., & Jackson, R. J. (1999). Prospective evaluation of anxiety sensitivity in the pathogenesis of panic: Replication and extension. *Journal of Abnormal Psychology, 108*, 532–537.

Simms, L. J., Watson, D., & Doebbeling, B. N. (2002). Confirmatory factor analyses of posttraumatic stress symptoms in deployed and non-deployed veterans of the Gulf War. *Journal of Abnormal Psychology, 111*, 637–647.

Taylor, S. (1999). *Anxiety sensitivity: Theory, research, and treatment of the fear of anxiety.* Mahwah, NJ: Erlbaum.

Taylor, S., Koch, W. J., & Crockett, D. J. (1991). Anxiety sensitivity, trait anxiety, and the anxiety disorders. *Journal of Anxiety Disorders, 6*, 293–311.

Tellegen, A. (1985). Structures of mood and personality and their relevance to assessing anxiety, with an emphasis on self-report. In A. H. Tuma & J. D. Maser (Eds.), *Anxiety and the anxiety disorders* (pp. 681–706). Hillsdale, NJ: Erlbaum.

Tellegen, A. (in press). *Manual for the Multidimensional Personality Questionnaire.* Minneapolis: University of Minnesota Press.

Viken, R. J., Rose, R. J., Kaprio, J., & Koskenvuo, M. (1994). A developmental genetic analysis of adult personality: Extraversion and neuroticism from 18 to 59 years of age. *Journal of Personality and Social Psychology, 66*, 722–730.

Vollebergh, W. A. M., Iedema, J., Bijl, R. V., de Graaf, R., Smit, F., & Ormel, J. (2001). The structure and stability of common mental disorders: The NEMESIS Study. *Archives of General Psychiatry, 58*, 597–603.

Watson, D. (2000). *Mood and temperament.* New York: Guilford Press.

Watson, D. (2005). Rethinking the mood and anxiety disorders: A quantitative hierarchical model for *DSM-V. Journal of Abnormal Psychology, 114*, 522–536.

Watson, D., & Clark, L. A. (1991). *The Mood and Anxiety Symptom Questionnaire.* Unpublished manuscript, University of Iowa, Iowa City.

Watson, D., & Clark, L. A. (1992). On traits and temperament: General and specific factors of emotional experience and their relation to the five-factor model. *Journal of Personality, 60*, 441–476.

Watson, D., & Clark, L. A. (1993). Behavioral disinhibition versus constraint: A dispositional perspective. In D. M. Wegner & J. W. Pennebaker (Eds.), *Handbook of mental control* (pp. 506–527). New York: Prentice-Hall.

Watson, D., & Clark, L. A. (1995). Depression and the melancholic temperament. *European Journal of Personality, 9*, 351–366.

Watson, D., & Clark, L. A. (1997a). Extraversion and its positive emotional core. In R. Hogan, J. Johnson, & S. Briggs (Eds.), *Handbook of personality psychology* (pp. 767–793). San Diego: Academic Press.

Watson, D., & Clark, L. A. (1997b). Measurement and mismeasurement of mood: Recurrent and emergent issues. *Journal of Personality Assessment, 68*, 267–296.

Watson, D., & Clark, L. A. (1999). *The PANAS-X: Manual for the Positive and Negative Affect Schedule—Expanded Form.* Retrieved from University of Iowa, Department of Psychology website: www.psychology.uiowa.edu/Faculty/Watson/Watson.html.

Watson, D., Clark, L. A., & Carey, G. (1988). Positive and negative affectivity and their relation to anxiety and depressive disorders. *Journal of Abnormal Psychology, 97,* 346–353.

Watson, D., Clark, L. A., & Harkness, A. R. (1994). Structures of personality and their relevance to psychopathology. *Journal of Abnormal Psychology, 103,* 18–31.

Watson, D., Clark, L. A., & Tellegen, A. (1988). Development and validation of brief measures of positive and negative affect: The PANAS Scales. *Journal of Personality and Social Psychology, 54,* 1063–1070.

Watson, D., Gamez, W., & Simms, L. J. (2005). Basic dimensions of temperament and their relation to anxiety and depression: A symptom-based perspective. *Journal of Research in Personality, 39,* 46–66.

Watson, D., Wiese, D., Vaidya, J., & Tellegen, A. (1999). The two general activation systems of affect: Structural findings, evolutionary considerations, and psychobiological evidence. *Journal of Personality and Social Psychology, 76,* 820–838.

Watson, D., & Wu, K. D. (2005). Development and validation of the Schedule of Compulsions, Obsessions, and Pathological Impulses (SCOPI). *Assessment, 12,* 50–65.

Watson, D., Wu, K. D., & Cutshall, C. (2004). Symptom subtypes of obsessive–compulsive disorder and their relation to dissociation. *Journal of Anxiety Disorders, 18,* 435–458.

Widiger, T. A., & Costa, P. T., Jr. (1994). Personality and the personality disorders. *Journal of Abnormal Psychology, 103,* 78–91.

Widiger, T. A., Verheul, R., & van den Brink, W. (1999). Personality and psychopathology. In L. A. Pervin & O. P. John (Eds.), *Handbook of personality* (2nd ed., pp. 347–366). New York: Guilford Press.

Chapter 3

The Five-Factor Model of Personality Disorder

A Translation across Science and Practice

STEPHANIE N. MULLINS-SWEATT
THOMAS A. WIDIGER

The theme of this text is "building bridges" across the domains of personality and psychopathology. Constructing a bridge across the domains of personality and personality disorder may also in turn construct another bridge, that between the basic science of personality and the clinical understanding of personality disorders. For some time, the National Institute of Mental Health (NIMH) has been encouraging the development of "translational" research. "NIMH has developed a number of initiatives designed to foster and speed the translation of basic behavioral and neuroscience work into research that addresses the etiology and treatment of mental disorders" (Cuthbert, 2002, p. 6). One intention of this compelling effort is to have the clinical understanding of mental disorders be guided more heavily by basic scientific understanding of psychological functioning. Additionally, these initiatives are intended to encourage laboratory research to have a more direct and clear impact on clinical practice. NIMH is investing considerable effort and funding to build the bridge across science and clinical practice. "These initiatives include large-scale and comprehensive translational research centers in neuroscience and behavioral science that are designed to encourage large-scale, hypothesis-driven integration of basic and clinical research" (Cuthbert, 2002, p. 6). One potential exemplification of this effort would be the integration of basic science research on personality structure with the psychiatric classification of personality disorders (Widiger & Costa, 1994).

"The application of personality trait models to the conceptualization of personality disorders has forged a much needed integration of what were separate areas of scientific study for most of the 20th century" (Ball, 2001, p. 151). The American Psychiatric Association's (2000) classification of personality disorders within the *Diagnostic and Statistical Manual of Mental Disorders* (DSM-IV-TR; American Psychiatric Association, 2000) has been derived from clinical experiences and research that have been largely divorced from the study of general personality structure (Millon et al., 1996). DSM-IV currently includes 10 personality disorder diagnostic categories (i.e., antisocial, avoidant, borderline, dependent, histrionic, narcissistic, obsessive–compulsive, paranoid, schizoid, and schizotypal). The theoretical and clinical origins of these diagnoses are diverse (Frances & Widiger, 1986; Livesley, 2001), but none traces its history to basic science research of general personality functioning.

The limitations of the DSM-IV personality disorder diagnoses have been well documented in a number of prior papers. These limitations include an inadequate scientific base, excessive diagnostic co-occurrence, arbitrary and inconsistent diagnostic boundaries, and inadequate coverage (First et al., 2002; Livesley, 2003; Shedler & Westen, 2004; Widiger, 1993). The purpose of this chapter is to understand the structure of maladaptive personality functioning from the perspective of general personality research. We present a brief summary of the conceptual and empirical support for the five-factor model of general personality functioning, followed by an indication of how the DSM-IV personality disorders can be understood from the perspective of the five-factor model (FFM). We conclude with a discussion of how personality disorders could be diagnosed with the FFM.

LEXICAL FOUNDATION OF THE FIVE-FACTOR MODEL

Most models of personality and personality disorder have been developed through the speculations and insights of prominent theorists (e.g., Cloninger, 2000; Millon et al., 1996). The development of the five-factor model was more consistently empirical, specifically, through empirical studies of trait terms within existing languages. This lexical paradigm is guided by the compelling hypothesis that what is of most importance, interest, or meaning to persons will be encoded within the language. Language can be understood as a sedimentary deposit of the observations of persons over the thousands of years of the language's development and transformation. The most important domains of personality functioning will be those with the greatest number of terms to describe and differentiate their various manifestations and nuances, and the structure of personality will be evident in the empirical relationship among these trait terms (Ashton & Lee, 2001; Goldberg, 1990, 1993).

The initial lexical studies were conducted, not surprisingly, within the English language, and these investigations converged well onto a five-factor structure (Goldberg, 1990). The five broad domains have been identified (in their order of size and therefore importance) as extraversion (or surgency), agreeableness, conscientiousness (or constraint), emotional instability (or neuroticism), and openness (or intellect, imagination, or unconventionality). There has been some disagreement as to the single best term to describe each domain, due in part to the fact that it is understandably difficult to identify one single term to adequately characterize the entire range of personality functioning included within a particular domain (Digman, 1990).

Subsequent lexical studies have been conducted on many additional languages, and these have confirmed well the existence of the five broad domains. De Raad, Perugini, Hrebiekova, and Szarota (1998) conducted a quantitative comparison of lexical studies conducted across seven languages (English, Dutch, German, Hungarian, Italian, Czech, and Polish). The first four domains of the FFM were found consistently. While the fifth factor (openness) was not identified as consistently, the researchers still concluded that the findings supported "the general contours of the Big Five model as the best working hypothesis of an omnipresent trait structure" (p. 214). Saucier and Goldberg (2001) summarized the results of lexical studies in English and 12 additional languages (German, Dutch, Czech, Polish, Russian, Italian, Spanish, Hebrew, Hungarian, Turkish, Korean, and Filipino). They concluded that the first three FFM domains (i.e., extraversion, agreeableness, and conscientiousness) were well replicated with the next two, smaller domains (i.e., neuroticism [negative affectivity] and openness [unconventionality]) replicating, but not as consistently. Ashton and Lee (2001) provided a systematic review of all of the lexical studies to date, and concluded that the studies which used the most credible procedures for language sampling "have repeatedly produced variances of surgency (I), agreeableness (II), conscientiousness (III), and emotional stability (IV), the first four factors of the well-known Big Five" (p. 328). The differences in findings for openness may reflect, in large part, cultural variations in the expression or appearance of this domain (Ashton, Lee, & Goldberg, 2004; McCrae, 2001). For example, openness "appears in various guises, ranging from pure Intellect (in German) to Unconventionality and Rebelliousness (in Dutch and Italian)" (John & Srivastava, 1999, p. 109).

The five-factor model does not suggest or imply that virtually every personality trait is included somewhere within the five broad domains. It only suggests that the five domains provide reasonably comprehensive coverage of the most important personality traits for describing oneself and other persons. There are personality traits and psychological attributes that exist beyond the Big Five. Lexical researchers disagree on whether it is useful to extract additional factors. Additional attributes that have been emphasized include religiosity, physical attractiveness, and judgmental evaluations (Ashton, Lee, & Goldberg, 2004), none of which might be necessary or useful to include in a dimensional model of personality disorder. It is even questionable whether all of these attributes should be included within a model of personality structure. For example, physical attractiveness is a very important individual differences variable that can have a significant impact on a wide range of social, occupational, and personal experiences. Nevertheless, it may not refer to differences in how a person characteristically thinks, feels, behaves, and relates to others.

The sixth domain of personality functioning that appears to have the most lexical support is an "honesty–humility" factor (sincere, fair, and honest vs. deceitful, sly, pretentious, and egotistical) identified by Ashton and his colleagues (e.g., Ashton, Lee, Perugini, et al., 2004). However, as a sixth factor, it is even smaller and less stable in its emergence than the fifth factor of openness (which itself is not as stable as the first four domains). In addition, this sixth factor does not describe traits that currently lie outside of the FFM. It is defined largely by traits included within the FFM domain of agreeableness (Costa & McCrae, 1992). Additionally important to note is that the first five domains of the Ashton six-factor model otherwise correspond well to the five domains of the FFM (Ashton, Lee, & Goldberg, 2004; Ashton, Lee, Perugini, et al., 2004).

Tellegen and Waller (1987) proposed additional dimensions of "personality" that concern how persons generally feel about or evaluate others. Terms with strong evaluative content (e.g., "excellent," "evil," "worthy," "superior," "impressive," "awful," and "cruel") have typically been excluded from lexical studies (Goldberg, 1990). Tellegen and Waller (1987) suggested that when one includes such evaluative terms, two additional broad domains of positive valence and negative valence are obtained. They further suggested that these two additional domains are particularly important in accounting for the psychopathology of personality disorders. It is evident that some of these terms are used explicitly in descriptions of some personality disorders (e.g., "evil" and "cruel" are used to describe antisocial persons). However, these terms do not appear to be describing a coherent domain of personality traits. The negative valence domain, for example, includes being dangerous, violent, insane, senile, retarded, stupid, or dumb, terms that clearly refer to a number of quite different areas of psychological dysfunction. This domain at best refers to a nonspecific social deviance

(Saucier, 2002) and is perhaps best understood as providing evaluative descriptions of, or attitudes toward, basic personality traits included within the first five domains of the FFM (Ashton & Lee, 2001). For example, being impressive, evil, or awful are evaluative judgments of personality traits; they themselves do not necessarily refer to particular traits. Persons would be considered to be excellent, evil, impressive, or awful because of their personality traits. For example, antisocial persons will be considered to be evil because of their callous exploitation of others, which is represented explicitly within facets of the FFM domain of antagonism (Lynam, 2002; Widiger & Lynam, 1998).

A universal appearance of the FFM is not surprising when one considers the domains of personality functioning that are being described (Ashton & Lee, 2001). The first two and largest domains are extraversion and agreeableness, which account largely for all manner of interpersonal relatedness. It is perhaps self-evident that a domain of personality functioning considered to be important across all cultures and languages would concern how persons relate to one another. Many personality disorder theorists have in fact placed considerable emphasis on interpersonal relatedness as providing the core features of personality and personality disorder (Benjamin, 1993; Kiesler, 1996; Plutchik & Conte, 1997; Wiggins, 2003). All forms of interpersonal relatedness are described well by the interpersonal circumplex (Kiesler, 1996), which is generally defined in terms of the two broad domains of agency (dominance vs. submission) and communion (affiliation, or love, vs. hate). These two dimensions have been shown in many studies to be equivalent to 45 degree rotations of the FFM domains of extraversion and agreeableness (Wiggins, 2003).

The third domain of the FFM is conscientiousness. This domain concerns the control and regulation of behavior, and contrasts being disciplined, compulsive, dutiful, conscientious, deliberate, workaholic, and achievement-oriented with being irresponsible, lax, impulsive, disinhibited, negligent, and hedonistic. It is again perhaps self-evident that all cultures would consider it to be important to describe the likelihood a person will be responsible, conscientious, competent, and diligent as a mate, parent, friend, employee, or colleague (versus being negligent, lax, disinhibited, and impulsive). The fourth domain, emotionality instability, is of considerable importance in the fields of clinical psychology and psychiatry, saturating most measures of personality disorder (Lilienfeld, 1994). It is again not surprising that most, and perhaps all, cultures consider the emotional stability (anxiousness, depressiveness, irritability, hostility, and vulnerability) of its partners, children, friends, and employees to be of considerable importance. In fact, the first four domains of the FFM (extraversion, agreeableness, conscientiousness, and emotional instability) distinctly define the fundamental domains of impairment that are used to diagnose personality (and other) mental disorders (i.e., impairment in social and occupational functioning, and personal distress; American Psychiatric Association, 2000). The fifth domain, openness, intellect, or unconventionality, reflects a culture or society's interest in creativity, intellect, imagination, and conventionality.

In sum, lexical studies have reported strong support for the universality of the first four domains of the FFM (extraversion, agreeableness, conscientiousness, and emotional instability) and somewhat less but still compelling support for the fifth and smallest domain, openness, intellect, or unconventionality. As Church (2001) concluded on the basis of his review of the cross-cultural research that the "Big-Five-like dimensions appear to be ubiquitous even in relatively indigenous lexical and inventory measures" (p. 987).

CONSTRUCT VALIDITY OF THE FIVE-FACTOR MODEL

One of the compelling features of the FFM as a dimensional model of personality disorders is its substantial empirical support as a dimensional model of general personality functioning. This research includes, but is not confined to, studies concerning convergent and discriminant validity, temporal stability, heritability, cross-cultural replication, and robustness. Each of these will be discussed briefly in turn.

Convergent and Discriminant Validity

The predominant measure of the FFM is the NEO Personality Inventory—Revised (NEO PI-R; Costa & McCrae, 1992). The NEO PI-R includes six facet scales within each of the five domains. Table 3.1 provides descriptors for each of the 60 poles of the 30 facets of the FFM, taken from the Five-Factor Model Rating Form that was modeled after the NEO PI-R (Mullins-Sweatt, Jamerson, Samuel, Olson, & Widiger, in press). Convergent and discriminant validity at both the domain and facet level have been well documented in quite a few studies conducted with the NEO PI-R (Costa & McCrae, 1992, 1995). This research includes convergent and discriminant validity among the respective scales of self-reports, peer reports, and spouse reports (e.g., McCrae, Stone, Fagan, & Costa, 1998) and the stability of the five-factor structure across gender, race, and age groups (e.g., Costa, McCrae, & Dye, 1991). Countless studies have also documented the convergent and discriminant validity of the NEO PI-R assessment of the domains and facets of the FFM with respect to constructs assessed by other inventories (Costa & McCrae, 1992; John & Srivastava, 1999).

TABLE 3.1. Domains and Facets of the Five-Factor Model

Extraversion versus Introversion

	High Extraversion	*Low Extraversion*
Warmth	Cordial, affectionate, attached	Cold, aloof, indifferent
Gregariousness	Sociable, outgoing	Withdrawn, isolated
Assertiveness	Dominant, forceful	Unassuming, quiet, resigned
Activity	Vigorous, energetic, active	Passive, lethargic
Excitement-Seeking	Reckless, daring	Cautious, monotonous, dull
Positive Emotions	High-spirited	Placid, anhedonic

Agreeableness versus Antagonism

	High Agreeableness	*Low Agreeableness*
Trust	Gullible, naive, trusting	Skeptical, cynical, paranoid
Straightforwardness	Confiding, honest	Cunning, manipulative, deceitful
Altruism	Sacrificial, giving	Stingy, greedy, exploitative
Compliance	Docile, cooperative	Combative, aggressive
Modesty	Meek, self-effacing, humble	Confident, boastful, arrogant
Tender-Mindedness	Soft, empathic	Tough, callous, ruthless

Conscientiousness versus Undependability

	High Conscientiousness	*Low Conscientiousness*
Competence	Perfectionist, efficient	Lax, negligent
Order	Ordered, methodical, organized	Haphazard, disorganized, sloppy
Dutifulness	Rigid, reliable, dependable	Casual, undependable, unethical
Achievement	Workaholic, ambitious	Aimless, desultory
Self-Discipline	Dogged, devoted	Hedonistic, negligent
Deliberation	Ruminative, reflective	Hasty, careless, rash

Neuroticism versus Emotional Stability

	High Neuroticism	*Low Neuroticism*
Anxiousness	Fearful, apprehensive	Relaxed, unconcerned, cool
Angry Hostility	Angry, bitter	Even-tempered
Depressiveness	Pessimistic, glum	Optimistic
Self-Consciousness	Timid, embarrassed	Self-assured, glib, shameless
Impulsivity	Tempted, urgent	Controlled, restrained
Vulnerability	Helpless, fragile	Stalwart, fearless, unflappable

Openness versus Closedness to Experience

	High Openness	*Low Openness*
Fantasy	Dreamer, unrealistic, imaginative	Practical, concrete
Aesthetics	Aberrant interests, aesthetic	Uninvolved, no aesthetic interest
Feelings	Sensitive, responsive	Constricted, alexithymic
Actions	Unconventional, adventurous	Predictable, stubborn, habitual
Ideas	Strange, odd, peculiar, creative	Pragmatic, rigid
Values	Permissive, broad-minded	Traditional, inflexible, dogmatic

Note. Descriptors taken from the Five-Factor Model Rating Form (Mullins-Sweatt, Jamerson, Samuel, Olson, & Widiger, in press).

The FFM, as assessed by the NEO PI-R, does not obtain a perfect simple structure. The domains and some of the facets of the FFM do correlate with other domains and with facet scales within other domains. These findings could suggest fundamental flaws of the FFM structural model. On the other hand, the findings may also represent understandable complexities of personality structure that are addressed reasonably well by the NEO PI-R FFM structure. Two illustrations from the domain of neuroticism will be provided: angry hostility and impulsiveness.

Angry Hostility

The NEO PI-R neuroticism facet of angry hostility often correlates significantly with the domain of antagonism (e.g., a significant correlation of .48 is reported in the NEO PI-R test manual, along with the correlation of .63 with the domain of neuroticism). This correlation is reasonable, as "hostile people are generally antagonistic" (Costa & McCrae, 1992, p. 45). Angry hostility is included within the domain of neuroticism because it refers to one of the fundamental components of negative affectivity (along with anxiousness and depressiveness; Watson & Tellegen, 1985). "Angry hostility represents the tendency to experience anger and related states such as frustration and bitterness" (Costa & McCrae, 1992, p. 16), whereas antagonism would refer to the interpersonal expression of this anger.

An alternative approach to the FFM is to shift much, if not all, of antagonism into the domain of negative affectivity, an approach taken by the three-factor models of Clark (1993) and Tellegen (Tellegen & Waller, 1987). These three-factor models do not include a separate domain of antagonism versus agreeableness. A limitation of this model, however, is that it loses an explicit representation of the two agency and affiliation dimensions that define the interpersonal circumplex (McCrae & Costa, 1989; Wiggins & Pincus, 1989). The interpersonal circumplex is a compelling structure of general personality functioning that has substantial conceptual and empirical support as a model of personality disorder (Benjamin, 1993; Kiesler, 1996; Plutchik & Conte, 1997; Wiggins, 2003). The agency and affiliation dimensions of the interpersonal circumplex are not recovered well by the three-factor models, whereas it is represented quite well by the two extraversion and agreeableness interpersonal domains of the FFM. In addition, factor analyses of personality disorder symptoms generally yield a separate antagonism factor (Livesley, Jang, & Vernon, 1998). For example, Clark's (1993) Schedule for Nonadaptive and Adaptive Personality (SNAP) includes scales for mistrust, manipulativeness, and aggression in order to represent all of the maladaptive personality traits included within DSM-IV (American Psychiatric Association, 2000). These scales are included within the negative affectivity domains of the three-factor model. However, factor analyses of the SNAP with other measures of personality disorder symptoms (with or without a measure of the FFM) have typically resulted in a separate antagonism factor (Clark & Livesley, 2002).

A complementary alternative is to shift the angry hostility facet of neuroticism to the domain of antagonism, a move that would be more consistent with the existing behavioral genetic research discussed later in this chapter (Jang, Livesley, Angleitner, Reimann, & Vernon, 2002). A limitation of this proposal is that it would dismantle the conceptually coherent domain of negative affectivity (Watson & Tellegen, 1985), separating the negative affects of anger and rage from anxiousness and depressiveness. Some of this difficulty, of course, reflects the fact that the optimal structural arrangement does not necessarily correspond to a factorial simple structure, with some axes occupying perhaps an interstitial location (McCrae & Costa, 1989).

Impulsiveness

The NEO PI-R neuroticism facet of impulsiveness often correlates with extraversion and conscientiousness. For example, in the NEO PI-R test manual, the neuroticism facet of impulsiveness correlated .49 with the domain of neuroticism (the lowest correlation obtained by any one of the facets of neuroticism), −.32 with conscientiousness and .35 with extraversion. Extraversion includes a facet of excitement-seeking, which will itself correlate with impulsiveness (Costa & McCrae, 1995). Additionally, some have suggested that impulsiveness instead should be confined largely to the domain of conscientiousness, titled perhaps as disinhibition, impulsive sensation seeking, or constraint (Clark, 1993; Zuckerman, 2002).

However, the approach taken by the NEO PI-R may in fact be advantageousness, as it is apparent from the literature that there are quite a few different meanings of the terms "impulsivity," "sensation seeking," "novelty seeking," "constraint," and "disinhibition." "Impulsivity comprises a heterogeneous cluster of lower-order traits that includes terms such as impulsivity, sensation seeking, risk-taking, novelty seeking, boldness, adventuresomeness, boredom susceptibility, unreliability, and unorderliness" (Depue & Collins, 1999, p. 495). "The term impulsiveness is used by many theorists to refer to many different and unrelated traits" (Costa & McCrae, 1992, p. 16). Whiteside and Lynam (2001) used the NEO PI-R to distinguish among four different variants of impulsivity: urgency, low premeditation, low perseverance, and sensation seeking.

The impulsiveness facet of the NEO PI-R is perhaps best described as urgency. "It refers to the tendency to experience strong impulses, frequently under conditions of negative affect" (Whiteside & Lynam, 2001, p. 685). As indicated by Costa and McCrae (1992), "NEO PI-R impulsiveness should not be confused with spontaneity, risk-taking, or rapid decision time" (p. 16). The disposition to act on the spur of the moment and without regard to consequences is represented by the NEO PI-R conscientiousness facet of deliberation, "the tendency to think carefully before acting" (Costa & McCrae, 1992, p. 18). Persons who are low in deliberation "are hasty and often speak or act without considering the consequences" (p. 18). Whiteside and Lynam (2001) refer to this variant of impulsivity as a lack of premeditation. "Premeditation refers to the tendency to think and reflect on the consequences of an act before engaging in that act" (Whiteside & Lynam, 2001, p. 685). NEO PI-R self-discipline refers to "the ability to begin tasks and carry them through to completion despite boredom and other distractions" (Costa & McCrae, 1992, p. 18). Whiteside and Lynam refer to this disposition as perseverance. The fourth and final variant of impulsivity is NEO PI-R excitement-seeking, which involves an enjoyment in taking risks and engaging in dangerous activities.

Whiteside and Lynam (2001) demonstrated empirically that these four different variations of the meaning of impulsivity have quite different correlations with existing impulsivity measures. Their inclusion within three different domains of the FFM is consistent with their different meaning and empirical correlates. Nevertheless, their distinction would probably be facilitated by using the term "urgency" for the facet of neuroticism rather than the more general term "impulsivity."

Temporal Stability

The temporal stability of the domains and facets of the FFM has been well documented through a number of studies, including longitudinal, prospective studies of 7–10 years in duration (McCrae & Costa, 2003). This does not imply that there are no changes in personality functioning. The studies of McCrae and Costa (2003) instead suggest that there are, on average, notable changes in neuroticism and extraversion (declining) and agreeableness and conscientiousness (increasing) between adolescence and age 30. They also suggest that there is a continuing (but lesser) decline in neuroticism, extraversion, and openness after age 30 (Costa, Herbst, McCrae, & Siegler, 2000; McCrae et al., 1999), although others suggest that the data indicate instead an increasing continuity of personality as one ages (Roberts & DelVecchio, 2000). In any case, the data do clearly support the fundamental principle of stability and continuity of personality functioning. This is in contrast to the weak temporal stability of personality disorder diagnoses and assessments, leading some to even question whether personality disorders are stable over time (Shea & Yen, 2003).

Heritability

There have been a number of univariate and multivariate heritability analyses of the FFM (e.g., Jang, McCrae, Angleitner, Riemann, & Livesley, 1998; Loehlin, McCrae, Costa, & John, 1998; Riemann, Angleitner, & Strelau, 1997). In comparison, there have been relatively few heritability studies of most of the DSM-IV personality disorders. It is evident that "the current DSM system of overlapping and arbitrary categorical diagnoses . . . yields obscure phenotypes that have limited value in genetic research" (Jang, Vernon, & Livesley, 2001, p. 242). In fact, reviews of the heritability of the personality disorders have relied substantially on the behavioral genetic research of the FFM personality traits (McGuffin & Thapar, 1992; Nigg & Goldsmith, 1994).

The behavioral genetic research has supported the heritability of the domains and facets of the FFM, as well as much of the FFM structural relationships among the domains and facet scales (e.g., McCrae, Jang, Livesley, Riemann, & Angleitner, 2001). Jang et al. (1998) conducted analyses of the raw and residual NEO PI-R (Costa & McCrae, 1992) facet scales (i.e., common variance shared with the domain scales removed), and demonstrated genetic and environmental influences of the same type and magnitude across both Canadian and German twin samples. The facet scales not only shared common variance with the domain scales but also demonstrated unique genetic variance. "These findings provide strong support for hierarchical models of personality that posit a large number of narrow traits as well as a few broader trait factors" (Jang et al., 1998, p. 1563). They further proposed that the findings suggest other specific traits (e.g., dependency and compulsiveness) that are currently not fully represented by the existing facet scales might also be included within the respective domains of the FFM.

Jang et al. (2002) subsequently used the same data to explore whether the heritability data support the specific hierarchical structure of the FFM provided by the NEO PI-R (Costa & McCrae, 1992). "For most domains there is a single common genetic factor that influences all the facets in a domain" (Jang et al., 2002, p. 99), "supporting the observed coherence of the NEO PI-R facet sets" (Jang et al., 2002, p. 83). Nevertheless, there was some fractionation, although not as extensive as has occurred using other measures of the FFM (e.g., Johnson & Krueger, 2004). Some of this fractionation is consistent with phenotypic studies, as for instance the finding that NEO PI-R impulsivity shares genetic variance with the domain of conscientiousness and angry hostility shares genetic variance with antagonism.

The search for the genes of personality functioning has produced mixed results (Plomin & Caspi, 1998). Jang et al. (2001) suggest that "most of the inconsistencies in the serotonin–neuroticism literature come from studies that do not use the NEO PI-R" (p. 235). In an extensive meta-analysis involving 5,629 subjects, Sen, Burmeister, and Ghosh (2004) concluded "that there is a strong association between the serotonin transporter promoter variant and neuroticism as measured in the NEO personality inventory and that non-replications are largely due to small sample size and the use of different inventories" (p. 85). Nevertheless, it is also apparent that the complex relationships between phenotypic traits and multiple genetic contributions will be difficult to isolate (Hamer, Greenberg, Sabol, & Murphy, 1999).

Cross-Cultural Replication

A common distinction in cross-cultural research is between etic and emic studies (Church, 2001). Etic studies use constructs and measures from one culture imported into another, determining (in part) whether the importation reproduces the nomological net of predictions previously obtained in other cultures. Emic studies use constructs and measures that are indigenous to a particular culture, determining whether a particular model of personality structure is evident from the perspective of that culture.

Etic studies are considered by many to be less compelling than emic studies. "The fact that researchers using different structural models of personality have been equally successful in replicating these structures across cultures suggests that imported measures do 'impose,' to some extent, their structure in new cultural contexts" (Church, 2001, p. 986). For example, one of the few etic studies of the universality of the DSM-IV personality disorder nomenclature was provided by the World Health Organization's International Pilot Study of Personality Disorders (WHO, 1992). This study determined whether the DSM-III-R (American Psychiatric Association, 1987) personality disorder nomenclature could be applied reliably in 11 different countries of North America, Europe, Africa, and Asia (Loranger et al., 1994). Loranger et al. reported problems for only two of the DSM-III-R personality disorder diagnostic criteria (i.e., the antisocial criterion pertaining to monogamous relationships and the sadistic criterion pertaining to harsh treatment of spouses and children). "Otherwise, the clinicians viewed [DSM-III-R] as applicable to their particular cultures" (Loranger et al., 1994, p. 223). However, a limitation of this etic study is evident by the fact that persons could meet the diagnostic criteria for a disorder that lacks any validity within the culture in which the criteria set was applied (Rogler, 1999). One can develop diagnostic criteria for an entirely illusory disorder and still find that a proportion of the population are beyond the threshold for its diagnosis. For example, one of the WHO findings was that passive–aggressive personality disorder was diagnosed in approximately 5% of the patients assessed in the different countries; yet, this diagnosis subsequently lost its official recognition in DSM-IV (American Psychiatric Association, 1994).

The lexical studies are emic approaches, as they determine whether particular domains of personality are evident within the indigenous languages of a particular society. Another emic approach is to study the structure found within inventories indigenous to a particular culture. Such studies have been conducted on inventories developed for Filipinos, Indians, and Chinese (Church, 2001). For example, Katigbak, Church, Guanzon-Lapena, Carlota, and del Pilar (2002) studied personality inventories and constructs indigeneous to the Filipino collectivist culture. They concluded that "most of the dimensions measured by Philippine personality inventories overlap considerably with, and are adequately encompassed by, dimensions of the five-factor model" (p. 97). They identified only a few scales that were less well accounted for (i.e., social curiosity, risk-taking, and religiosity), but they noted that the constructs assessed by these scales might not be entirely outside the realm of the FFM. Equally importantly, the Philippine inventories did not generally outperform an imported measure of the FFM in predicting scores on culture-relevant criteria, and the incremental validity provided by the indigenous scales was modest.

A criticism of the emic lexical paradigm is that it's essentially a series of studies of folk concepts (Rogler, 1999; Tellegen, 1993; Westen, 1995). For example, it is unlikely to be the case that all cultures or societies will have equally valid conceptualizations of personality structure or personality disorder. Simply because a personality trait (e.g., negative affectivity) or a disorder (e.g., schizophrenia) is not recognized within a particular culture or language does not necessarily imply that the trait or the disorder does not exist within that culture (Wakefield, 1994). Etic studies, then, can provide compelling support for the universal validity of a personality disorder nomenclature. For example, the perceptual experiences of a person who might be diagnosed, per DSM-IV, with the disorder of schizophrenia can be considered by some cultures or societies as partaking in a religious experience (Kirmayer, 1994). However, if this person genuinely met the DSM-IV criteria for schizophrenia, including insidious deterioration in functioning (e.g., in self-care or work for at least 6–months and a 1–month period of disorganized speech, grossly disorganized behavior, and negative symptoms (along with seemingly hearing the voice of God), one might in fact be correct in diagnosing this person with the mental disorder of schizophrenia rather than concluding that he or she did indeed hear the voice of God. This need not reflect a culturally biased perspective of a culture that is imposing its nomenclature onto another culture; instead, it may reflect the substantial amount of scientific research that supports the validity of the diagnosis of schizophrenia and the lack of comparable research to support the validity of the religious explanation (Widiger, 2002).

McCrae and Costa (1997) summarized the results of an extensive etic cross-cultural study of personality structure using translations of the NEO PI-R. The languages were from five different families: German (Germanic branch of the Indo-European), Portuguese (Italic branch of Indo-European), Hebrew (Hamito-Semitic), Chinese (Sino-Tibetan), Korean (not classified but shares features of Altaic languages), and Japanese (not classified but shares features of Austronesian and Austro-Asiatic languages). "When rotation was guided by a hypothesized target, virtually identical structures were found in all seven samples" (p. 514), with median cross-language factor congruence coefficients .94 or above for each domain; only 2 of the 105 coefficients failed to reach .90 (both were equal to .89). Replications of the cross-cultural stability of the FFM structure using translations of FFM measures have been provided in quite a number of additional languages (McCrae & Allik, 2002).

Robustness

An additional strength of the FFM is its robustness. "Personality psychology has been long beset by a chaotic plethora of personality constructs that sometimes differ in label while measuring nearly the same thing, and sometimes have the same label while measuring very different things" (Funder, 2001, p. 2000). The FFM has been used effectively in many prior studies and reviews as a basis for comparing, contrasting, and integrating seemingly diverse sets of personality scales (Funder, 2001; McCrae & Costa, 2003). "One of the apparent strengths of the Big Five taxonomy is that it can capture, at a broad level of abstraction, the commonalities among most of the existing systems of personality traits, thus providing an integrative descriptive model for research" (John & Srivastava, 1999, p. 122). Examples include the personality literature concerning gender (Feingold, 1994), temperament (Shiner, 1998; Shiner & Caspi, 2003), temporal stability (Roberts & Del Vecchio, 2000), health psychology (Segerstrom, 2000), and even animal species (Gosling & John, 1999).

O'Connor (2002) conducted interbattery factor analyses with previously published correlations involving FFM variables and the scales of 28 other personality inventories published in approximately 75 studies. He concluded that "the factor structures that exist in the scales of many popular inventories can be closely replicated using data derived solely from the scale associations with the FFM" (O'Connor, 2002, p. 198). "Exceptions to this finding occurred for only two of 28 personality inventories" (p. 188), and these were attributed at least in part to methodological artifacts. O'Connor (2002) concluded that "the basic dimensions that exist in other personality inventories can thus be considered 'well captured' by the FFM" (p. 198).

THE FIVE-FACTOR MODEL
OF PERSONALITY DISORDER

Given the robustness of the FFM as an integrative model of personality structure across a variety of domains of theory and research (Funder, 2001; Ozer & Reise, 1994; John & Srivastava, 1999), it is hardly a stretch of the imagination to suggest that the DSM-IV personality disorders could be understood as maladaptive variants of the domains and facets of the FFM. Widiger, Trull, Clarkin, Sanderson, and Costa (1994) provided an FFM description of each of the DSM-III-R personality disorders by coding each of the respective diagnostic criteria in terms of the FFM. Widiger, Trull, Clarkin, Sanderson, and Costa (2002) updated these descriptions using the DSM-IV criterion sets. Lynam and Widiger (2001) asked personality disorder researchers to describe each of the DSM-IV personality disorders in terms of the FFM. Samuel and Widiger (2004) asked practicing clinicians to do the same. Table 3.2 provides the DSM-IV-based FFM descriptions of Widiger, Costa, and McCrae (2002), the researchers' FFM descriptions (Lynam & Widiger, 2001), and the clinicians' descriptions (Samuel & Widiger, 2004) for the antisocial, borderline, and obsessive–compulsive personality disorders.

It is apparent that there is considerable consistency across these different approaches to generating FFM descriptions of the personality disorders. Across all of the personality disorders, the convergent validity coefficients for the clinicians' and researchers' descriptions ranged from .90 (dependent) to .97 (antisocial). This substantial agreement did not reflect simply the provision of a common profile for each personality disorder, as the FFM descriptions also demonstrated considerable discriminant validity. For example, the clinicians' dependent and antisocial FFM profiles correlated –.82, the histrionic and schizoid correlated –.61, and the dependent and paranoid were virtually uncorrelated (Samuel & Widiger, 2004).

There is also strong convergent validity for the clinicians' (Samuel & Widiger, 2004) and researchers' (Lynam & Widiger, 2001) descriptions with the descriptions developed by Widiger et al. (2002). Convergent validity for the clinicians' and the researchers' descriptions with Widiger et al. (1994, 2002) were all above .60 for the schizoid, schizotypal, antisocial, borderline, avoidant, and dependent personality disorders. Convergent validity coefficients for the paranoid, histrionic, narcissistic, and obsessive–compulsive personality disorders ranged from .40 to .60.

Sprock (2002) sent 89 licensed psychologists brief descriptions of prototypic and nonprototypic cases of the schizoid, antisocial, and obsessive–compulsive personality disorders (each psychologist received three case vignettes) and asked them to describe the patient in terms of the 30 facets of the FFM. Internal consistency of the FFM descriptions was excellent for

TABLE 3.2. FFM Descriptions of DSM-IV Personality Disorders

	Antisocial			Borderline			Obsessive–compulsive		
	W	R	C	W	R	C	W	R	C
Neuroticism									
Anxiousness		_1.82_	2.00	H	**4.04**	4.25		**4.00**	4.49
Angry Hostility	H	**4.14**	3.93	H	**4.75**	4.56		3.00	3.24
Depressiveness		2.45	2.70	H	**4.17**	4.03		3.18	3.76
Self-Consciousness		_1.36_	_1.63_		3.17	2.94		3.29	3.86
Impulsivity		**4.73**	**4.22**	H	**4.79**	4.38		_1.53_	2.18
Vulnerability		2.27	2.07	H	**4.17**	4.03		3.12	3.49
Extraversion									
Warmth		2.14	_2.00_		3.21	2.69		2.06	2.24
Gregariousness		3.32	3.48		2.92	3.28		2.18	2.40
Assertiveness		**4.23**	4.07		3.17	3.69	H	3.00	3.03
Activity		**4.00**	4.00		3.29	3.56		3.35	3.31
Excitement-Seeking	H	**4.64**	4.30		3.88	**4.06**		_1.59_	1.88
Positive Emotions		2.86	3.52		2.63	3.16		2.41	2.29
Openness									
Fantasy		2.82	3.48		3.29	**4.00**		2.06	2.52
Aesthetic		2.36	2.78		2.96	3.19		2.59	2.56
Feelings		2.27	2.41		**4.00**	3.84		_1.82_	2.22
Actions		**4.23**	4.07		**4.00**	3.78		_1.53_	1.76
Ideas		2.91	3.26		3.21	3.69		_1.76_	2.48
Values		3.00	3.48		2.88	3.00	L	_1.76_	1.82
Agreeableness									
Trust		_1.45_	1.70	L	2.21	_1.69_		2.65	2.20
Straightforwardness	L	_1.41_	1.41		2.08	_1.94_		3.47	3.06
Altruism	L	_1.41_	1.41		2.46	2.31		2.76	2.63
Compliance	L	_1.77_	1.81	L	2.00	_1.81_		3.18	2.82
Modesty		_1.68_	1.70		2.83	2.56		3.06	3.17
Tender-Mindedness	L	_1.27_	1.52		2.79	2.47		2.82	2.76
Conscientiousness									
Competence		2.09	2.52	L	2.71	2.78	H	**4.53**	4.41
Order		2.41	2.74		2.38	2.31		**4.76**	**4.59**
Dutifulness	L	_1.41_	1.52		2.29	2.22	H	**4.76**	4.20
Achievement		2.09	2.33		2.50	2.72	H	**4.29**	4.03
Self-Discipline	L	_1.81_	1.85		2.33	2.34		**4.53**	4.06
Deliberation	L	_1.64_	1.96		_1.88_	2.09		**4.59**	4.37

Note. W, FFM description of Widiger et al. (2002); R, FFM descriptions by personality disorder researchers in Lynam and Widiger (2001); C, FFM descriptions by practicing clinicians in Samuel and Widiger (2004). H, high; L, low.

each of the personality disorders, and average interrater reliability correlations ranged from a low of .51 for the two schizoid cases to .64 for the obsessive–compulsive and antisocial cases. The descriptions of the prototypic cases also converged significantly with the Widiger et al. (1994) FFM descriptions that were based on the coding of the DSM-III-R criterion sets, obtaining correlations of .44 for the schizoid, .60 for the antisocial, and .66 for the obsessive–compulsive. The convergence was much better with the more extensive Lynam and Widiger (2001) FFM descriptions provided by the researchers, obtaining correlations of .84, .87, and .86, respectively. Sprock (2002) concluded that "practicing clinicians can directly apply the dimensions of the FFM to cases of disordered personality with a moderate level of reliability" (p. 417).

Inspection of the profiles indicates that much of the disagreement between the researchers' and clinicians' FFM descriptions with Widiger et al. (1994, 2002) reflects the fact that the latter descriptions are much more limited (see Table 3.2). Widiger et al. confined their descriptions to FFM facets suggested by each respective DSM-III-R and DSM-IV diagnostic criterion, whereas the clinicians and researchers used many more of the FFM facets. For example, the clinicians' description of a prototypic obsessive–compulsive patient correlated .53 ($p < .001$) with the DSM-IV-based description of this personality disorder by Widiger et al. (2004). Both the clinicians and Widiger et al. (2002) described the prototypic obsessive–compulsive as being very high in the dutifulness, order, competence, and achievement-striving facets of conscientiousness, and low in openness to values (see Table 2). What was appreciably different in the two descriptions is that the clinicians also described the prototypic obsessive–compulsive as being high in the conscientiousness facets of self-discipline and deliberation; high in depressiveness and self-consciousness; low in the neuroticism facet of impulsiveness; low in openness to feelings and actions; low in the agreeableness facet of trust; and low in warmth and excitement-seeking. In sum, clinicians' FFM descriptions are providing a more comprehensive and rich description of this personality disorder.

It has long been recognized that it is difficult to represent the complex personality traits that constitute a personality disorder in terms of a small set of behaviorally specific diagnostic criteria (Hare, Hart, & Harpur, 1991; Livesley, 1985; Westen, 1997; Widiger & Frances, 1985). The existing criterion sets are an inconsistent mixture of behaviorally specific acts and general personality traits (Clark, 1992; Shea, 1992). A more comprehensive description of each personality disorder is provided by the FFM. For example, included within the researchers' and clinicians' FFM description of a prototypic case of antisocial personality disorder (see Table 3.2) were the low self-consciousness (glib charm), low modesty (arrogance), and low tender-mindedness (callousness) that are present within the traditional

conceptualizations of psychopathy (Lilienfeld, 1994) but have been excluded from the DSM-IV criterion set for antisocial personality disorder
(Hare et al., 1991). The FFM description of antisocial personality disorder
even includes the low anxiousness recognized by Cleckley (1941) that is not
included in the PCL-R (Hare, 2003).

Empirical Support

There is also considerable empirical support for understanding the DSM-IV
personality disorders as maladaptive variants of the personality traits included within the FFM. Widiger and Costa (2002) distinguished between
two waves of FFM personality disorder research. The first wave includes
the many studies of Costa, McCrae, and their colleagues that indicated
how the traits included within existing personality inventories can be well
accounted for by the FFM (Costa & McCrae, 1992; O'Connor, 2002).
Much of this extensive research is relevant to determining whether the FFM
can account for personality disorder symptoms, as most of the instruments
and scales they investigated were used, and continue to be used, within clinical populations to assess maladaptive personality traits.

Consider, for example, McCrae, Costa, and Busch (1986). McCrae et
al. demonstrated how the 100 items within the California Q-Set (CQS;
Block, 1961) can be readily understood from the perspective of the FFM.
The CQS items were developed by successive panels of psychodynamically
oriented clinical psychologists seeking a common language for the description of psychological functioning. McCrae et al. administered the CQS and
the NEO-PI (Costa & McCrae, 1992) to participants in the Baltimore Longitudinal Study of Aging. A factor analysis of the complete set of items (N – 403)
yielded five factors that corresponded empirically to the five domains of the
FFM. The results of McCrae et al. demonstrated a close correspondence of
a sophisticated psychodynamic nomenclature with the FFM. The CQS
"represents a distillation of clinical insights, and the fact that very similar
factors can be found in it provides striking support for the five-factor
model" (McCrae et al., 1986, p. 442).

A second wave of FFM personality disorder research has focused specifically on the American Psychiatric Association personality disorder nomenclature. Widiger and Costa (2002) identified over 50 such studies that
have used a variety of measures and have sampled from a variety of clinical
and nonclinical populations (e.g., Ball, Tennen, Poling, Kranzler, & Rounsaville, 1997; Blais, 1997; Clarkin, Hull, Cantor, & Sanderson, 1993; Costa
& McCrae, 1990; Dyce & O'Connor, 1998; Trull, 1992; Wiggins &
Pincus, 1989). All but a few of the authors of these studies concluded that
the personality disorders are well understood from the perspective of the
FFM. Livesley (2001) concluded on the basis of his review of the research

that "multiple studies provide convincing evidence that the DSM personality disorders diagnoses show a systematic relationship to the five factors and that all categorical diagnoses of DSM can be accommodated within the five-factor framework" (p. 24). Saulsman and Page (2004) conducted a meta-analysis of a subset of these studies and concluded that "the results showed that each [personality] disorder displays a five-factor model profile that is meaningful and predictable given its unique diagnostic criteria" (p. 1055).

Consider, for example, O'Connor and Dyce (1998). This research examined the ability of dimensional models of personality functioning in adequately explaining the covariation among personality disorders reported in nine previously published studies. They conducted independent principal-axes confirmatory analyses of seven alternative dimensional models on the 12 correlation matrices provided by the nine studies, and obtained highly significant congruence coefficients for all 12 correlation matrices for two of the dimensional models. "The personality disorder configurations that were most strongly supported . . . were the two that are based on attempts to identify basic dimensions of personality that exist in both clinical and nonclinical populations" (p. 15), specifically, the five-factor model of general personality (McCrae & Costa, 2003) and the seven-factor model of Cloninger (2000).

Quite a few additional studies not covered in the Widiger and Costa (2002) and Saulsman and Page (2004) reviews have since been published (e.g., De Clercq & De Fruyt, 2003; Huprich, 2003; Reynolds & Clark, 2001; Trull, Widiger, & Burr, 2001). Several of these studies will be noted here. For example, Hicklin and Widiger (in press) demonstrated the effectiveness of the FFM for understanding the convergence and divergence among six measures of antisocial and psychopathic personality disorder. The six measures had high convergent validity coefficients (Widiger & Coker, 2001), but, from the perspective of the FFM, they also clearly diverged with respect to their representation of core traits of psychopathy. The FFM includes not only the traits common to the antisocial and psychopathy constructs (e.g., exploitation, deception, impulsivity, irresponsibility, and aggression) but also the psychopathic personality traits of glib charm, low anxiousness, fearlessness, and arrogance not included within DSM-IV (Brinkley, Newman, Widiger, & Lynam, 2004; see Table 3.2). Facets of the FFM that represent these components of psychopathy (e.g., anxiousness, self-consciousness, vulnerability, and modesty; Lynam, 2002) were effective in clarifying fundamental distinctions among the antisocial and psychopathy measures.

Warner et al. (2004) considered the role of FFM personality traits in accounting for the temporal stability of personality disorder symptoms. Using data obtained from the Collaborative Longitudinal Study of Personality Disorders (CLPS; Gunderson et al., 2000), they reported considerable temporal stability in the FFM personality trait profiles. In addition, the researchers stated that "there is a specific temporal relationship between traits and disorder whereby changes in the [FFM] personality traits hypothesized to underlie personality disorders lead to subsequent changes in the disorder [but] this relationship does not seem to hold in the opposite direction" (Warner et al., 2004, pp. 222–223). Changes in FFM personality trait profiles predicted changes in the borderline, schizotypal, and avoidant personality disorder symptoms, but changes in the personality disorder symptoms had no comparable predictive validity for personality trait structure. "That is, trait changes are required to alter personality disorder, but personality disorder changes . . . do not necessarily lead to a change in traits" (Warner et al., 2004, p. 223). Warner et al. (2004) concluded that their finding "supports the contention that personality disorders stem from particular constellations of personality traits" (pp. 222–223).

Morey et al. (2002) used the CLPS data to address the discriminant validity of the FFM. They reported the FFM scores of 86 patients diagnosed with schizotypal, 175 with borderline, 157 with avoidant, and 153 with obsessive–compulsive personality disorders in the CLPS project. A discriminant function analysis indicated that the four personality disorders were differentiated significantly in terms of the 30 facets of the FFM, "demonstrating that variation in patient diagnoses could be explained in part by personality trait combinations" (p. 221). Nevertheless, it was also apparent from a visual inspection of the profiles that "all four of the disorders displayed a similar configuration of FFM traits" (p. 229). Much of the similarity, however, was due to the substantial diagnostic co-occurrence. Morey et al. repeated the analyses using a subsample of 24 schizotypals, 72 borderlines, 103 avoidants, and 105 obsessive–compulsives who did not meet criteria for one of the three other respective personality disorders. "The elimination of patients with comorbid study diagnoses did appear to sharpen the distinction between the personality disorder groups, whereas only 18 facets revealed substantive differences (i.e., effect sizes larger than .50) among the cell-assigned personality disorder diagnoses; 31 facets achieved this threshold using the noncomorbid groups" (pp. 224–225). The differentiation might further increase if the additional diagnostic co-occurrence with the six other personality disorders was also excluded.

Excessive diagnostic co-occurrence is a considerable problem for the construct validity of the DSM-IV personality disorder nomenclature (First et al., 2002; Livesley, 2003; Widiger, 1993). Lynam and Widiger (2001) indicated that much of this diagnostic co-occurrence can be accounted for by the FFM. They aggregated the personality disorder co-occurrence reported in 15 previous studies, and then demonstrated that this covariation was largely explained by the facets of the FFM that are common to the respective personality disorders. For example, the FFM understanding of the antisocial personality disorder accounted for 85% of its diagnostic occurrence reported in nine DSM-III (American Psychiatric Association, 1980) studies and 76% of its diagnostic co-occurrence reported in the six DSM-III-R (1987) studies obtained for the authors of the DSM-IV criterion sets. "Under the FFM account, disorders appear comorbid to the extent that they are characterized by the same [FFM] facets" (Lynam & Widiger, 2001, p. 409).

Coker, Samuel, and Widiger (2002) conducted one of the few lexical studies of personality disorder. They evaluated social desirability ratings of the 1,710 trait terms included within Goldberg's (1982) lexical sample to indicate that both poles of all five domains include maladaptive personality traits, many of which clearly refer to DSM-IV personality disorder symptoms (e.g., dependent, conscienceless, violent, reckless, deceitful, introverted, and flaunty). High neuroticism is generally less adaptive than low neuroticism, antagonism is generally less adaptive than agreeableness, introversion is generally less adaptive than extraversion, and low conscientiousness is generally less adaptive than high conscientiousness, but both poles of every domain do appear to include at least some maladaptive personality functioning, consistent with prior studies of low neuroticism (e.g., Costa & McCrae, 1990; Miller, Lynam, Widiger, & Leukefeld, 2001; Soldz, Budman, Denby, & Merry, 1993; Wiggins & Pincus, 1989), high agreeableness (e.g., Blais, 1997; Costa & McCrae, 1990; Dyce & O'Connor, 1998; Wiggins & Pincus, 1989), high extraversion (e.g., Blais, 1997; Soldz et al., 1993; Trull et al., 1998; Wiggins & Pincus, 1989), and high conscientiousness (e.g., Blais, 1997; Costa & McCrae, 1990; Dyce & O'Connor, 1998; Soldz et al., 1993; Wiggins & Pincus, 1989).

Most existing FFM instruments have been developed for the study of general personality functioning (De Raad & Perugini, 2002). Therefore, these instruments might not provide adequate fidelity for the assessment and description of the maladaptive variants of the FFM. For example, although many studies have verified that FFM agreeableness is associated with dependent personality traits (e.g., Blais, 1997; Costa & McCrae, 1990; Dyce & O'Connor, 1998; Wiggins & Pincus, 1989), conscientiousness is associated with obsessive–compulsive personality traits (e.g., Blais, 1997; Costa & McCrae, 1990; Dyce & O'Connor, 1998; Soldz et al., 1993; Wiggins & Pincus, 1989), and openness is associated with schizotypal traits (e.g., Trull et al., 1998; Wiggins & Pincus, 1989), additional studies have failed to confirm these associations (e.g., Bornstein & Cecero, 2000; Ball et al., 1997; Yeung, Lyons, Waternaux, Faraone, & Tsuang, 1993). Haigler and Widiger (2001) demonstrated empirically that the negative findings could be due largely to the absence of adequate representation of the maladaptive variants of the domains of agreeableness, conscientiousness, and openness within the predominant measures of the FFM.

Haigler and Widiger (2001) first replicated the insignificant to marginal correlations of NEO PI-R (Costa & McCrae, 1992) agreeableness, conscientiousness, and openness with the dependent, obsessive–compulsive, and schizotypal personality disorders (each of the latter were assessed by three independent measures). They then revised existing NEO PI-R items by inserting words to indicate that the behavior described within the item was excessive, extreme, or maladaptive. The content of the items was not otherwise altered. This experimental manipulation of the NEO PI-R items resulted in quite substantial correlations of agreeableness with dependency, conscientiousness with the obsessive–compulsive personality disorder, and (to a somewhat lesser extent) openness with schizotypal personality disorder. Haigler and Widiger (2001) concluded that their findings "offer further support for the hypothesis that personality disorders are maladaptive variants of normal personality traits by indicating that correlations of NEO PI-R Conscientiousness, Agreeableness, and Openness scales with obsessive–compulsive, dependent, and schizotypal symptomatology would . . . be obtained by simply altering existing NEO PI-R . . . items that describe desirable, adaptive behaviors or traits into items that describe undesirable, maladaptive variants of the same traits" (p. 356).

Miller and colleagues (Miller & Lynam, 2003; Miller et al., 2001) demonstrated that a quantitative measure of the extent to which a person's FFM personality trait profile matches the hypothesized FFM profile of psychopathy resonated with those findings commonly reported for psychopathy, including drug usage, delinquency, risky sex, aggression, and several laboratory assessments of pathologies hypothesized to underlie psychopathy (including willingness to delay gratification in a time-discounting task and a preference for aggressive responses in a social-information processing paradigm). Similarly, Trull, Widiger, Lynam, and Costa (2003) demonstrated that the extent to which an individual's FFM personality trait profile matched the hypothesized FFM profile of borderline personality disorder correlated as highly with measures of borderline personality disorder as the latter correlated with one another. Furthermore, this FFM borderline index demonstrated incremental validity in accounting for borderline psychopathology beyond the variance that was explained by a 2–hour semistructured interview devoted to the assessment of this personality disorder. Such studies suggest that the extent to which an individual's FFM profile of personality traits matches profiles of a respective personality disorder reproduces the nomological net of predictions that have been hypothesized for that personality disorder.

Sprock (2003) addressed the potential clinical utility of the FFM descriptions in a survey of clinicians. She asked one group of psychologists to rate brief case vignettes of prototypic and nonprototypic cases of three personality disorders with respect to the FFM (as well as other dimensional models of personality disorder), to indicate the confidence of their rating, and to estimate the potential usefulness of the descriptions for professional communication, case conceptualization, and treatment planning. Another group of psychologists provided the same ratings for the DSM-IV personality disorder diagnostic categories. Diagnostic confidence was higher for the DSM-IV diagnostic categories, as were the ratings of utility for professional communication, case conceptualization, and treatment planning. However, Sprock acknowledged that much of her results could simply reflect the fact that the clinicians had been trained with, and were much more familiar with, the DSM-IV diagnostic categories. She suggested that "it may take a new cohort of clinicians, trained in a dimensional approach to diagnosis, to obviate the need to translate back to the categories" (Sprock, 2003, p. 1010). In addition, an important methodological limitation of her study was that the vignettes provided to the clinicians were written to represent explicitly DSM-III-R and DSM-IV personality disorder diagnostic criteria. It is perhaps hardly surprising that DSM-IV diagnoses were more easily applied to case studies written explicitly to represent their diagnostic criterion sets. Nevertheless, the findings of her study do suggest that further work is needed on developing the clinical utility of the FFM if, in fact, it is to become a viable replacement for the DSM-IV diagnostic categories.

Five-Factor Model Personality Disorder Diagnosis

Widiger, Costa, and McCrae (2002) have proposed a four-step procedure for clinicians to use to diagnose a personality disorder from the perspective of the FFM. The first step is to provide a comprehensive assessment of personality functioning with an existing measure of the FFM (De Raad & Perugini, 2002). The second step is to identify the social and occupational impairments and distress associated with the individual's characteristic personality traits. Widiger et al. identified common impairments that would likely be associated with each of the 60 poles of the 30 facets of the FFM, including (but not limited to) DSM-IV personality disorder symptomatology. The third step is to determine whether the dysfunction and distress reach a clinically significant level of impairment. The fourth step is a quantitative matching of the individual's personality profile to prototypic profiles of diagnostic constructs. This last step is provided for clinicians and researchers who wish to continue to provide single diagnostic labels to characterize a person's personality profile. To the extent that an individual's profile does match the FFM profile of a prototypic case, a single term (e.g., psychopathic) would provide a succinct means of communication (Lynam, 2002). However, prototypic profiles are likely to be quite rare within clinical practice. In such cases, the matching can serve to indicate the extent to which any particular diagnostic category would be adequately descriptive.

We expect that an FFM diagnosis of personality disorder will ulti-mately prove to have considerable clinical utility. A five-factor description of maladaptive personality functioning could facilitate treatment recom-mendations, as each domain may have more differentiated implications for functioning and treatment planning than the existing diagnostic categories. In fact, the structure of the FFM corresponds well with the basic compo-nents of personality impairment. A personality disorder is diagnosed when the personality traits lead to "clinically significant distress or impairment in social, occupational, or other important areas of functioning" (American Psychiatric Association, 2000, p. 689). FFM extraversion and agreeable-ness provide the domains of maladaptive interpersonal relatedness (social impairment). Dysfunction within these domains will be of particular inter-est and concern to clinicians specializing in marital, family, or other forms of interpersonal dysfunction. The domain of conscientiousness involves, at the low end, disorders of impulse dysregulation and disinhibition for which there is a considerable amount of specific treatment literature. Disorders within this realm would be particularly evident in behavior that affects work, career, and parenting (occupational impairment), with laxness, irre-sponsibility, and negligence at one pole and a maladaptively excessive per-fectionism and workaholism at the other pole. The domain of neuroticism or negative affectivity provides the domain of distress, and would be most suggestive of pharmacotherapy (as well as psychotherapy) for the treatment of various forms of affective dysregulation that are currently spread across the diagnostic categories, including anxiousness, depressiveness, anger, and instability of mood. Finally, high levels of the domain of openness would have specific implications for impaired reality testing, magical thinking, and perceptual aberrations (i.e., cognitive dysfunction), whereas at the other pole would be alexithymia, prejudice, closed-mindedness, and a ster-ile absence of imagination.

CONCLUSIONS

The purpose of this chapter was to build a bridge between basic science re-search on general personality structure with the clinical diagnosis of per-sonality disorder. We suggest that the FFM provides a compelling basis for this bridge. Advantages of the FFM approach to the diagnosis of personal-ity disorders include the provision of a precise yet comprehensive descrip-tion of both normal and abnormal personality functioning, the avoidance of the many limitations and problems inherent to the categorical diagnostic system, and the incorporation of basic science research on general personal-ity functioning into our understanding of personality disorders.

REFERENCES

American Psychiatric Association. (1980). *Diagnostic and statistical manual of mental disorders* (3rd ed.). Washington, DC: Author.

American Psychiatric Association. (1987). *Diagnostic and statistical manual of mental disorders* (3rd ed., rev.). Washington, DC: Author.

American Psychiatric Association. (1994). *Diagnostic and statistical manual of mental disorders* (4th ed.). Washington, DC: Author.

American Psychiatric Association. (2000). *Diagnostic and statistical manual of mental disorders* (4th ed., text rev.). Washington, DC: Author.

Ashton, M. C., & Lee, K. (2001). A theoretical basis for the major dimensions of personality. *European Journal of Personality, 15,* 327–353.

Ashton, M. C., Lee, K., & Goldberg, L. R. (2004). A hierarchical analysis of 1,710 English personality-descriptive adjectives. *Journal of Personality and Social Psychology, 87*(5), 707–721.

Ashton, M. C., Lee, K., Perugini, M., Szarota, P., de Vries, R. E., Di Blas, L., et al. (2004). A six-factor structure of personality descriptive adjectives: Solutions from psycholexical studies in seven languages. *Journal of Personality and Social Psychology, 86,* 356–366.

Ball, S. A. (2001). Reconceptualizing personality disorder categories using personality trait dimensions: Introduction to special section. *Journal of Personality, 69,* 147–153.

Ball, S. A., Tennen, H., Poling, J. C., Kranzler, H. R., & Rounsaville, B. J. (1997). Personality, temperament, and character dimensions and the DSM-IV personality disorders in substance abusers. *Journal of Abnormal Psychology, 106,* 545–553.

Benjamin, L. S. (1993). Dimensional, categorical, or hybrid analyses of personality: A response to Widiger's proposal. *Psychological Inquiry, 4,* 91–95.

Blais, M. (1997). Clinician ratings of the five-factor model of personality and DSM-IV personality disorders. *Journal of Nervous and Mental Diseases, 185,* 388–393.

Block, J. (1961). *The Q-sort method in personality assessment and psychiatric research.* Springfield, IL: Thomas.

Bornstein, R. F., & Cecero, J. J. (2000). Deconstructing dependency in a five-factor world: A meta-analytic review. *Journal of Personality Assessment, 74,* 324–343.

Brinkley, C. A., Newman, J. P., Widiger, T. A., & Lynam, D. R. (2004). Two approaches to parsing the heterogeneity of psychopathy. *Clinical Psychology Science and Practice, 11,* 69–94.

Church, A. T. (2001). Personality measurement in cross-cultural perspective. *Journal of Personality, 69,* 979–1006.

Clark, L. A. (1992). Resolving taxonomic issues in personality disorders: The value of large-scale analyses of symptom data. *Journal of Personality Disorders, 6,* 360–376.

Clark, L. A. (1993). *Manual for the Schedule for Nonadaptive and Adaptive Personality.* Minneapolis: University of Minnesota Press.

Clark, L. A., & Livesley, W. J. (2002). Two approaches to identifying the dimensions of personality disorder: Convergence on the five-factor model. In T. A. Widiger

& P. T. Costa (Eds.), *Personality disorders and the five-factor model of personality* (2nd ed., pp. 161–176). Washington, DC: American Psychological Association.

Clarkin, J. F., Hull, J. W., Cantor, J., & Sanderson, C. (1993). Borderline personality disorder and personality traits: A comparison of SCID-II BPD and NEO-PI. *Psychological Assessment, 5,* 472–476.

Cleckley, H. (1941). *The mask of sanity.* Oxford, UK: Mosby.

Cloninger, C. R. (2000). A practical way to diagnose personality disorder: A proposal. *Journal of Personality Disorders, 14,* 98–108.

Coker, L. A., Samuel, D. B., & Widiger, T. A. (2002). Maladaptive personality functioning within the Big Five and the five-factor model. *Journal of Personality Disorders, 16,* 385–401.

Costa, P. T., Herbst, J. H., McCrae, R. R., & Siegler, I. C. (2000). Personality at midlife: Stability, intrinsic maturation, and response to life events. *Assessment, 7,* 365–378.

Costa, P. T., Jr., & McCrae, R. R. (1990). Personality disorders and the five-factor model of personality. *Journal of Personality Disorders, 4,* 362–371.

Costa, P. T., Jr., & McCrae, R. R. (1992). *The NEO PI-R professional manual.* Odessa, FL: Psychological Assessment Resources.

Costa, P., & McCrae, R. R. (1995). Domains and facets: Hierarchical personality assessment using the Revised NEO Personality Inventory. *Journal of Personality Assessment, 64,* 21–50.

Costa, P. T., McCrae, R. R., & Dye, D. A. (1991). Facet scales for agreeableness and conscientiousness: A revision of the NEO Personality Inventory. *Personality and Individual Differences, 12,* 887–898.

Cuthbert, B. N. (2002). Social anxiety disorder: Trends and translational research. *Biological Psychiatry, 51,* 4–10.

De Clercq, B., & De Fruyt, F. (2003). Personality disorder symptoms in adolescence: A five-factor model perspective. *Journal of Personality Disorders, 17,* 269–292.

DePue, R. A., & Collins, P. F. (1999). Neurobiology of the structure of personality: Dopamine, facilitation of incentive motivation, and extraversion. *Behavioral and Brain Sciences, 22,* 491–569.

De Raad, B., & Perugini, M. (2002). *Big five assessment.* Ashland, OH: Hogrefe & Huber.

De Raad, B., Perugini, M., Hrebiekova, M., & Szarota, P. (1998). Lingua franca of personality: Taxonomies and structures based on the psycholexical approach. *Journal of Cross Cultural Psychology, 29,* 212–232.

Digman, J. M. (1990). Personality structure: Emergence of the five-factor model. *Annual Review of Psychology, 41,* 417–470.

Dyce, J. A., & O'Connor, B. P. (1998). Personality disorder and the five-factor model: A test of facet level predictions. *Journal of Personality Disorders, 12,* 31–45.

Feingold, A. (1994). Gender differences in personality: A meta-analysis. *Psychological Bulletin, 116*(3), 429–456.

First, M. B., Bell, C. B., Cuthbert, B., Krystal, J. H., Malison, R., Offord, D. R., et al. (2002). Personality disorders and relational disorders: A research agenda for addressing crucial gaps in DSM. In D. J. Kupfer, M. B. First, & D. A. Regier (Eds.),

A research agenda for DSM-V (pp. 123–199). Washington, DC: American Psychiatric Association.

Frances, A., & Widiger, T. A. (1986). Methodological issues in personality disorder diagnosis. In G. L. Klerman & T. Millon (Eds.), *Contemporary directions in psychopathology: Toward the DSM-IV* (pp. 381–400). New York: Guilford Press.

Funder, D. C. (2001). Personality. *Annual Review of Psychology, 52,* 197–221.

Goldberg, L. R. (1982). From Ace to Zombie: Some explorations in the language of personality. In C. D. Spielberger & J. N. Butcher (Eds.), *Advances in personality assessment* (Vol. 1, pp. 203–234). Hillsdale, NJ: Erlbaum.

Goldberg, L. R. (1990). An alternative "description of personality": The Big-Five-factor structure. *Journal of Personality and Social Psychology, 59,* 1216–1229.

Goldberg, L. R. (1993). The structure of phenotypic personality traits. *American Psychologist, 48,* 26–34.

Gosling, S. D., & John, O. P. (1999). Personality dimensions in nonhuman animals: A crossspecies review. *Current Directions in Psychological Science, 8,* 69–75.

Gunderson, J. G., Shea, M. T., Skodol, A. E., McGlashan, T. H., Morey, L. C., Stout, R. L., et al. (2000). The Collaborative Longitudinal Personality Disorders Study: I. Development, aims, design, and sample characteristics. *Journal of Personality Disorders, 14,* 300–315.

Haigler, E. D., & Widiger, T. A. (2001). Experimental manipulation of NEO PI-R items. *Journal of Personality Assessment, 77,* 339–358.

Hamer, D. H., Greenberg, B. D., Sabol, S. Z., & Murphy, D. L. (1999). Role of the serotonin transporter gene in temperament and character. *Journal of Personality Disorders, 13,* 312–328.

Hare, R. D. (2003). *Hare Psychopathy Checklist Revised (PCL-R): Technical manual.* North Tonawanda, NY: Multi-Health Systems.

Hare, R. D., Hart, S. D., & Harpur, T. J. (1991). Psychopathy and the DSM-IV criteria for antisocial personality disorder. *Journal of Abnormal Psychology, 100,* 391–398.

Hicklin, J., & Widiger, T. A. (in press). Similarities and differences among antisocial and psychopathic self-report inventories from the perspective of general personality functioning. *European Journal of Psychology.*

Huprich, S. K. (2003). Evaluating facet-level predictions and construct validity of depressive personality disorder. *Journal of Personality Disorders, 17,* 219–232.

Jang, K. L., Livesley, W. J., Angleitner, A., Riemann, R., & Vernon, P. A. (2002). Genetic and environmental influences on the covariance of facets defining the domains of the five-factor model of personality. *Personality and Individual Differences, 33,* 83–101.

Jang, K. L., McCrae, R. R., Angleitner, A., Riemann, R., & Livesley, W. J. (1998). Heritability of facet-level traits in a cross-cultural twin sample: Support for a hierarchical model of personality. *Journal of Personality and Social Psychology, 74,* 1556–1565.

Jang, K. L., Vernon, P. A., & Livesley, W. J. (2001). Behavioural-genetic perspectives on personality function. *Canadian Journal of Psychiatry, 46,* 234–244.

John, O. P., & Srivastava, S. (1999). The Big Five trait taxonomy: History, measurement, and theoretical perspectives. In L. A. Pervin & O. P. John (Eds.), *Hand-*

book of personality: Theory and research (2nd ed., pp. 102–138). New York: Guilford Press.

Johnson, W., & Krueger, R. F. (2004). Genetic and environmental structure of adjectives describing the domains of the Big Five Model of personality: A nationwide U.S. twin study. *Journal of Research in Personality, 38,* 448–472.

Katigbak, M. S., Church, A. T., Guanzon, L. M., Carlota, A. J., & del Pilar, G. H. (2002). Are indigenous personality dimensions culture specific? Philippine inventories and the five-factor model. *Journal of Personality and Social Psychology, 82,* 89–101.

Kiesler, D. J. (1996). *Contemporary interpersonal theory and research: Personality, psychopathology, and psychotherapy.* New York: Wiley.

Kirmayer, L. J. (1994). Is the concept of mental disorder culturally relative? In S. A. Kirk & S. D. Einbinder (Eds.), *Controversial issues in mental health* (pp. 2–9). Boston: Allyn & Bacon.

Lilienfeld, S. O. (1994). Conceptual problems in the assessment of psychopathy. *Clinical Psychology Review, 14,* 17–38.

Livesley, W. J. (1985). The classification of personality disorder: II. The problem of diagnostic criteria. *Canadian Journal of Psychiatry, 30,* 359–362.

Livesley, W. J. (2001). Conceptual and taxonomic issues. In W. J. Livesley (Ed.), *Handbook of personality disorders: Theory, research, and treatment* (pp. 3–38). New York: Guilford Press.

Livesley, W. J. (2003). Diagnostic dilemmas in classifying personality disorder. In K. A. Phillips, M. B. First, & H. A. Pincus (Eds.), *Advancing DSM. Dilemmas in psychiatric diagnosis* (pp. 153–190). Washington, DC: American Psychiatric Association.

Livesley, W. J., Jang, K. L., & Vernon, P. A. (1998). Phenotypic and genetic structure of traits delineating personality disorder. *Archives of General Psychiatry, 55,* 941–948.

Loranger, A. W., Sartorius, N., Andreoli, A., Berger, P., Buchheim, P., Channabasavanna, S. M., et al. (1994). The International Personality Disorder Examination. The World Health Organization/Alcohol, Drug Abuse, and Mental Health Administration international pilot study of personality disorders. *Archives of General Psychiatry, 51,* 215–224.

Lynam, D. R. (2002). Fledgling psychopathy: A view from personality theory. *Law and Human Behavior, 26,* 255–259.

Lynam, D. R., & Widiger, T. A. (2001). Using the five-factor model to represent the DSM-IV personality disorders: An expert consensus approach. *Journal of Abnormal Psychology, 110,* 401–412.

McCrae, R. R. (2001). Trait psychology and culture: Exploring intercultural comparisons. *Journal of Personality, 69,* 819–846.

McCrae, R. R., & Allik, J. (2002). *The five-factor model of personality across cultures.* New York: Plenum Publishers.

McCrae, R. R., & Costa, P. T. (1989). The structure of interpersonal traits: Wiggins's circumplex and the five-factor model. *Journal of Personality and Social Psychology, 56,* 586–595.

McCrae, R. R., & Costa, P. T. (1997). Personality trait structure as a human universal. *American Psychologist, 52,* 509–516.

McCrae, R. R., & Costa, P. T. (2003). *Personality in adulthood. A five-factor theory perspective* (2nd ed.). New York: Guilford Press.

McCrae, R. R., Costa, P. T., & Busch, C. M. (1986). Evaluating comprehensiveness in personality systems: The California Q-Set and the five-factor model. *Journal of Personality, 54,* 430–446.

McCrae, R. R., Costa, P. T., de Lima, M. P., Simoes, A., Ostendorf, F., Angleitner, A., et al. (1999). Age differences in personality across the adult life span: Parallels in five cultures. *Developmental Psychology, 35,* 466–477.

McCrae, R. R., Jang, K. L., Livesley, W. J., Riemann, R., & Angleitner, A. (2001). Sources of structure: Genetic, environmental, and artifactual influences on the covariation of personality traits. *Journal of Personality, 69,* 511–535.

McCrae, R. R., Stone, S. V., Fagan, P. J., & Costa, P. T. (1998). Identifying causes of disagreement between self-reports and spouse ratings of personality. *Journal of Personality, 66,* 285–313.

McGuffin, P., & Thapar, A. (1992). The genetics of personality disorder. *British Journal of Psychiatry, 160,* 12–23.

Miller, J. D., & Lynam, D. R. (2003). Psychopathy and the five-factor model of personality: A replication and extension. *Journal of Personality Assessment, 81,* 168–178.

Miller, J. D., Lynam, D. R., Widiger, T. A., & Leukefeld, C. (2001). Personality disorders as extreme variants of common personality dimensions: Can the Five-Factor Model adequately represent psychopathy? *Journal of Personality, 69,* 253–276.

Millon, T., Davis, R. D., Millon, C. M., Wenger, A., Van Zuilen, M. H., Fuchs, M., et al. (1996). An evolutionary theory of personality disorders. In M. F. Lenzenweger & J. F. Clarkin (Eds.), *Major theories of personality disorder* (pp. 221–346). New York: Guilford Press.

Morey, L. C., Gunderson, J. G., Quigley, B. D., Shea, M. T., Skodol, A. E., McGlashan, T. H., et al. (2002). The representation of borderline, avoidant, obsessive–compulsive, and schizotypal personality disorders by the five-factor model. *Journal of Personality Disorders, 16,* 215–234.

Mullins-Sweatt, S. N., Jamerson, J. E., Samuel, D. B., Olson, D. R., & Widiger, T. A. (in press). *Psychometric properties and implications of an abbreviated instrument of the five-factor model.* Unpublished manuscript, University of Kentucky, Lexington.

Nigg, J. T., & Goldsmith, H. H. (1994). Genetics of personality disorders: Perspectives from personality and psychopathology research. *Psychological Bulletin, 115,* 346–380.

O'Connor, B. P. (2002). A quantitative review of the comprehensiveness of the five-factor model in relation to popular personality inventories. *Assessment, 9,* 188–203.

O'Connor, B. P., & Dyce, J. A. (1998). A test of personality disorder configuration. *Journal of Abnormal Psychology, 107,* 3–16.

Ozer, D. J., & Reise, S. P. (Eds.). (1994). Personality assessment. *Annual Review of Psychology, 45,* 357–388.

Plomin, R., & Caspi, A. (1998). DNA and personality. *European Journal of Personality, 12,* 387–407.

Plutchnik, R., & Conte, H. R. (1997). *Circumplex models of personality and emotions.* Washington, DC: American Psychological Association.

Reynolds, S. K., & Clark, L. A. (2001). Predicting dimensions of personality disorders from domains and facets of the five-factor model. *Journal of Personality, 69,* 199–222.

Riemann, R., Angleitner, A., & Strelau, J. (1997). Genetic and environmental influences on personality: A study of twins reared together using the self- and peer-report NEO-FFI scales. *Journal of Personality, 65,* 449–475.

Roberts, B. W., & DelVecchio, W. F. (2000). The rank-order consistency of personality traits from childhood to old age: A quantitative review of longitudinal studies. *Psychological Bulletin, 126,* 3–25.

Rogler, L. H. (1999). Methodological sources of cultural insensitivity in mental health research. *American Psychologist, 54,* 424–433.

Samuel, D. B., & Widiger, T. A. (2004). Clinicians' personality descriptions of prototypic personality disorders. *Journal of Personality Disorders, 18,* 286–308.

Saucier, G. (2002). Gone too far—or not far enough? Comments on the article by Ashton and Lee (2001). *European Journal of Personality, 16,* 55–62.

Saucier, G., & Goldberg, L. R. (2001). Lexical studies of indigenous personality factors: Premises, products, and prospects. *Journal of Personality, 69,* 847–880.

Saulsman, L. M., & Page, A. C. (2004). The five-factor model and personality disorder empirical literature: A meta-analytic review. *Clinical Psychology Review, 23,* 1055–1085.

Segerstrom, S. C. (2000). Personality and the immune system: Models, methods, and mechanisms. *Annals of Behavioral Medicine, 22,* 180–190.

Sen, S., Burmeister, M., & Ghosh, D. (2004). Meta-analysis of the association between a serotonin transporter polymorphism (5–HTTLPR) and anxiety-related personality traits. *American Journal of Medical Genetics Part B, 127B,* 85–89.

Shea, M. T. (1992). Some characteristics of the Axis II criteria sets and their implications for assessment of personality disorders. *Journal of Personality Disorders, 6,* 377–381.

Shea, M. T., & Yen, S. (2003). Stability as a distinction between Axis I and Axis II disorders. *Journal of Personality Disorders, 17,* 373–386.

Shedler, J., & Westen, D. (2004). Refining DSM-IV personality disorder diagnosis: Integrating science and practice. *American Journal of Psychiatry, 161,* 1350–1365.

Shiner, R. (1998). How shall we speak of children's personalities in middle childhood?: A preliminary taxonomy. *Psychological Bulletin, 124,* 308–332.

Shiner, R., & Caspi, A. (2003). Personality differences in childhood and adolescence: Measurement, development, and consequences. *Journal of Child Psychology and Psychiatry, 44,* 2–32.

Soldz, S., Budman, S., Demby, A., & Merry, J. (1993). Representation of personality disorders in circumplex and five-factor space: Explorations with a clinical sample. *Psychological Assessment, 5,* 41–52.

Sprock, J. (2002). A comparative study of the dimensions and facets of the five-factor model in the diagnosis of cases of personality disorder. *Journal of Personality Disorders, 16,* 402–423.

Sprock, J. (2003). Dimensional versus categorical classification of prototypic and nonprototypic cases of personality disorder. *Journal of Clinical Psychology, 59,* 992–1014.

Tellegen, A. (1993). Folk concepts and psychological concepts of personality and personality disorder. *Psychological Inquiry, 4,* 122–130.

Tellegen, A., & Waller, N. G. (1987). *Exploring personality through test construction: Development of the Multidimensional Personality Questionnaire.* Unpublished manuscript, Minneapolis, MN.

Trull, T. J. (1992). DSM-III-R personality disorders and the five-factor model of personality: An empirical comparison. *Journal of Abnormal Psychology, 101,* 553–560.

Trull, T. J., Useda, J. D., Doan, B. T., Vieth, A. Z., Burr, R. M., Hanks, A. A., et al. (1998). Two year stability of borderline personality measures. *Journal of Personality Disorders, 12,* 187–197.

Trull, T. J., Widiger, T. A., & Burr, R. (2001). A structured interview for the assessment of the five-factor model of personality: Facet-level relations to the Axis II Personality Disorders. *Journal of Personality, 69,* 175–198.

Trull, T. J., Widiger, T. A., Lynam, D. R., & Costa, P. T. (2003). Borderline personality disorder from the perspective of general personality functioning. *Journal of Abnormal Psychology, 112,* 193–202.

Wakefield, J. C. (1994) Is the concept of mental disorder culturally relative? In S. A. Kirk & S. D. Einbinder (Eds.), *Controversial issues in mental health* (pp. 11–17). Boston: Allyn & Bacon.

Warner, M. B., Morey, L. C., Finch, J. F., Gunderson, J. G., Skodol, A. E., Sanislow, C. A., et al. (2004). The longitudinal relationship of personality traits and disorders. *Journal of Abnormal Psychology, 113,* 217–227.

Watson, D., & Tellegen, A. (1985). Toward a consensual structure of mood. *Psychological Bulletin, 98,* 219–235.

Westen, D. (1995). A clinical–empirical model of personality: Life after the Mischelian Ice age and the NEO-lithic era. *Journal of Personality, 63,* 495–524.

Westen, D. (1997). Divergences between clinical and research methods for assessing personality disorders: Implications for research and the evolution of Axis II. *American Journal of Psychiatry, 154,* 895–903.

Whiteside, S. P., & Lynam, D. R. (2001). The five-factor model and impulsivity: Using a structural model of personality to understand impulsivity. *Personality and Individual Differences, 30,* 669–689.

Widiger, T. A. (1993). The DSM-III-R categorical personality disorder diagnoses: A critique and an alternative. *Psychological Inquiry, 4,* 75–90.

Widiger, T. A. (2002). Values, politics, and science in the construction of the DSMs. In J. Sadler (Ed.), *Descriptions and prescriptions: Values, mental disorders and the DSMs* (pp. 25–41). Baltimore: Johns Hopkins University Press.

Widiger, T. A., & Coker, L. A. (2001). Assessing personality disorders. In J. N. Butcher (Ed.), *Clinical personality assessment: Practical approaches* (2nd ed., pp. 407–434). New York: Oxford University Press.

Widiger, T. A., & Costa, P. T. (1994). Personality and personality disorders. *Journal of Abnormal Psychology, 103,* 78–91.

Widiger, T. A., & Costa, P. T. (2002). Five-factor model personality disorder research. In T. A. Widiger & P. T. Costa (Eds.), *Personality disorders and the five-factor model of personality* (2nd ed., pp. 59–87). Washington, DC: American Psychological Association.

Widiger, T. A., Costa, P. T., & McCrae, R. R. (2002). A proposal for Axis II: Diagnosing personality disorders using the five-factor model. In T. A. Widiger & P. T. Costa (Eds.), *Personality disorders and the five-factor model of personality* (2nd ed., pp. 431–456). Washington, DC: American Psychological Association.

Widiger, T. A., & Frances, A. (1985). The DSM-III personality disorders: Perspectives from psychology. *Archives of General Psychiatry, 42,* 615–623.

Widiger, T. A., & Lynam, D. R. (1998). Psychopathy and the five-factor model of personality. In E. Simonsen & T. Millon (Eds.), *Psychopathy: Antisocial, criminal, and violent behavior* (pp. 171–187). New York: Guilford Press.

Widiger, T. A., Trull, T. J., Clarkin, J. F., Sanderson, C., & Costa, P. T. (1994). A description of the DSM-III-R and DSM-IV personality disorders with the five-factor model of personality. In P. T. Costa & T. A. Widiger (Eds.), *Personality disorders and the five-factor model of personality* (pp. 41–56). Washington, DC: American Psychological Association.

Widiger, T. A., Trull, T. J., Clarkin, J. F., Sanderson, C., & Costa, P. T. (2002). A description of the DSM-IV personality disorders with the five-factor model of personality. In P. T. Costa & T. A. Widiger (Eds.), *Personality disorders and the five-factor model of personality* (2nd ed., pp. 89–99). Washington, DC: American Psychological Association.

Wiggins, J. S. (2003). *Paradigms of personality assessment.* New York: Guilford Press.

Wiggins, J. S., & Pincus, A. L. (1989). Conceptions of personality disorders and dimensions of personality. *Psychological Assessment, 1,* 305–316.

World Health Organization. (1992). *The ICD-10 classification of mental and behavioural disorders. Clinical descriptions and diagnostic guidelines.* Geneva, Switzerland: Author.

Yeung, A. S., Lyons, M. J., Waternaux, C. M., Faraone, S. V., & Tsuang, M. T. (1993). Empirical determination of the thresholds for case identification: Validation of the Personality Diagnostic Questionnaire—Revised. *Comprehensive Psychiatry, 34,* 384–391.

Zuckerman, M. (2002). Zuckerman–Kuhlman Personality Questionnaire (ZKPQ): An alternative five-factorial model. In B. de Raad & M. Perugini (Eds.), *Big five assessment* (pp. 377–397). Kirkland, WA: Hogrefe & Huber.

Chapter 4

Perceptions of Self and Others Regarding Pathological Personality Traits

THOMAS F. OLTMANNS
ERIC TURKHEIMER

People with personality disorders are frequently unable to view themselves realistically and sometimes unaware of the effect that their behavior has on other people. There is, at best, only a modest correlation between the ways in which people describe themselves and the ways in which they are perceived by others (John & Robins, 1993; Wilson, 2002). Unfortunately, most knowledge of personality disorders—in both clinical and research settings—is based on evidence obtained from self-report measures. The study that we will describe in this chapter began as an exploration of discrepancies between self-report and informant measures in the assessment of personality disorders. It has evolved into a more broadly based investigation of interpersonal perception for pathological personality traits. We are studying ways in which people see themselves, ways in which they are seen by other people, and their beliefs about what other people think of them. This research project lies directly at the intersection of basic science and clinical research. It depends heavily on methods and concepts developed by investigators studying interpersonal perception. It is also concerned with the impact of pathological personality traits on functional outcomes in people's lives.

PERSON PERCEPTION

The typical emphasis given to self-report measures (questionnaires and interviews) for the assessment of personality disorders is somewhat surprising in light of the fact that many personality disorders involve distortions of self-perception and an inability to realistically assess one's effect on others (Westen, 1997; Westen & Shedler, 1999). Several reviews have recognized the importance of obtaining information from informants (e.g., Grove & Tellegen, 1991; Zimmerman, 1994). Unfortunately, these data are seldom collected. Studies that have compared self-report data with descriptions provided by other people almost always rely on a single informant and usually report low levels of agreement between sources (e.g., Bernstein et al., 1997; Dreessen, Hildebrand, & Arntz, 1998; Lara, Ferro, & Klein, 1997; Mann et al., 1999). Very few empirical studies have compared relations between, and the relative merits of, self-reports and peer reports in the assessment of personality disorders (cf. Klein, 2003).

Social and personality psychologists have been concerned with questions regarding similar issues for many years. Working with normal subjects, they have developed research paradigms and quantitative methods to address complex questions regarding interpersonal perception. The field of interpersonal perception has seen major progress in the past 20 years on basic science issues that are extremely relevant to the study of personality disorders (Funder, 1995; Kenny, 1991).

The strongest method employed in studies of interpersonal perception is a "round-robin" design in which every member of a group rates or judges everyone else in the group. Everyone serves as both a judge and a target. This is the design we used in our peer nomination study. Kenny's social relations model analyzes person perception in terms of three components: perceiver effects, target effects, and relationship effects. These effects can also be described in terms of types of agreement. One involves consensus. Do two judges agree in their judgments about another person's personality? Our interest in self–other agreement provided the original motivation for our study. In other words, do people see themselves in the same way that they are perceived by other people? Target accuracy and self-accuracy refer to the validity of self- and other judgments. And then, finally, another important topic involves "meta-accuracy." If people disagree with the perceptions that others have of them, is it because they know what the other people think and simply disagree? Or are they completely oblivious to the others' point of view?

Studies of interpersonal perception indicate that there is a fair amount of consensus among lay people when making judgments of others' personality traits. There is also a considerable amount of disagreement between self-report and peer report. This is particularly true for evaluative traits (which are the kind included in definitions of personality disorders). For some traits, peers are more accurate judges than the self. We know that people do have some insight into what other people think of them, and this is more true for "generalized others" than for dyadic interactions (see Kenny & DePaulo, 1993; Funder, 1999; Kenny, 1994; John & Robins, 1993).

Perhaps the most important issue in the field of interpersonal perception involves accuracy, or validity. Kenny (1994) wrote, "The field of interpersonal perception needs to move beyond consensus and self–other agreement to study the relationship between behavior and perception." We feel the same way about disagreements between self and informant measures regarding personality disorders. The important question is no longer whether they agree. We know they don't. The ultimate question is: When do peer and self data tell us something meaningful about the person?

PARTICIPANTS IN THE PEER NOMINATION STUDY

In this chapter, we will review some of the most important findings from the Peer Nomination Study. We begin with an overview of the considerations that led to the selection of our samples and a more specific description of the people who participated in our study.

Military Recruits and College Dorm Residents

Our study included two large nonclinical samples of participants: military recruits and college freshmen. They were all identified and tested in groups (training flights and dorm floors). Most of the groups included both men and women. We chose these groups for several important reasons. Most importantly, they offered an opportunity to collect self-report and peer nomination data within groups composed of people who were relatively well acquainted with one another. We wanted to collect the data simultaneously from all members of the group (in one testing session) in order to minimize the potential for them to discuss their answers with one another. Two additional characteristics of the military and college samples were also important. Each group was composed of people who had known one another for the same amount of time, and they were assigned to live together on a more or less random basis. We had considered other sources of participants (such as church groups, recreational sports teams, and members of work-related teams), and we had collected our pilot data for this study using members of fraternities and sororities (Oltmanns, Turkheimer, & Strauss, 1998). In comparison to the recruits and dorm residents, the members of these other groups would have been much more heterogeneous in terms of the length of time that they had known each other. Furthermore, in many cases, the members of the other groups participate actively in the selection of their own members (thus introducing the possibility that they would select for or against various kinds of personality traits).

Our groups included previously unacquainted young adults who were assembled from a wide range of geographic areas and all lived together in close proximity for a fairly standard period of time (6 weeks for the recruits and 5–7 months for the students). All were going through a challenging period of adjustment. For most, this was the first time that they had lived for an extended period of time away from their parents' home. The participants were adapting to a completely new set of circumstances (living arrangements, educational or occupational demands) and also becoming acquainted with a new group of people. Individual differences might be expected to be exaggerated (and perhaps best studied) during this type of transition or period of social discontinuity (Caspi & Moffitt, 1993).

The fact that we collected data from both recruits and students allowed us to compare our results across samples and to check the generalizability of our findings. Each sample offered some advantages and disadvantages. In terms of gender distribution, more of the recruits were male (approximately 60%), while more of the students were female (approximately 60%). The students had known one another longer (a few months rather than a few weeks), and the military training groups were, on average, larger than the college student dorm groups. Although almost all of the military recruits were high school graduates, the college students were selected in terms of superior academic achievement (University of Virginia is a highly selective public university). Both samples were culturally and ethnically diverse.

These samples offer an opportunity to examine pathological personality traits in two nonclinical samples of young adults—relatively uncomplicated by additional mental health problems such as substance abuse, major mood disorders, or psychosis. Many studies of personality disorders have focused on clinical samples, often people who present for treatment with both personality problems and other significant co-occurring mental disorders (Dolan-Sewell, Krueger, & Shea, 2001). We did not expect to find many people with Axis I disorders in the military sample. Screening for obvious mental disorders takes place during enlistment and again at the outset of training. Furthermore, people with severe problems would be unlikely to complete this rigorous training experience. We did expect to find, however, people who meet the criteria for personality disorders, given estimates that somewhere around 10% of community samples will do so.

The age of our samples also deserves some comment. According to DSM-IV-TR, the pattern of inflexible and maladaptive personality traits that represent the core feature of a personality disorder "is stable and of long duration, and its onset can be traced back at least to adolescence or early adulthood" (p. 686). The characteristic features of the personality disorder are presumably evident by early adulthood. Therefore, anyone in our samples who, upon more extended observation, would be qualified to receive a personality disorder diagnosis would be expected to exhibit features of these problems by the time they participated in our study. On the other hand, we also know that many people who show evidence of maladaptive personality traits during adolescence do not necessarily continue to experience these problems later in life (e.g., Johnson et al., 2000; Lenzenweger, Johnson, & Willett, 2004; Tickle, Heatherton, & Wittenberg, 2001; Zanarini, Frankenberg, Hennen, & Silk, 2003). Because the participants in our study were relatively young, we should not assume that everyone who exhibited pathological personality traits would definitely meet the full criteria for a clinical diagnosis of a personality disorder, which requires that the pattern be pervasive across a broad range of personal and social situations and that the pattern be stable and of long duration.

Specific Features of Study Participants

The first set of participants included 2,026 Air Force recruits (1,265 males, 761 females) completing their basic military training at Lackland Air Force Base in San Antonio, Texas. The recruits were enlisted personnel (not pilots) who were being trained for a wide variety of jobs, ranging from positions such as security police and cooks to assignments as electronics technicians and language specialists. On the first day of basic training, recruits are assigned to groups, known as "flights." Each flight includes approximately 40–45 recruits. For the next 6 weeks, members of a flight do virtually everything together. Recruits observe one another's behavior during many challenging situations, and they become very well acquainted. The median number of recruits in each group, or "flight," was 42 (range = 27–53). Fifty flights were included in the study; 17 of the flights (13 male, 4 female) were single-sex. In the mixed-sex flights, on average 54% were males (range = 43–62%). Participants' ages ranged from 18 to 35 years, with a median age of 19 years. Ninety percent of participants were between 18 and 25. All recruits signed informed consent statements and participated on a voluntary basis.

Our second sample of participants included 1,686 freshman students (564 males, 1,122 females) at the University of Virginia. These were people who had lived together for at least 5 months on the same floor of a dormitory (approximately 12–22 individuals per group). In comparison to our military participants, the students lived in smaller groups and had known one another for a longer period of time. On the other hand, most members of the dorm groups spent less time with one another on a day-to-day basis.

Participants' ages ranged from 17 to 27 years, with 98% being either 18 or 19 years of age. We recruited students through their resident advisors.

ASSESSMENT PROCEDURES

Our assessment process proceeded in two stages. In the first stage, the members of each group completed a set of questionnaires as well as a peer nomination procedure. We tested members of each group simultaneously in a single 2-hour session. Each participant was seated in front of his or her own computer terminal. The assessment battery began with a demographics form, the Beck Depression Inventory, the Beck Anxiety Inventory, and the Schedule for Nonadaptive and Adaptive Personality (SNAP; Clark, 1993), a 375-item self-report inventory.[1] The SNAP measures trait dimensions that are related to personality disorders, and it also includes diagnostic scales for each specific type of personality disorder. Following the SNAP, participants completed the peer nomination process (described below), which was developed for the purpose of this study.

After all members of a group had completed the SNAP and the peer nomination process, we selected a subset of the group's members (approximately 25%) to be interviewed using the Structured Interview for DSM-IV Personality (SIDP-IV).[2] Approximately one-third of these people were chosen on the basis of elevated self-report scores regarding personality disorder features, one-third were chosen because their peers had identified them as exhibiting personality disorder features, and the other third were chosen at random from the remaining people in the group (so that the interviewer would not know whether the person was expected to exhibit pathological personality traits). In the military sample, the semistructured interviews were conducted on the same day as the first phase of assessment. In the college student sample, the interviews were conducted within a few weeks after the person's dorm floor had gone through the first phase of assessment.

Peer Nomination

The Multi-source Assessment of Personality Pathology (MAPP)[3] is composed of 103 items, including 79 items based on the features of 10 personality disorders listed in DSM-IV as well as 24 supplementary items based on additional personality traits (mostly positive characteristics, such as "trustworthy and reliable"). The items are presented to participants in a quasi-random order. For each item, the participant is asked to nominate members of his or her group who exhibit the characteristic in question. We decided to use a nomination procedure because our list of items was quite long. If the participants had been required to rate every member of their group on each item, the assessment procedure would have been prohibitively time-consuming.

Items for the MAPP were constructed by translating the DSM-IV criterion sets for personality disorders into lay language. All of the 78 DSM-IV personality disorder features were rewritten into words that avoided the use of technical psychopathological terms and psychiatric jargon. One of the diagnostic criteria (narcissistic personality disorder criterion #8) was split into two separate items ("is often envious of others or believes that others are envious of him or her" became "is jealous of other people" and "thinks other people are jealous of him/her." One item ("has little, if any, interest in having sexual experiences with another person") was excluded from the MAPP presented to recruits due to military regulations.[4]

The MAPP is presented on a computer screen. For each item, the personality trait or feature is listed at the top of the screen. The names of all other members of the group (excluding the name of the participant completing the MAPP) appear below the trait description. The numbers "0" (never like this), "1" (sometimes like this), "2" (usually like this), and "3" (always like this) are listed to the right of each person's name, with the default selection being "0." Instructions tell the participants:

> "We are interested in your perceptions of other people in your group. You will be presented with descriptions of various personal characteristics. For each characteristic, you will be asked to click the mouse button when the cursor is pointing to the names of the people in your group who best fit that description. You may click as many names as you want, but you must select at least one person for each characteristic. If you have an especially difficult time identifying even one person who fits the description, select the person who comes closest to the description and then indicate that your choice was difficult or problematic by clicking the mouse on the word 'yes' next to the box that says 'It was difficult to select anyone for this item.' "[5]

This process represents a combination of both nominations and ratings. In other words, judges could nominate as many people as they saw fit for each particular item, but they did not have to rate each person in their group. When they did nominate someone, however, they were required to indicate the extent to which the target person showed the feature in question. Judges used the full range of the scale, with approximately 50% of the nominations being rated "1," 25% rated "2," and 25% rated "3." Item scores were calculated by summing across judges for each target and then dividing by the number of judges. Scale scores were calculated by summing the items associated with each personality disorder and dividing by the number of items for that personality disorder.

Rater reliabilities for peer nominations were computed using generalizability theory (Cronbach, Gleser, Nanda, & Rajaratnam, 1971). For each diagnosis within each group of judges, an analysis of variance was conducted, producing mean squares attributable to targets, judges, items, and interactions among the main effects. The mean squares were transformed to variance components. The ratio of target variance to total variance is the reliability of a single judge rating a single item, and can be interpreted as the average correlation between pairs of judges on a single item. The Spearman–Brown formula was then used to calculate the reliability of a nine-item composite (i.e., a sum of criteria for a single Axis II diagnosis), and the mean of 20 judges on a nine item composite (Table 4.1). A sample size of 20 was selected as a compromise between the size of the military groups and the college groups, so the reliabilities could be compared. In practice, the larger military groups were slightly more reliable than indicated by the values in the table, and the smaller college groups were slightly less reliable. Although the reliabilities of individual criteria are quite low, the composites of judges and items that form the basis for our analysis are highly reliable. The reliability of scores based on any single judge is quite low, but the scores that we used in subsequent analyses are highly reliable because they are based on composite scores taken from several judges.

Self-Report and Expected Peer Scores

In addition to the peer nomination items, the MAPP includes a section that asks participants to describe themselves by using exactly the same items that are included in the peer nomination section of the instrument. Identical

TABLE 4.1. Reliabilities of Peer-Based PD Scores for Military and University Samples

Scale	Air Force			University of Virginia		
	1 item/ 1 rater	9 items/ 1 rater	9 items/ 20 raters	1 item/ 1 rater	9 items/ 1 rater	9 items/ 20 raters
Paranoid	.04	.30	.89	.07	.38	.91
Schizoid	.03	.23	.84	.10	.48	.92
Schizotypal	.05	.33	.89	.09	.44	.92
Antisocial	.08	.43	.93	.13	.56	.95
Borderline	.05	.31	.89	.09	.45	.95
Histrionic	.06	.37	.91	.10	.49	.94
Narcissistic	.09	.49	.95	.13	.56	.96
Avoidant	.06	.33	.88	.09	.45	.89
Dependent	.07	.37	.90	.07	.41	.91
Obsessive–compulsive	.04	.28	.87	.05	.30	.87

questions were used because we wanted to be sure that, when we compared self and other data, inconsistencies could be attributed specifically to a difference of opinion rather than to the fact that the two different sources were being asked different questions.[6]

The self-report section of the MAPP also included questions that were concerned with metaperception (self-knowledge regarding the ways in which other people view the self). Our pilot data led us to believe that the correlations between self and others would be low. We added the metaperception items because we wanted to be able to distinguish between two different explanations for low self–other agreement. One explanation would be that the target person understands but disagrees. The other would be that he or she does not even know what other people think.

After they completed the peer nomination items, the participants were once again presented with each item from the inventory. They were asked two additional questions about each item: (1) "How do you think most other people in your group rated you on this characteristic?" and (2) "What do you think you are really like on this characteristic?" For each question, they were required to select a response from four options: Never like this ("0"), sometimes like this ("1"), usually like this ("2"), or always like this ("3").

We explored the convergent validity of the MAPP self-report scores by computing correlations with the diagnostic scales and the trait scales derived from the SNAP. The SNAP diagnostic scales that were available at the time were based on a previous version of the diagnostic manual (DSM-III-R), while our MAPP self-report scores were based on DSM-IV. Therefore, we did not expect that correlations between scores for the same personality disorder category would be extremely high. These values are presented in Tables 4.2 and 4.3 (for the military and college samples, respectively). Notice that the scores on the diagonal (convergent validity) are consistently higher than scores between other scales, suggesting that the MAPP self-report scores did measure the same construct identified by the SNAP diagnostic scales. Of course, these tables also indicate that there is quite a bit of overlap among different personality disorder categories, a phenomenon that has been noted frequently in the literature (e.g., Clark, Livesley, & Morey, 1997).

Correlations between the MAPP self-report personality disorder scores and SNAP trait scales also support the conclusion that, in comparison to other self-report measures, the MAPP scores are valid indices of the constructs that they were intended to measure. For example, the SNAP trait scales with the highest correlations to the MAPP paranoid personality disorder scale were Mistrust ($r = .48$) and Negative Temperament ($r = .44$). For the MAPP schizoid personality disorder scale, the highest correlation was with Detachment ($r = .47$). For the MAPP antisocial personality disorder scale, the

TABLE 4.2. Correlations between MAPP Self-Report Personality Disorder Scores and SNAP Diagnostic Scales in the Military Sample

SNAP	MAPP-report									
	1.	2.	3.	4.	5.	6.	7.	8.	9.	10.
1. Paranoid	.55	.33	.44	.30	.36	.27	.22	.32	.22	.22
2. Schizoid	.26	.48	.25	.14	.16	.02	.06	.20	.03	.16
3. Schizotypal	.47	.35	.53	.27	.39	.26	.20	.36	.23	.24
4. Antisocial	.31	.21	.34	.49	.37	.36	.33	.20	.23	.07
5. Borderline	.43	.27	.47	.45	.50	.39	.33	.34	.30	.20
6. Histrionic	.15	−.06	.17	.20	.21	.38	.30	.05	.16	.09
7. Narcissistic	.32	.18	.36	.30	.31	.38	.40	.14	.20	.22
8. Avoidant	.36	.35	.35	.15	.27	.10	.09	.44	.20	.21
9. Dependent	.26	−.01	.31	.23	.36	.29	.19	.43	.42	.13
10. Obsessive–compulsive	.16	.12	.14	−.01	.10	.07	.10	.11	.04	.31

Note. N = 1,504.

highest correlations were with Disinhibition ($r = .46$), Manipulativeness ($r = .43$), Impulsiveness ($r = .40$), and Aggression ($r = .40$).

Semistructured Diagnostic Interviews

A subset of people from each group was invited to participate in the second phase of our assessment process. They were interviewed using the Structured Interview for DSM-IV Personality, the latest edition of a well-validated semistructured interview for personality disorders (Pfohl, Blum, & Zimmerman, 1997). Questions on the SIDP-IV are arranged by themes rather than by disorders (e.g., work style, emotions, interests and activities). The interview includes 101 questions that correspond to the diagnostic criteria for 10 forms of personality disorder. Because the SIDP-IV is not accompanied by a formal training or reference manual, we relied extensively on the manual that accompanies another semistructured interview for personality disorders, the Personality Disorder Interview–IV (Widiger, Magine, Corbitt, Ellis, & Thomas, 1995). During training and throughout the rest of the data collection process, we relied heavily on the detailed and thoughtful descriptions of personality disorders and diagnostic dilemmas that are provided in the PDI-IV manual.

Twelve carefully trained people conducted interviews with 433 recruits (Jane, Pagan, Turkheimer, Fiedler, & Oltmanns, 2006). The interviewers were three licensed, doctoral-level clinical psychologists (the authors of this chapter and Edna Fiedler) as well as nine graduate students in clinical psychology. Five of the graduate students had master's-level clinical experience before they were trained to use the SIDP-IV. Ten of the interviewers were trained by Nancee Blum, one of the authors of the SIDP-IV. All interviewers

TABLE 4.3. Correlations between MAPP Self-Report Personality Disorder Scores SNAP Diagnostic Scales in the College Sample

SNAP	MAPP self-report									
	1.	2.	3.	4.	5.	6.	7.	8.	9.	10.
1. Paranoid	.49	.38	.45	.38	.45	.30	.30	.37	.29	.27
2. Schizoid	.18	.51	.35	.13	.16	.02	.10	.30	.02	.23
3. Schizotypal	.38	.46	.51	.27	.39	.23	.22	.37	.24	.26
4. Antisocial	.26	.21	.30	.51	.37	.33	.28	.03	.14	−.02
5. Borderline	.40	.27	.41	.46	.52	.36	.32	.24	.34	.19
6. Histrionic	.16	−.07	.09	.25	.25	.39	.32	−.01	.22	.03
7. Narcissistic	.34	.20	.31	.37	.37	.40	.40	.13	.21	.17
8. Avoidant	.30	.43	.37	.10	.27	.06	.11	.49	.23	.31
9. Dependent	.26	.03	.16	.11	.30	.23	.11	.33	.46	.16
10. Obsessive– compulsive	.28	.28	.24	.07	.22	.15	.23	.31	.21	.43

Note. N = 693.

watched a number of videotapes of interviews together before beginning the study in order to improve reliability through discussion of the interviews and ratings. After the study began, 20 videotaped interviews, 2 from each interviewer, were sent to Ms. Blum for her ratings and comments on interview style. This was done in an effort to maintain fidelity with ratings made by the original lab and in order to continue to improve the quality of our interviewing skills.

All interviewers were blind to the status of the people they interviewed (i.e., whether or not they had been chosen for an interview based on self-report information, peer report information, or randomly from the other people in the group). All diagnostic interviews were recorded on videotape. Every interview was subsequently viewed and rated a second time by an independent judge (one of the other interviewers). Interrater reliability for each of the personality disorder criteria was high, except for the observational items. For most of the specific personality disorder criteria, our reliabilities were over .70 (see Table 4.4). Reliability estimates were higher when diagnostic agreement was computed using dimensional scores rather than categorical scores. Avoidant and dependent personality disorders demonstrated the highest interrater reliability, while schizoid and schizotypal personality disorders showed the lowest.

Nineteen percent (82 of 433) of the participants who were interviewed qualified for at least one personality disorder diagnosis on the SIDP. Of the 82 who did qualify for at least one diagnosis, 52 met the DSM-IV criteria for one type of personality disorder, 26 met the criteria for two personality disorders, 3 met the criteria for 3 personality disorders, and 1 was above the diagnostic threshold for four types of personality disorder. Another 10% of the sample qualified for a "probable" personality disorder, defined

as falling one criterion short of the threshold for a diagnosis without qualifying for any other definite diagnosis. Information regarding the number of
people who qualified for either definite or probable diagnosis is presented
in Table 4.4. The disorder most frequently diagnosed in the military sample
was obsessive–compulsive personality disorder. The disorders least frequently diagnosed were schizoid and schizotypal personality disorders.
These data suggest that, using semistructured diagnostic interviews (the
generally accepted gold standard in this field), personality disorders were
present in this nonclinical sample. The exact prevalence rate in the overall
sample is difficult to compute because we did not select people for interviews using a specific cut-off score on any of our screening measures. The
prevalence rates found in our interviewed sample are, of course, higher
than we would find in the entire sample, because most of the people we selected for interviews had shown either self- or peer indications of personality problems. Working backward, we expect that approximately 9.4% of
the overall military sample would have qualified for a definite personality
disorder diagnosis. That figure is approximately the same as other estimates based on community samples (Mattia & Zimmerman, 2001; Weissman, 1993).

SUBJECTIVE DISTRESS AND SOCIAL IMPAIRMENT

We included self-report measures of anxious and depressed mood (the Beck
Depression Inventory [BDI] and the Beck Anxiety Inventory [BAI]) as well
as social adjustment because we wanted to know whether the personality

TABLE 4.4. Frequency of Personality Disorder Diagnosis and Interrater Reliability

	Definite		Probable		Interrater reliability		
Diagnosis	Freq (%)		Freq (%)		Categorical	No. of criteria	Continuous
Paranoid	12	(2.8)	31	(7.2)	.57	.75	.84
Schizoid	1	(0.6)	9	(2.1)	−.01	.77	.81
Schizotypal	0	(0.0)	8	(1.8)	.03	.65	.79
Antisocial	13	(3.0)	20	(4.6)	.62	.79	.84
Borderline	12	(2.8)	17	(3.9)	.60	.79	.85
Histrionic	4	(0.9)	8	(1.8)	.55	.72	.77
Narcissistic	8	(1.8)	18	(4.2)	.35	.77	.82
Avoidant	17	(3.9)	25	(5.8)	.85	.90	.93
Dependent	4	(0.9)	8	(1.8)	.84	.85	.88
Obsessive–compulsive	43	(9.9)	80	(18.5)	.55	.75	.84

Note. N = 433 military recruits who were interviewed with the SIDP-IV. Freq, number of people with the diagnosis; (%), percentage of people with the diagnosis; Probable, one criterion short of diagnosis.

disorder data that we collected were able to identify people whose patho-logical personality characteristics were also associated with subjective dis-tress or social and occupational impairment. We used the self-report ver-sion of the Social Adjustment Scale (SAS-SR; Weissman, Olfson, Garneroff, Feder, & Fuentes, 2001) and the Social Functioning Questionnaire (Tyrer, 1993) as indices of social and occupational impairment. The SAS-SR in-cludes questions related to six role areas, and we included three in our study: occupational performance (as a student), social and leisure function-ing, and relations with extended family. The SAS-SR was used only with our college student sample. We did not include this measure with the mili-tary recruits because of the special circumstances in which they had been living for the preceding 6 weeks.

Depressed and Anxious Mood

Personality disorder scores based on self-report were, in fact, correlated with higher scores on both depressed and anxious mood. This pattern was relatively consistent for both the military and the college sample (see Table 4.5). People who described themselves as showing features of personality disorders were more depressed and anxious than participants who pro-duced lower self-report personality disorder scores. The highest correla-tions in both samples were between the BDI and self-report scores on our scale for borderline personality disorder (.39 in the military sample and .45 in the college sample). The lowest correlations with the BDI were for the self-report scale for narcissistic personality disorder (.14 in the military sample and .21 in the college sample). These patterns suggest that, in these nonclinical samples, people who report that their experience is consistent

TABLE 4.5. Correlations between Self-Report Personality Disorder Scores (from the MAPP) and Self-Report Measures of Subjective Distress (Depression and Anxiety)

	Air Force sample		University of Virginia sample	
Self-report	Beck Depression	Beck Anxiety	Beck Depression	Beck Anxiety
1. Paranoid	.34	.20	.35	.28
2. Schizoid	.21	.14	.29	.12
3. Schizotypal	.35	.33	.38	.26
4. Antisocial	.21	.24	.21	.12
5. Borderline	.39	.19	.45	.33
6. Histrionic	.34	.23	.25	.19
7. Narcissistic	.14	.17	.21	.14
8. Avoidant	.38	.35	.35	.27
9. Dependent	.19	.28	.32	.24
10. Obsessive–compulsive	.38	.20	.24	.24

with the DSM-IV features of personality disorders are also experiencing at least modest levels of subjective distress.

Peer scores on the personality disorder scales were less likely to be correlated with subjective distress, either in terms of the BDI or the BAI (see Table 4.6). There were a couple of exceptions. In the military sample, people whose peers described them as exhibiting features of avoidant and dependent personality disorder did produce higher scores on the BDI and the BAI. The same pattern was found for those described by their peers as showing features of schizotypal and borderline personality disorder. In the college sample, only peer scores for schizotypal and borderline personality disorder were significantly correlated with the BDI. The fact that mood is more closely related to self-report scores for personality disorders can be attributed most easily to method variance (i.e., people who are unhappy are more likely to describe themselves in other negative ways, as on the MAPP self-report personality disorder items).

Social Functioning and Interpersonal Problems

Our measures of personality pathology were also related to problems in social functioning, if we measure these adjustment problems using self-report measures (the SAS-SR and the SFQ). In the college student sample, we found that both self-reported and peer-based personality disorder scores contributed to the prediction of impairment in social functioning above and beyond the influence of depressed mood (Oltmanns, Melley, & Turkheimer, 2002). The relation between personality disorders and social impairment was generally more striking when personality disorders were measured by

TABLE 4.6. Correlations between Peer Personality Disorder Scores and Self-Report Measures of Subjective Distress (Depression and Anxiety)

Self-report	Air Force sample		University of Virginia sample	
	Beck Depression	Beck Anxiety	Beck Depression	Beck Anxiety
1. Paranoid	.12	.11	.09	.00
2. Schizoid	.10	.06	.09	−.03
3. Schizotypal	.18	.17	.13	.01
4. Antisocial	.07	.03	.07	−.03
5. Borderline	.18	.17	.14	.04
6. Histrionic	.06	.04	.03	−.05
7. Narcissistic	.01	−.01	−.01	−.06
8. Avoidant	.18	.18	.04	−.03
9. Dependent	.15	.15	.05	−.02
10. Obsessive–compulsive	.02	.01	−.01	−.08

self-report. All of the self-report personality disorder categories showed significant correlations with reduced social functioning scores,

The one exception with regard to personality pathology and self-reported social functioning was found in relation to symptoms of histrionic personality disorder. People who described themselves as having more histrionic features also described themselves as having *better* functioning in their social and family roles. We doubt that histrionic personality disorder is actually associated with improved adjustment. Instead, this unexpected finding points toward limitations with existing measures of social adjustment in this area. The SAS-SR was developed and tested for use with depressed outpatients, and it is focused on forms of impairment that are associated with that disorder. People with histrionic personality disorder would be expected to have *superficial* relationships with other people (not necessarily *fewer* social relationships). This finding has stimulated our interest in developing more specific measures of social and occupational impairment that might be uniquely associated with specific forms of personality disorder (rather than with all forms of psychopathology).

The data that we collected with regard to mood and social adjustment support two conclusions. First, at the level of self-report measures, most forms of personality pathology in these nonclinical samples are associated with both subjective distress and social impairment. Second, the strength of this association is much less obvious when peer measures are used as an index of personality pathology. We suspect that better measures are needed to measure social and occupational problems, both in terms of finding tools that do not depend on self-report and also in terms of developing measures that focus more specifically on the kinds of impairment that might be uniquely related to personality pathology, rather than relying on measures that were intended to identify impairment associated with other kinds of mental disorders, such as depression, psychosis, and substance use disorders.

In order to explore these issues, we added the Inventory of Interpersonal Problems (IIP; Horowitz, Alden, Wiggins, & Pincus, 2000) to our assessment battery for the college sample. The IIP was originally developed as a tool for the measurement of interpersonal problems described by outpatients when they are seeking psychological treatment. They are written in two formats. One type of item is focused on things that are difficult to do. Examples include "Get along with other people," and "Open up and tell my feelings to another person." The other type of item is focused on "*things I do too much.*" Examples include "I manipulate other people too much to get what I want" and "I argue with other people too much." In contrast to questionnaires such as the SAS-SR, which focus on subjective dissatisfaction with work performance and the quantity of social interactions, the interpersonal problems that are included in the IIP seem to capture the more subtle quality of social impairment that is presumably associated with personality disorders.

We included the self-report IIP and a peer nomination version of the same instrument during 1 year of data collection with our college student sample. We tested 393 students who were living in dorm groups that ranged in size from 7 to 19 people. Our analyses focused on the connections between features of personality disorders and interpersonal problems. One set of analyses examined these connections as viewed from the same source (self-report of both domains and peer report of both domains). The other set of analyses focused on connections across sources (e.g., self-report of personality disorder features related to peer report of interpersonal problems). We found significant relations between personality disorder features and interpersonal problems, but these patterns were most obvious when they were seen from the same perspective—either the self or the peers (Clifton, Turkheimer, & Oltmanns, 2005). Some interesting patterns did appear in our across-source analyses. For example, people who described themselves as having features of narcissistic and antisocial personality disorders were viewed by their peers as being domineering, vindictive, and intrusive.

COMPARISON OF SELF-REPORT AND PEER DATA

The most important analyses in the peer nomination project involve the correspondence between self-report (from the MAPP) and peer nominations for characteristic features of personality disorders. Tables 4.7 and 4.8 show correlations between peer-report and self-report for the military recruits and college students. The correlations range from low to moderate. In all but one case, the within-trait cross-method correlation (e.g., self-report for avoidant personality disorder with peer nomination for avoidant personality disorder) is higher than any of the cross-trait correlations. The correlations in the college sample are, on average, somewhat higher than the military correlations, probably because the groups were better acquainted and somewhat more reliable. Of course, alternative explanations may involve a number of factors, such as the length of time for which the group members had known each other, the relative proportion of men and women in each sample, and the average IQ of the people in each group.

These tables suggest a modest level of convergent and discriminant validity for peer and self-perception on these particular traits. The correlations are all statistically significant, but they are also consistently low. In fact, they are a bit lower than correlations typically reported in studies of self–other agreement on personality traits using systems such as the five-factor model. Remembering that the reliabilities of the peer nomination

TABLE 4.7. Correlations between MAPP Self-Report Personality Disorder Scores and Peer Nomination Personality Disorder Scores in the Military Sample

MAPP PEER	MAPP self-report									
	1.	2.	3.	4.	5.	6.	7.	8.	9.	10.
1. Paranoid	**.15**	.12	.11	.11	.11	.05	.09	−.01	.00	.10
2. Schizoid	.10	**.21**	.16	.12	.12	.04	.08	.08	.03	.10
3. Schizotypal	.13	.13	**.24**	.12	.18	.09	.07	.14	.10	.11
4. Antisocial	.15	.15	.15	**.23**	.16	.14	.18	.00	.07	.06
5. Borderline	.14	.09	.19	.14	**.20**	.12	.10	.08	.09	.08
6. Histrionic	.09	.04	.09	.12	.10	**.17**	.18	−.05	.05	.04
7. Narcissistic	.06	.06	.02	.10	.04	.09	**.16**	−.11	−.03	.07
8. Avoidant	.09	.08	.19	.05	.15	.04	.01	**.21**	.14	.06
9. Dependent	.11	.07	.18	.11	.16	.11	.06	.16	**.18**	.04
10. Obsessive–compulsive	.00	.05	.00	.00	−.02	−.02	.03	−.09	−.07	**.13**

Note. N = 2,028.

scales are close to .90, these correlations raise important questions about whether research based exclusively on self-report provides a complete perspective on the nature of personality disorders and pathological personality traits. They suggest that a person's own description of his or her personality problems may provide a rather limited—indeed, perhaps a distorted—view of this type of mental health problem.

The pattern of correlations between self and other were quite similar in men and women. Relevant data are presented in Table 4.9. We had ex-

TABLE 4.8. Correlations between MAPP Self-Report Personality Disorder Scores and Peer Nomination Personality Disorder Scores in the College Sample

MAPP PEER	MAPP self-report									
	1.	2.	3.	4.	5.	6.	7.	8.	9.	10.
1. Paranoid	**.11**	.18	.17	.22	.18	.18	.24	.03	.15	.05
2. Schizoid	.04	**.35**	.23	.09	.08	.03	.10	.09	.02	.07
3. Schizotypal	.06	.30	**.26**	.15	.14	.11	.15	.06	.07	.05
4. Antisocial	.08	.09	.12	**.35**	.21	.25	.27	−.05	.14	−.03
5. Borderline	.06	.14	.15	.23	**.19**	.17	.20	.00	.14	−.01
6. Histrionic	.04	.06	.08	.21	.13	**.26**	.26	−.06	.13	−.02
7. Narcissistic	.03	.04	.04	.18	.09	.22	**.28**	−.07	.10	.00
8. Avoidant	.03	.22	.15	.03	.05	.03	.08	**.12**	.10	.07
9. Dependent	.00	.04	.05	.10	.09	.14	.13	−.02	**.17**	−.01
10. Obsessive–compulsive	−.02	.17	.08	.04	.00	.03	.16	.02	.04	**.12**

Note. N = 1,691.

pected, based on previous results aimed primarily at positive personality traits, that women would show higher rates of agreement between their own descriptions of themselves and opinions provided by peers (Kenny, 1994). In fact, we found only two cases in which women showed significantly higher agreement than men—both in the military sample. Female recruits were more likely to agree with their peers' perceptions of features for paranoid and narcissistic personality disorders. Male recruits showed higher levels of self–other agreement for avoidant personality disorder. In the college student sample, men were more likely to agree with their peers' perceptions regarding features of antisocial personality disorder. Because the significant differences were not observed in both samples, we are reluctant to suggest that gender plays an important role in moderating the connection between self-report and peer perceptions.

Acquaintance Moderates Self–Other Agreement

Previous studies regarding self–other agreement for personality traits have reported correlations that are somewhat higher than we found in our study. Several factors may account for these differences. One is the nature of the relationship between the target person and the people who made nominations. Many other investigations have employed close friends or family members as informants, while our study focused on people who were members of the same training groups or who lived on the same dorm floors. Some of these people undoubtedly knew one another well, but others did not. Congruence between self- and other reports for personality pathology

TABLE 4.9. Correlations between MAPP Self-Report Scores and Peer Nomination Scores by Gender

	Air Force sample		University of Virginia sample	
Peer report	Male	Female	Male	Female
1. Paranoid	.09*	.25	.10	.11
2. Schizoid	.19	.25	.33	.35
3. Schizotypal	.25	.23	.25	.25
4. Antisocial	.22	.23	.41*	.28
5. Borderline	.21	.17	.17	.20
6. Histrionic	.17	.19	.31	.24
7. Narcissistic	.13†	.23	.30	.28
8. Avoidant	.25*	.14	.15	.11
9. Dependent	.20	.17	.13	.19
10. Obsessive–compulsive	.10	.18	.10	.14

Note. Military sample: 911 males, 592 females; college sample: 562 males, 1,122 females.
*$p < .05$; †$p < .10$.

might be expected to be higher when the informant is a person with whom the target person is well acquainted.

Before they completed the MAPP, all of our participants had been asked to *rate* how well they knew and liked each member of the group.[7] We found considerable variability within our groups with regard to these "knowing" and "liking" variables. In the military sample, 62% of the ratings indicated that the rater knew the target, and about half of these said that they knew the target well or very well. In the college student sample 87% of the ratings indicated that the rater knew the target, and two-thirds of these said they knew the target well or very well. In the military sample, 19% of the ratings indicated that the rater disliked the target very much, 20% indicated the rater liked the target very much, with the rest in between. In the college sample, 6% of the ratings indicated that the rater disliked the target, 36% of the ratings indicated the rater liked the target, with the remainder in between.

Social network techniques can be used to examine the role of acquaintance as a moderator of self–other agreement (Clifton, Turkheimer, & Oltmanns, 2006). Focusing on our military sample, these quantitative procedures were used to identify more cohesive subgroups on the basis of each person's indications of the extent to which he or she knew every other person in the group. The training flights were generally composed of two informal and loosely organized subgroups of people who were better acquainted with one another than with members of the other group. In some cases, these groups broke down along gender lines. Within social networks, peer nominations were more reliable, and they were more closely associated with self-report personality disorder scores.

While social network analyses suggest that level of acquaintance is related to the extent of self–other agreement, it should also be noted that these correlations remain quite modest, even when we consider only data within groups of people who know one another well. The median correlation within clusters (i.e., training groups subdivided into groups that are better acquainted) was approximately .20, which is roughly the same as the level of agreement found for the group as a whole. In other words, peer scores obtained within a cluster did not produce *greater* than average agreement between self- and peer report. Rather, peer scores that were obtained between clusters were associated with *poorer* agreement.

Positive versus Negative Content and Nominations versus Ratings

Two other factors might have had an impact on the magnitude of agreement between self- and other scores that were obtained in our study. One is the nomination method that we used for our assessments. Peer nomination has been demonstrated to be more reliable and valid than other forms of peer assessment (Kane & Lawler, 1978; Schwarzwald, Koslowsky, & Mager-Bibi, 1999), and it has been used in several previous studies of normal personality (Norman, 1963; Passini & Norman, 1966; Waters & Waters, 1970; Mervielde & De Fruyt, 2000). The nomination process required each participant to identify one or more members of the group who were best described by each criterion. An alternative procedure, used in many other studies, has been to use *ratings*, such that each target person would be rated on each item by all of the judges in the group. These different methods of peer assessment have not been compared directly using the same participants. Despite its high reliability and validity, peer nomination often produces a skewed distribution in which information is obtained only for people who exhibit the most examples of each characteristic or trait. This skewed distribution could produce a decreased self–other correlation because the majority of participants would have little variance in their peer scores.

Another important consideration involves the extent to which the characteristics in question are considered to be undesirable or maladaptive, as in the case of features of personality disorders. Previous reports suggest that higher levels of agreement are found for positive or less evaluative traits (Fuhrman & Funder, 1995; Kenny, 1994). It seems possible that, in our study, the level of agreement between self- and other assessments can be attributed partially to the fact that the personality features in question are undesirable. In other words, they are behaviors and experiences that people might be expected to deny, and they are things that friends could be reluctant to describe.

We conducted a separate investigation, using college students who were not part of the primary study, in order to consider these possible explanations for low self–other agreement (Turkheimer, Chan, Clifton, & Oltmanns, 2006). Participants were 40 members of the same sorority. All served as both targets and judges. They were asked to describe themselves and the other members of their group with regard to features of one positive personality feature (extraversion) and one negative or pathological personality trait (narcissism). To compare the effects of nomination and rating methodologies, half of the women were randomly assigned to a condition in which they described their peers using nominations, while the other half described the same peers using Q-sort ratings. The Q-sort methodology forces a roughly normal distribution of scores for each target and has been used in the assessment of both normal personality (Adams & John, 1997) and personality pathology (Shedler & Westen, 1998). Each participant completed a self-report measure and one of two peer assessment measures. Twenty-three items were included in each measure: 12 were concerned with extraversion (items from the NEO Personality Inventory [NEO-PI]), and 11 were narcissistic personality disorder items taken from the MAPP. Using this process, each person in the group received scores on both traits (extraversion and narcissism) from three sources (self-report, peer nominations from half of her sorority sisters, and peer ratings from the other half of her sisters).

Correlations among the three sources of personality data are presented in Table 4.10. Correlations between self-report and peer report were higher for extraversion than for narcissism, and slightly higher for nominations than for Q-sort ratings. The correlations between the two peer-based assessment procedures administered to independent groups of raters were quite high for both extraversion and narcissism. To investigate whether the differences in self–peer correlations between extraversion and narcissism or the two peer report methods might be attributable to differences in the reliability of either self- or peer report, we disattenuated the correlations by dividing the observed correlations by the square roots of the reliabilities. The disattenuated correlations are above the diagonals in Table 4.10. If the differences in self–peer correlations among traits and rating methods are attributable to reliability differences, differences among the self–peer correlations should be reduced when they are disattenuated for reliability. This does not appear to be the case for our data.

This study replicated the fundamental findings it was designed to investigate: correlations between self- and peer report were of moderate magnitude for the normal personality trait of extraversion, but they were lower for items measuring the pathological trait of narcissism. Although the mean, variance, and reliability of the nomination-based narcissism measure were attenuated relative to the other measures, correlations with self-report were actually higher for the nomination-based measure than for the measure based on Q-sort ratings.

Even more striking were the correlations between the peer descriptions

TABLE 4.10. Correlations among Self-Report, Peer Nominations, and Q-Sorts

	Self-report	Nominations	Q-sort
Extraversion			
Self-Report	—	.57	.42
Nominations	.46	—	1.0
Q-sort	.34	.88	—
Narcissism			
Self-Report	—	.26	.20
Nominations	.21	—	.94
Q-sort	.18	.77	—

Note. Raw correlations below diagonal, disattenuated correlations above diagonal.

using the two methodologies: the participants' total narcissism scores based on peer nominations and Q-sorts correlated at $r = .77$. Although this is precisely what we would have predicted based on the reliability analysis, it is worth considering this result carefully. Two completely separate groups of raters, using different methods, agreed on the narcissism levels of the group members at $r = .77$. The correlations of the two peer methods with self-report were both exactly $r = .21$. Independent groups of raters agree with one another but not with self-report. Whatever the reason for low self–peer agreement is, it is not that the nomination method is crude or that peers are responding in the absence of knowledge. Assessing negative traits does appear to contribute to low self–peer agreement, however, because correlations for extraversion were significantly higher, at $r = .35$.

Systematic Relations between Self- and Other Report

Peers are able to identify reliably people who exhibit features of specific types of personality disorder. Unfortunately, the descriptions provided by peers often stand in marked contrast to descriptions that the target persons provide of themselves. Having identified this same pattern in two large samples, we wondered whether we could find systematic connections between self- and other reports, even if the descriptions point to different perspectives on the same person. In other words, if peers describe the person as being paranoid, and if the person does not endorse the same view, how *does* he describe himself? Similarly, if an individual endorses certain traits using a self-report procedure, but peers do not agree, how do the peers perceive that person? We decided to look for *systematic* differences between self- and other report rather than dismissing the lack of congruence as being the product of measurement error. By studying the similarities and differences in perception between self and peers, we hoped to find discrepancies that are predictable (Clifton, Turkheimer, & Oltmanns, 2004).

We used data from the first two years of our military sample for these analyses. To avoid capitalizing on chance, we randomly divided the participants into two samples: an experimental sample ($n = 796$) and a cross-validation sample ($n = 397$). Using the experimental sample, we performed regressions predicting the peer-based personality disorder scales using the corresponding SNAP scales. The residuals from these regressions represent the unexplained variance after the corresponding SNAP scales are partialled out. In order to find the SNAP items that explain the greatest amount of variance in the peer scale, over and above the corresponding SNAP scale, these residuals were correlated with the entire set of SNAP items. The 10 SNAP items that were most highly correlated with these residuals were designated the self-reported "supplemental items" for the appropriate diagnostic scale. This procedure was repeated, predicting SNAP scales from the peer nomination scores, and determining 10 peer-reported "supplemental items." Using the cross-validation sample, unit-weighted scales made up of these supplemental items were added to the appropriate diagnostic scales and were found to increase the amount of variance explained.

Several interesting findings emerged from qualitative examination of the supplemental items. Some were items that were similar in content to the corresponding personality disorder scale, but were not included in the original scale. For example, peer supplemental items for schizoid personality disorder consist of negatively correlated histrionic and narcissism items. A second type of supplemental item was based on a systematic difference between self and other in the perception of a trait. For example, the peer supplemental items for paranoid personality disorder indicate that a person who describes himself as paranoid is actually viewed by others as being cold and unfeeling. Working in the other direction (from peers to self), people who are described by their peers as being paranoid tend to describe themselves as being angry (but not suspicious or hypervigilant).

A third type of supplemental item is an example of what the test construction literature refers to as a "subtle item." These are self-reported items that are less obvious, nonpejorative examples of personality disorder traits. For example, people who were described by peers as being narcissistic tended to describe themselves as being extremely outgoing, gregarious, and likeable. In other words, the participants put a positive spin on their own extremely positive view of themselves. In so doing, they may have displayed—in a more subtle or flattering way—the same narcissism that their peers had tried to describe.

METAPERCEPTION

The MAPP allows us to answer another important question about the nature of agreement and disagreement between self- and peer reports. Is the target person aware of what other people think of him or her, even if those two perspectives are at odds with each other? What happens if we ask people to indicate what they think most other people in their group said about them with regard to the same features of personality pathology? For each item, the MAPP asked participants to provide two responses: (1) how they thought their peers described them and (2) what they are really like. We refer to the former set of items as "expected peer" scores. Kenny (1994) used the term "metaperception" to describe the same phenomenon. One reason that self- and peer report may disagree is that people may know how they are viewed by others but disagree systematically with that view in their self-report.

We found very high correlations between self-scores and expected peer scores. These correlations ranged from .77 to .87 in the military sample (Oltmanns, Gleason, Klonsky, & Turkheimer, 2005). The results show that, to a large extent, people believe that others share the same view that they hold of their own personality characteristics. The fact that these correlations are not perfect, however, also suggests that expected peer scores are not *the same* as self scores.

We then examined how self-report and expected peer personality disorder scores function as joint predictors of peer report for the same personality disorder features. Expected peer scores are positively associated with actual peer scores. In other words, if you think that your peers will give you higher ratings on personality pathology, they will, in fact, give you higher scores. Expected peer scores did predict variability in peer report over and above self-report for all 10 diagnostic traits. This pattern shows that people do have some incremental knowledge of how they are viewed by others, but they don't tell you about it unless you ask them to do so; the knowledge is not reflected in ordinary self-report data.

When self-report and expected peer report are used simultaneously as predictors of actual peer report in a multiple regression, expected peer report contributes unique variance for every diagnostic category. Self-report generally does not. The joint prediction of peer report from self-report and expected peer report is modest, but it is statistically significant for each category. To the extent that this prediction can be uniquely attributed to one or the other source, it is almost always expected peer report that is doing the work. The effect size for expected peer is substantially higher than that for the self score, so to whatever extent we are interested in knowing about what the peers actually think of the person, we learn more from the expected peer scores.

INFORMANTS

Some studies of personality disorders have collected data from informants in addition to using self-report measures (see Klonsky, Oltmans, & Turkheimer, 2002, for a review). Typically, the target persons have been asked to provide the name of a friend or family member who knows them well. This person is then interviewed or asked to fill out a questionnaire in order to describe the target participant. In most research settings, this is the only way to obtain data from informants. It is often difficult to collect data from a large number of people who know the target person, and it is almost always impossible to collect informant data from people who are not selected by (and may not like) the target person. Most researchers will continue to rely on single informants chosen by the subject. It therefore becomes important to understand the biases such informants may bring with them to the lab. Specifically, how are data provided by selected informants different than those that might also be provided by informants who are not selected by the subject? We have examined this issue in two ways.

Hypothetical Informants within Peer Groups

Before they began to complete our questionnaires, we asked each partici-pant to select from his or her group of peers one person who would make the best "hypothetical informant." We asked each participant, "If we wanted to talk to someone who knows you well, in order to better under-stand your personality, which member of your group would make the best informant?" Remember that our "knowing" and "liking" ratings indicate a range of scores within each group. In the military sample, 19% of the rat-ings indicated that the rater disliked the target person. Like everyone else, people with personality disorders are disliked by some people who know them well. These people might provide extremely useful information about the person if we could talk to them, but they are unlikely to be nominated to serve as an informant. Most informants are identified because the target person likes the informant and also believes that the informant likes him or her. Our groups provide an interesting opportunity to examine the general-izability of informant data. We can compare peer nominations from our "hypothetical informants" with nominations made by the rest of the group.

We conducted an analysis using a subset of the data collected from our military sample ($N = 1,581$). We compared descriptions of the target per-son that were provided by the designated hypothetical informant with the descriptions of the target person that were provided by other people in the group (whom we called "potential informants"). The latter group included only those people who indicated that they knew the target person well (i.e., rated the person with a "2" or a "3" when asked "how well do you know this person?"). We excluded those people who indicated that they did not know the target person, but we did not take into consideration whether or not the peer member *liked* the target person.

In general, nominations made by the hypothetical informants were in substantial agreement with those made by potential informants (Turk-heimer, Friedman, Klonsky, & Oltmanns, 2006). Correlations between nominations made by hypothetical and potential informants ranged from .32 (for paranoid personality disorder) to .46 (for borderline personality disorder). Furthermore, the level of self–other agreement was not sub-stantially different as a function of the type of informant. Viewed from this perspective, it would appear that informants who are identified by the target person do provide useful information that will approximate de-scriptions provided by a wider assortment of people who know the per-son well.

On the other hand, informants selected by the target person also showed a significant bias with regard to certain kinds of personality items. Target people were significantly more likely to be nominated by hypothetical informants on all 24 of the positive personality characteristics that were included as filler items in our inventory (such as "good sense of humor," "trustworthy and reliable," and "cheerful optimistic outlook on life"). With regard to features of personality pathology, our results showed that some crucial items were underreported by hypothetical informants, particularly those pertaining to friendship and sociability. In other words, the target person's best friend is unlikely to nominate him or her as someone who doesn't have any friends. This pattern held for a number of items that were related to disorders listed in Cluster A and Cluster B. In contrast to scores provided by other peers, the hypothetical informants also gave the target persons lower scores on items related to narcissism, paranoia, and antisocial personality disorder. A different picture emerged with regard to personality problems associated with Cluster C (where anxiety plays a more prominent role). Hypothetical informants provided the target people with higher scores on items related to avoidant and obsessive–compulsive personality disorder. These results suggest that the value of informant data varies as a function of the type of problem being assessed. Some Cluster A and Cluster B disorders will be underreported by informants who are selected by the target person. On the other hand, informant data may be better than data from unselected peers with regard to the assessment of "internalizing disorders," such as avoidant and obsessive–compulsive personality disorder.

The greatest shortcoming of nominations obtained from hypothetical informants was one they shared with self-report: compared to peer nominations, they are unreliable. Just as there is only one self for self-report, there was only one hypothetical informant in our analyses. Therefore, his or her nominations could not be balanced by those obtained from other unselected peers. This aspect of our analysis clearly points to the value of using multiple informants.

Family Members, Compared to Informants and Peer Groups

Previous studies that have collected personality data from informants have often selected family members—parents or siblings—to provide information about the target person. Family members have the advantage of knowing the person over an extended period of time. They are presumably able to provide a much more intimate view of the person than we might hope to obtain from peers, especially those who are not necessarily close friends. The low level of self–other agreement that we found in our college and military samples might be attributed to the fact that we had not obtained data from more traditional sources. We conducted a follow-up study, using college students who had been tested in one particular year, in order to compare levels of self–other agreement using different sources of information.

We began with a sample of students (75% female) who completed the peer nomination study while they were living in 1-year dormitories. They were recontacted one year later and asked to complete the self-report version of the MAPP again. We also asked for their permission to contact at least one family member (a parent or sibling) who would be able to complete an informant version of the MAPP that would be used to describe the target person's personality. We asked for the name of a family member with whom the person had lived for at least 5 years. At the time of follow-up, we also obtained the target person's permission to contact again the student who had been designated (1 year earlier) as his or her hypothetical informant. If that person was not available, we selected another former member of the dorm group who had indicated that he or she was well acquainted with the target person. From the original sample of 393 target persons, 294 completed all of the self-report follow-up measures. Follow-up peer information was obtained for 151 of these people, and follow-up family information was collected for 141 target persons.

The 1-year test–retest stability of the self-report MAPP personality disorder scales was quite good. Correlations were mostly in the range of .50 to .60. There was also a fair amount of consistency between the original peer scores, based on nominations obtained from all members of the person's first-year dorm floor, and follow-up informant scores (based only on informants selected by the target person). These correlations fell in the range between .30 and .45. As in the case of our hypothetical informant analyses (described above), this pattern suggests that informant scores do provide an approximation of the perspective afforded by descriptions based on a larger and more broadly representative sample of peers.

Similar to our previous findings, self–other correlations based on reports obtained from family members were modest at best. Correlations between self-report scores on the MAPP personality disorder scales (from Time 2) and MAPP informant scores from family members fell in the range between .20 and .40. This pattern resembled closely the pattern of correlations that were obtained between the same self-report scores and informant scores obtained from designated peers at follow-up. The results of this study point to two general conclusions. First, different kinds of informants provide differing perspectives on the target person's personality. Second, there appears to be an upper limit to the level of agreement that can be expected between a person's own description of his or her personality and the view that would be provided by someone else who has had an opportunity to get to know the person well. None of the correlations between self- and informant report exceeded .50.

VALIDITY OF SEMISTRUCTURED
DIAGNOSTIC INTERVIEWS

Semistructured diagnostic interviews have come to be accepted as the gold standard for the diagnosis of personality disorders. This state of affairs seems a bit surprising when considered in light of the limitations of self-report measures. In many ways, semistructured diagnostic interviews are quite similar to questionnaires. A fixed series of questions are read aloud to the person. Unlike the situations with questionnaires, the target person does have an opportunity to provide an open-ended response. The interviewer is allowed to ask follow-up questions, probing for more information on the basis of the target person's answers to opening questions. Unlike the situations with questionnaires, the person's score is based on the interviewer's observation of the target person's behavior (speech patterns, facial expressions, posture, and so on). Nevertheless, the results of interviews are based heavily on the content of the person's own description. If he or she is unable or unwilling to acknowledge personality problems, the interviewer probably will not identify the presence of a personality disorder. For this reason, we believe that interviews should be considered primarily another form of self-report.

For the subset of people in our study who completed the SIDP-IV, we were able to compare the results of these interviews to the data that we obtained using peer and self-report scores from the MAPP. Table 4.11 presents correlations between the interviews (using continuous scores with regard to symptoms for each type of personality disorder) and the other sources. In both the military and college samples, the SIDP was more closely correlated with self-report scores from the MAPP than it was with the description provided by peer nominations. This is not surprising because the questionnaire and the interview depend on the person both being able to recognize his or her own personality problems and also being willing to acknowledge these problems when asked about them. Many of the problems that were described by the peers may be issues of which the target person has little awareness.

The discrepancy between information provided by peers and results from diagnostic interviews indicates that there are occasions when these interviews "miss." Although the peers are telling us that someone does exhibit features of a particular form of personality disorder, when that person is given an opportunity to describe himself in the context of an interview, he does not acknowledge the same problems. This observation is consistent with some results of studies that have attempted to determine the prevalence of personality disorders in nonclinical samples using semistructured interviews. Narcissistic personality disorder is an interesting example. Very few cases of this disorder have been identified in community studies (Mattia & Zimmerman, 2001).

TABLE 4.11. Correlations between Scores Based
on Semistructured Interview and Scores Based on Peer
Nominations and a Self-Report Questionnaire

| | Correlation of SIDP with: | |
	MAPP peer	MAPP self-report
	Military	
Paranoid	.15	.43
Schizoid	.15	.32
Schizotypal	.19	.39
Antisocial	.19	.43
Borderline	.12	.44
Histrionic	.24	.33
Narcissistic	.26	.36
Avoidant	.23	.41
Dependent	.19	.32
Obsessive–compulsive	.12	.22
	College	
Paranoid	.03	.46
Schizoid	−.02	.04
Schizotypal	.15	.32
Antisocial	.35	.47
Borderline	.3	.43
Histrionic	.13	.38
Narcissistic	.18	.37
Avoidant	.08	.49
Dependent	−.01	.41
Obsessive–compulsive	.00	.36

In an informal attempt to explore the discrepancy between peer reports and diagnostic interviews, we reviewed the videotapes of several interviews. We intentionally selected people who had received very high
scores for narcissism on our peer nomination index and who had also received no indication of narcissistic personality disorder from the interviewers who conducted the interview. Our impressions, based on this experience, suggested some interesting hypotheses. Viewed with the knowledge
of what the peers had told us, it seemed that some of the target persons
did exhibit characteristics—such as arrogance and indifference to the feelings of others—that are consistent with a diagnosis of narcissistic personality disorder. These indications were often subtle and did not rise to the
level of definitive symptoms. If the original interviews had noticed them,
they would not have rated them because the target person did not acknowledge or endorse their presence. Nevertheless, it seemed that the videotapes might contain subtle evidence that would corroborate the impressions conveyed by the person's peers. In other words, the results obtained

from the interviews and the peer nominations might be less discrepant than they originally appeared to be.

In order to examine this impression empirically, we took advantage of the videotapes of our semistructured interviews. From the sample of 433 military recruits who had completed the SIDP-IV, we were able to identify 8 who had been identified by the peers as having strong features of narcissistic personality disorder but who nevertheless had received very low scores on the basis of the semistructured interviews. These people might be considered "false negatives." In other words, their peer scores suggested that they do have issues with regard to narcissistic personality disorder, but they did not report any recognizable symptoms of narcissism during the interview. These interviews were compared to those conducted with another set of 8 people who were selected because they matched the targets for gender and race. The comparison interviews also showed no evidence of narcissism. The only obvious difference between the two sets of interviews was that the target people had received a large number of nominations for features of narcissistic personality disorder, while the people in the comparison sample had not. The videotape of each interview was viewed by six undergraduate students. These raters knew nothing about personality disorders, and they knew nothing about the people on the tapes. Each rater watched two tapes (one target and one control). After watching each tape, the rater was asked to rate the person on the tape, using the 30 facets of the five-factor model of personality. They also rated the person with regard to 24 features of personality pathology taken from the peer version of the MAPP (including all narcissistic personality disorder items).

The ratings made by naive undergraduates identified several significant differences between the target and control interviews (Gruber, Oltmanns, Turkheimer, & Fiedler, 2002). With regard to facets of the Five Factor Model, the most obvious differences appeared with regard to agreeableness. This trait and its facets are clearly associated with the DSM-IV description of narcissistic personality disorder (Widiger, Trull, Clarkin, Sanderson, & Costa, 2002). The target people (false negatives) were rated as being lower on modesty, tendermindedness, and compliance. With regard to the specific DSM-IV features of NPD, the targets were rated as being higher on grandiosity, arrogance, and "believes he or she is special." The naive undergraduate raters did see something on these tapes; they detected subtle arrogance and grandiosity as it was displayed by target persons, whose peers had recognized these same features when they made their nominations. In that sense, the results of the interviews may be seen as somewhat less discrepant from the descriptions that were provided by other people.

What do these results suggest about the value of semistructured diagnostic interviews? This is a difficult question. Laypersons who viewed the tapes were able to identify some potential personality problems that were also identified by peers in basic military training. On the other hand, lack of modesty does not imply that a person should qualify for a diagnosis of personality disorder. Structured diagnostic interviews have become the gold standard in psychiatric assessment because they produce reliable results, and increased reliability of diagnostic decisions has set the stage for many advances in the study of psychopathology. The results of our study point to possible problems regarding the concurrent validity of self-report measures— including structured interviews—for the diagnosis of personality disorder because they do not identify some people who appear to suffer from personality pathology, based on other sources of information. The sensitivity of the interviews could be raised by training interviewers to rely more heavily on their subjective impressions of personality traits, such as arrogance and grandiosity. Unfortunately, changes of that sort could easily lead to a decrease in reliability. Further exploration of these alternatives does seem to be warranted.

PREDICTIVE VALIDITY OF PEER NOMINATIONS

Disagreement between sources of information (self and other) does not suggest that one kind of measure is more valid than the other. Moving beyond the demonstration of inconsistencies, we have begun to ask which source of data (self or peer) is most useful, and for what purpose? In the military sample, we have been able to follow our recruits by using electronic data provided (on an anonymous basis) by the Defense Manpower Data Center. This information provides evidence regarding real-life outcomes, such as health care problems, drug testing, disciplinary reports, and promotion records. One issue that we have examined in relation to personality pathology is adjustment and job success following the successful completion of basic military training.

Four years after we began to collect personality data in our military sample, we examined the job status of all participants (see Fiedler, Oltmanns, & Turkheimer, 2004, for a preliminary report of these findings). All of the recruits had enlisted for a period of 4 years. At the time of follow-up, we divided the recruits into two groups: (1) those still engaged in active-duty employment, and (2) those who had been given an early discharge from the military (after completion of basic training but before the end of their expected 4-year tour of duty). An early discharge is typically granted by a superior officer on an involuntary basis, and is most often justified by repeated disciplinary problems, serious interpersonal difficulties, a poor performance record, or some combination of these considerations.

Two hundred and twenty-six of the 2,116 recruits had been discharged. Their records indicated the following reasons for early separation: character or behavior disorder, pattern of minor disciplinary infractions, unsatisfactory performance, unqualified for active duty, misconduct (reason unknown), or commission of a serious offense. Only separations that were given a code indicating poor performance were used in this study. Individuals separated through a "no-fault separation" who had parenthood-related issues, medical, or other nonbehavioral reasons were not included in the separation number. The mean length of time from the start of basic training to the point of involuntary discharge was 13 months ($SD = 9$ months).

The data were analyzed using survival analysis because the recruits had not completed our initial personality assessment process simultaneously. At the time that survival analyses were performed, the mean length of time that had elapsed since entry to basic training was 2.2 years (range from 1.3 years to 3.7 years). We used dimensional scores on each of the SNAP diagnostic and trait scales because they are more reliable than categorical scores. Each recruit received a score based on the number of items that he or she endorsed for each scale. For the peer nomination measure, we added scores for a given personality disorder feature across all judges and divided by the number of members in the group.

Univariate contributions to the survival analysis model from SNAP diagnostic scales are presented in Table 4.12. For these self-report scales, the strongest relationship was between scores on borderline personality disorder and early separation. When the diagnostic scales were considered together in a forward stepwise sequence of chi-squares, only the borderline scale made a significant independent contribution to the prediction of separation (chi-square increment 13.64, $p = .0002$). Univariate contributions to the model from SNAP trait scales are also included in Table 4.12. A forward stepwise sequence of chi-squares found that only the self-harm scale made significant contributions to the prediction of separation (chi-square increment 28.01, $p = .0001$). The strongest individual SNAP items predicting early separation were concerned with suicidal ideation (e.g., "I have hurt myself on purpose several times") and emotional distress (e.g., "I often have strong feelings such as anxiety or anger without really knowing why," and "My future looks very bright to me [false]").

A very different picture emerged when we considered data obtained using peer nominations. Univariate contributions to the survival analysis model from peer nomination covariates are presented in Table 4.13. The strongest relationship was found between peer nominations for antisocial characteristics and early separation from the military. The peers' information regarding features of borderline personality disorder was also related to discharge status. A forward stepwise sequence of chi-squares found that three different peer scores made significant independent contributions to

TABLE 4.12. Survival Analyses Using SNAP Self-Report Scales to Predict Early Separation from the Military

	Maximum likelihood chi-square	p
SNAP diagnostic scores		
Borderline	13.64	.0002
Antisocial	1.62	.0012
Paranoid	1.48	.0011
Schizotypal	6.84	.0089
Histrionic	4.34	.037
Dependent	3.92	.048
Narcissistic	3.73	.054
Avoidant	2.76	.096
Schizoid	0.44	.51
Obsessive–compulsive	0.01	.94
SNAP trait scores		
Self-harm (self-esteem + suicide)	28.01	<.0001
Suicide proneness (subscale of SH)	23.21	<.0001
Mistrust	10.95	.0009
Aggression	10.94	.0009
Impulsivity	10.77	.001
Disinhibition (temperament scale)	10.58	.001
Eccentric perceptions	8.27	.004
Manipulativeness	6.50	.011
Propriety (negative)	5.85	.016

the prediction model: antisocial, obsessive–compulsive (inverse relation), and borderline personality disorders. The best peer nomination items (from the MAPP) predicting early separation were concerned with recklessness, impulsivity, and irresponsibility (e.g., "Is irresponsible; can't be counted on to do his/her work or pay bills," "Has a reckless lack of concern for safety of self or other people," and "Does things without thinking; doesn't plan ahead"). When we combined the self-report and peer-based information to predict the survival function, the best predictor variable was the peer score for antisocial features (maximum likelihood chi-square increment 33.08, $p < .0001$). The SNAP self-harm score and the peer obsessive–compulsive score (inverse relation) also made significant contributions to the survival function. After those scores were entered, no other score made a significant contribution.

This set of results points to several general conclusions. One is that in this nonclinical sample personality pathology is associated with an objective index of occupational impairment. Various features of personality disorders appear to have a negative impact on adjustment to military life. This

TABLE 4.13. Survival Analyses Using Peer Nomination
Scores to Predict Early Separation from the Military

	Maximum likelihood chi-square	p
Diagnostic category		
Antisocial	29.79	<.0001
Borderline	2.51	<.0001
Histrionic	19.62	<.0001
Dependent	17.33	<.0001
Schizotypal	13.96	.0002
Avoidant	1.94	.0009
Schizoid	9.45	.002
Paranoid	5.82	.016
Obsessive–compulsive	4.75	.029
Narcissistic	4.01	.045

finding complements the results obtained in our college sample, where features of personality disorders were associated with self-report of impaired social functioning. The present study is important, in part, because most evidence regarding this issue has previously been obtained by using patients in treatment for psychiatric disorders.

Both self-report and peer nominations were able to identify meaningful connections between personality problems and early separation from the military. The self-report measures emphasized features that might be described as internalizing problems (subjective distress and self-harm), while the peer-report measure emphasized externalizing problems (antisocial traits). Considered together, the peer nomination scores were more effective than the self-report scales in predicting occupational outcome (i.e., who remained on active duty).

SUMMARY AND RECOMMENDATIONS

Peer nominations produce reliable and valid information that is largely independent of that obtained from self-report. Both sources of information were useful in predicting the ability of these recruits to succeed in their military careers. Although the correlation between self-report and peer report is consistently low, the independent information in peer reports does seem to tell us something important about personality. This finding is consistent with the previous suggestions that personality disorders are frequently defined and experienced in terms of interpersonal conflict and problems in person perception. Although most investigators rely on self-report measures to assess personality disorders, a more accurate description of personality problems would be obtained by collecting information from associates, friends, or family members.

The results of our study can be summarized by the following statements:

- Features of personality disorders can be identified reliably in non-clinical samples of young adults.
- These problems are associated with social and occupational impairment.
- People's own descriptions of their personality problems are frequently different from descriptions obtained from other people.
- Systematic patterns connect discrepant self- and peer reports (e.g., people who are viewed as being paranoid describe themselves as being angry).
- People do have some awareness of the ways that they are viewed by others, but they do not tell you about it if you only ask them for their own description of themselves.
- Informants provide useful information, but those who are selected by the target person may have some blind spots.
- Interviews sometimes miss aspects of a person's personality, but these aspects can sometimes be discerned from other sources.

Our data raise questions about the potential incremental value of obtaining information from sources that complement more traditional self-report measures. With regard to the use of informants, we would recommend two things. First, it is helpful to obtain information from more than one other person, in large part because data from multiple sources will be more reliable. Second, the clinician or investigator should keep in mind the biases that may influence ratings provided by informants who are selected by the target person. Self-selected informants will probably be a better source of information about internalizing disorders than about externalizing disorders.

The results of our study also lead us to make some suggestions about ways in which the sensitivity of semistructured diagnostic interviews might be raised. Because people do have some knowledge of the impressions that they form among other people, it may be useful to phrase questions in a way that probes specifically for the ways in which other people see the target person. Existing interviews do contain some questions of this type. For example, one question aimed at narcissistic personality disorder in the SIDP-IV asks "Have other people said that you have an attitude problem?" This is clearly a very different question than asking "Do you have an attitude problem?" Our analyses of systematic relations between self- and peer report also suggest that people whose peers see them as exhibiting personality problems may tend to put a positive spin on their own descriptions of these phenomena. People who are narcissistic, for example, will describe themselves in glowing terms (high positive affect) without acknowledging the more negative elements of these same characteristics (being grandiose or exploitative). Finally, our consideration of discrepant interviews suggests that there may be some value in training interviewers to attend more carefully to subjective impressions of the person being interviewed. Whether or not these kinds of changes in diagnostic interviews would lead to an increase in validity or simply a decrease in reliability remains an important topic for future investigations.

ACKNOWLEDGMENTS

We want to express our sincere appreciation to Edna Fiedler for her invaluable contributions to this study. Marci Gleason performed many of the quantitative analyses reported in this chapter. Several of our graduate students have played crucial roles in the study, including David Klonsky, Jacqueline Friedman, Allan Clifton, Susan South, Cannon Thomas, Serrita Jane, Alison Melley, Melissa Gruber, Jason Pagan, and Mayumi Okada. Our professional staff members, Maria Whitmore and Derek Ford, provided excellent assistance with data collection and management. We also want to thank Pat Kyllonen, Janice Hereford, Armando Lara, and Sgt. Randy John at Lackland Air Force Base for their assistance in testing participants and organizing data. Lee Anna Clark has provided invaluable advice on a number of issues. Roger Blashfield and Irv Gottesman helped us refine our lay translations of DSM-IV personality disorder features. Nancee Blum and Bruce Pfohl were generous with their time and expertise regarding the SIDP-IV. Many undergraduate research assistants participated actively in our study, including Sheri Towe, Laura Koepfler, Yi Lam Chan, Letty Lau, Fran Arnold, and Elizabeth Flanagan.

This study was supported by Grant No. MH51187 from the National Institute of Mental Health.

NOTES

1. During the final year of data collection at the University of Virginia, we replaced the SNAP with the Inventory of Interpersonal Problems (Horowitz et al., 2000), which was employed as a supplementary measure of social adjustment (to complement the Social Adjustment Scale-Self-Report [SAS-SR]).
2. Personality disorders are defined in terms of enduring personality traits and characteristic features that lead to clinically significant distress or impairment in social or occupational adjustment. We did not collect extensive information or make *clinical* judgments about the length of time for which these traits might have been present or the extent to which these traits interfered with the person's life. Therefore, we cannot determine whether our participants met the full diag-

nostic criteria for a personality disorder in the same way that a person seeking treatment would be evaluated by his or her therapist.

3. In some previous publications, we have referred to this instrument as the Peer Nomination Inventory (PNI; Thomas, Turkheimer, & Oltmanns, 2003). We believe the MAPP is a more useful name for two reasons. One is that PNI does not describe the content of the instrument. The other is that the instrument includes self-report and metaperception questions as well as peer nomination items. Therefore, MAPP provides a better description.

4. Air Force administrators requested these omissions in order to comply with their "don't ask, don't tell" policy. Questions concerning drug use and sexual orientation were also excluded. This limited the number of questions we could ask for the criterion concerning conduct disorder in antisocial personality disorder and for that concerning identity disturbance in borderline personality disorder. Items relevant to the optional research categories (depressive, negativistic, and self-defeating personalities) also were not asked.

5. Participants indicated that approximately 30% of their nominations were made when it was difficult to select anyone who fit the description of the item. In spite of these reservations, the people who were identified in these nominations were largely the same as those people selected without a difficult designation. Correlations between difficult to rate and not difficult items were calculated within diagnoses, with results ranging from .63 for schizoid personality disorder to .80 for avoidant personality disorder.

6. We expected that the self-report items from the MAPP would produce personality disorder scores that closely resemble scores obtained using other popular self-report personality disorder scales, such as the Personality Disorder Questionnaire (PDQ-IV; Hyler, 1994). We compared our MAPP self-report items with the PDQ-IV in a sample of 206 undergraduate students who were not otherwise part of the Peer Nomination Study (Okada & Oltmanns, unpublished manuscript). Correlations between scales ranged from .69 (dependent personality disorder) to .87 (paranoid, borderline, and antisocial personality disorder). The MAPP self-report scales were more conservative than the PDQ-IV, identifying 14% of this student sample as meeting criteria for at least one form of personality disorder, while the PDQ-IV identified 24% as having at least one personality disorder.

7. "Knowing" and "liking" were the only items in the inventory for which judges were required to rate every other member of their group. For all other items, they nominated *at least* one person but could avoid providing information about the others.

REFERENCES

Adams, S. H., & John, O. P. (1997). A Hostility Scale for the California Psychological Inventory: MMPI, observer Q-sort, and Big Five correlates. *Journal of Personality Assessment, 69,* 408–424.

Bernstein, D. P., Kasapis, C., Bergman, A., Weld, E., Mitropoulou, V., Horvath, T., et al. (1997). Assessing Axis II disorders by informant interview. *Journal of Personality Disorders, 11*, 158–167.

Caspi, A., & Moffitt, T. E. (1993). When do individual differences matter? A paradoxical theory of personality coherence. *Psychological Inquiry, 4*, 247–271.

Clark, L. A. (1993). *Manual for the Schedule for Nonadaptive and Adaptive Personality*. Minneapolis: University of Minnesota Press.

Clark, L. A., Livesley, W. J., & Morey, L. (1997). Personality disorder assessment: The challenge of construct validity. *Journal of Personality Disorders, 11*, 205–231.

Clifton, A., Turkheimer, E., & Oltmanns, T. F. (2004). Contrasting perspectives on personality problems: Descriptions from the self and others. *Personality and Individual Differences, 36*, 1499–1514.

Clifton, A., Turkheimer, E., & Oltmanns, T. F. (2005). Self and peer perspectives on pathological personality traits and interpersonal problems. *Psychological Assessment, 17*, 123–131.

Clifton, A., Turkheimer, E., & Oltmanns, T. F. (2006). *Improving assessment of pathological personality traits through social network analysis*. Manuscript under review.

Cronbach, L. J., Gleser, G. C., Nanda, H., & Rajaratnam, N. (1971). *The Dependability of Behavioral Measurements*. New York: Wiley.

Dolan-Sewell, R. T., Krueger, R. F., & Shea, M. T. (2001). Co-occurrence with syndrome disorders. In W. J. Livesley (Ed.), *Handbook of personality disorders: Theory, research, and treatment* (pp. 84–106). New York: Guilford Press.

Dreessen, L., Hildebrand, M., & Arntz, A. (1998). Patient–informant concordance on the Structured Clinical Interview for DSM-III-R personality disorders (SCID-II). *Journal of Personality Disorders, 12*, 149–161.

Fiedler, E. R., Oltmanns, T. F., & Turkheimer, E. (2004). Traits associated with personality disorders and adjustment to military life: Predictive validity of self and peer reports. *Military Medicine, 169*, 207–211.

Fuhrman, R. W., & Funder, D. C. (1995). Convergence between self and peer in the response-time processing of trait-relevant information. *Journal of Personality and Social Psychology, 69*, 961–974.

Funder, D. C. (1995). On the accuracy of personality judgment: A realistic approach. *Psychological Review, 102*, 652–670.

Funder, D. C. (1999). *Personality judgment: A realistic approach to person perception*. San Diego, CA: Academic Press.

Grove, W. M., & Tellegen, A. (1991). Problems in the classification of personality disorders. *Journal of Personality Disorders, 5*, 31–41.

Gruber, M., Oltmanns, T. F., Turkheimer, E., & Fiedler, E. (2002). *Structured Interviews and Informant Reports for the Assessment of Narcissistic Personality Disorder*. Unpublished manuscript.

Horowitz, L. M., Alden, L. E., Wiggins, J. S., & Pincus, A. L. (2000). *Inventory of Interpersonal Problems: Manual*. San Antonio, TX: Psychological Corporation.

Hyler, S. E. (1994). *The Personality Diagnostic Questionnaire 4* (PDQ-4). New York: New York State Psychiatric Institute.

Jane, J. S., Pagan, J. L., Turkheimer, E., Fiedler, E. R., & Oltmanns, T. F. (2006). *The interrater reliability of the structured interview for DSM-IV personality disorders.* Manuscript under review.

John, O. P., & Robins, R. W. (1993). Determinants of interjudge agreement on personality traits: The big five domains, observability, evaluativeness, and the unique perspective of the self. *Journal of Personality, 61,* 521–551.

Johnson, J. G., Cohen, P., Kasen, S., Skodol, A. E., Hamagami, F., & Brook, J. S. (2000). Age-related change in personality disorder trait levels between early adolescence and adulthood: A community-based longitudinal investigation. *Acta Psychiatrica Scandinavica, 102,* 265–275.

Kane, J. S., & Lawler, E. E. (1978). Methods of peer assessment. *Psychological Bulletin, 85,* 555–586.

Kenny, D. A. (1991). A general model of consensus and accuracy in interpersonal perception. *Psychological Review, 98,* 155–163.

Kenny, D. A. (1994). *Interpersonal perception: A social relations analysis.* New York: Guilford Press.

Kenny, D. A., & DePaulo, B. M. (1993). Do people know how others view them?: An empirical and theoretical account. *Psyschological Bulletin, 114,* 145–161.

Klein, D. N. (2003). Patients' versus informants' reports of personality disorders in predicting 7½ year outcome in outpatients with depressive disorders. *Psychological Assessment, 15,* 216–222.

Klonsky, E. D., Oltmanns, T. F., & Turkheimer, E. (2002). Informant reports of personality disorder: Relation to self-reports and future research directions. *Clinical Psychology: Science and Practice, 9,* 300–311.

Lara, M. E., Ferro, T., & Klein, D. N. (1997). Family history assessment of personality disorders: II. Association with measures of psychosocial functioning in direct evaluations with relatives. *Journal of Personality Disorders, 11,* 137–145.

Lenzenweger, M. F., Johnson, M. D., & Willett, J. B. (2004). Individual growth curve analysis illuminates stability and change in personality disorder features: The longitudinal study of personality disorders. *Archives of General Psychiatry, 61,* 1015–1024.

Mann, A. H., Raven, P., Pilgrim, J., Khanna, S., Velayudham, A., Suresh, K. P., et al. (1999). An assessment of the Standardized Assessment of Personality as a screening instrument for the International Personality Disorder Examination: A comparison of informant and patient assessment for personality disorder. *Psychological Medicine, 29,* 985–989.

Mattia, J. I., & Zimmerman, M. (2001). Epidemiology. In W. J. Livesley (Ed.), *Handbook of personality disorders: Theory, research, and treatment* (pp. 107–123). New York: Guilford Press.

Mervielde, I., & De Fruyt, F. (2000). The Big Five personality factors as a model for the structure of children's peer nominations. *Journal of Personality, 14,* 91–106.

Norman, W. T. (1963). Toward an adequate taxonomy of personality attributes: Replicated factor structure in peer nomination personality ratings. *Journal of Abnormal and Social Psychology, 66,* 574–583.

Oltmanns, T. F., Gleason, M., Klonsky, E. D., & Turkheimer, E. (2005). Metaperception for pathological personality traits. *Cognition and Consciousness, 14,* 739–751.

Oltmanns, T. F., Melley, A. H., & Turkheimer, E. (2002). Impaired social functioning and symptoms of personality disorders in a non-clinical population. *Journal of Personality Disorders, 16,* 438–453.

Oltmanns, T. F., Turkheimer, E., & Strauss, M. E. (1998). Peer assessment of personality traits and pathology. *Assessment, 5,* 53–65.

Passini, F. T., & Norman, W. T. (1966). Ratee relevance in peer nominations. *Journal of Applied Psychology, 53,* 185–187.

Pfohl, B., Blum, N., & Zimmerman, M. (1997). *Structural Interview for DSM-IV Personality Disorders.* Washington, DC: American Psychiatric Association.

Schwarzwald, J., Koslowsky, M., & Mager-Bibi, T. (1999). Peer ratings versus peer nominations during training as predictors of actual performance criteria. *Journal of Applied Behavioral Science, 35,* 360–372.

Shedler, J., & Westen, D. (1998). Refining the measurement of AXIS II: A Q-sort Procedure for assessing personality pathology. *Assessment, 5,* 333–353.

Thomas, C., Turkheimer, E., & Oltmanns, T. F. (2003). Factorial structure of pathological personality traits as evaluated by peers. *Journal of Abnormal Psychology, 112,* 1–12.

Tickle, J. J., Heatherton, T. F., & Wittenberg, L. G. (2001). Can personality change? In W. J. Livesley (Ed.), *Handbook of personality disorders: Theory, research, and treatment* (pp. 242–258). New York: Guilford Press.

Turkheimer, E., Chan, Y. L., Clifton, A., & Oltmanns, T. F. (2006). *Method and trait effects in peer assessment of personality.* University of Virginia, Charlottesville. Unpublished manuscript.

Turkheimer, E., Friedman, J. W., Klonsky, E. D., & Oltmanns, T. F. (2006). *Informants, friends, and peers in the assessment of personality disorders.* University of Virginia, Charlottesville. Unpublished manuscript.

Tyrer, P. (1993). Measurement of social function. In P. Tyrer & P. Casey (Eds.), *Social function in psychiatry: The hidden axis of classification exposed* (pp. 21–52). Petersfield, UK: Wrightson Biomedical.

Waters, L. K., & Waters, C. W. (1970). Peer nominations as predictors of short-term sales performance. *Journal of Applied Psychology, 54*(1, Pt. 1), 42–44.

Weissman, M. M. (1993). The epidemiology of personality disorders: A 1990 update. *Journal of Personality Disorders,* (Suppl. 1), 44–62.

Weissman, M. M., Olfson, M., Gameroff, M. J., Feder, A., & Fuentes, M. (2001). A comparison of three scales for assessing social functioning in primary care. *American Journal of Psychiatry, 158,* 460–466.

Westen, D. (1997). Divergences between clinical and research methods for assessing personality disorders: Implications for research and the evolution of Axis II. *American Journal of Psychiatry, 154,* 895–903.

Westen, D., & Shedler, J. (1999). Revising and assessing Axis II: Part II. Toward an empirically based and clinically useful classification of personality disorders. *American Journal of Psychiatry, 156,* 273–285.

Widiger, T. A., Mangine, S., Corbitt, E. M., Ellis, C. G., & Thomas, G. V. (1995). *Personality Disorder Interview—IV: A Semistructured Interview for the Assessment of Personality Disorders.* Odessa, FL: Psychological Assessment Resources.

Widiger, T. A., Trull, T. J., Clarkin, J. F., Sanderson, C., & Costa, P. T., Jr. (2002). A description of the DSM-IV personality disorders with the five-factor model of personality. In P. T. Costa, Jr., & T. A. Widiger (Eds.), *Personality disorders and the five-factor model of personality* (2nd ed., pp. 89–102). Washington, DC: American Psychological Association.

Wilson, T. D. (2002). *Strangers to ourselves: Discovering the adaptive unconscious.* Cambridge, MA: Harvard University Press.

Zanarini, M. C., Frankenberg, F. R., Hennen, J., & Silk, K. R. (2003). The longitudinal course of borderline psychopathology: 6–year prospective follow-up of the phenomenology of borderline personality disorder. *American Journal of Psychiatry, 160,* 274–283.

Zimmerman, M. (1994). Diagnosing personality disorders: A review of issues and research methods. *Archives of General Psychiatry, 51,* 225–245.

Chapter 5

Dispositional Dimensions and the Causal Structure of Child and Adolescent Conduct Problems

IRWIN D. WALDMAN
AMBER L. SINGH
BENJAMIN B. LAHEY

One problem with many existing models of psychopathology is that they do not readily translate into testable hypotheses. Our primary goal in this chapter is to present a developmental model of psychopathology that yields testable hypotheses regarding etiology, mediating psychological mechanisms, and later psychopathology. While our model is applicable to the broad spectrum of psychopathology, it is most fully developed with regard to child and adolescent conduct problems, which will be the focus of this chapter. Conduct problems include a range of correlated antisocial behaviors such as aggression, property offenses (e.g., vandalism), and status offenses (e.g., truancy). Lying, bullying, fighting, cruelty to animals, and violating family curfews are also considered conduct problems. These and other such behaviors constitute the symptoms of conduct disorder (CD) in DSM-IV (American Psychiatric Association, 1994). Conduct problems are considered part of a broader spectrum of externalizing behaviors (e.g., Krueger et al., 2002), which also includes substance abuse, and risk-taking behaviors (e.g., reckless driving, high-risk sexual behavior). In addition, these youths may meet diagnostic criteria for other associated disorders such as attention-deficit/hyperactivity disorder (ADHD), oppositional defiant disorder (ODD), and depressive and anxiety disorders.

An adequate developmental model must consider the full range of antisocial behaviors for at least two reasons. First, less severe conduct problems (e.g., those that do not warrant an arrest) constitute critical developmental aspects of later antisocial behavior. In order to understand the early developmental trajectory of antisocial behavior these less serious conduct problems must be considered. Second, we propose that the broad spectrum of externalizing behaviors (e.g., conduct problems, substance abuse, risky behavior, and adult antisocial acts) should be considered, given that they share many of their etiological influences (Krueger et al., 2002; Young et al., 2002).

OVERVIEW OF A DEVELOPMENTAL PROPENSITY MODEL OF CONDUCT PROBLEMS

Our model attempts to build on existing causal models by integrating and developing concepts extant in the relevant literature, as well as by introducing additional elements. For example, our model can be viewed as an extension of social learning approaches (Patterson, 1982; Patterson, Reid, & Dishion, 1992) in its inclusion of reinforcement, modeling, persuasion, and other social influence mechanisms. Our emphasis on the developmental trajectories of conduct problems also draws on existing developmental criminological models (Loeber, 1988; Loeber & LeBlanc, 1990; Moffitt, 1993). Like Moffitt (1993), we recognize the importance of characteristics of the child that are related to different trajectories of conduct problems. Gottfredson and Hirschi (1990) coined the term "antisocial propensity" and posited that this propensity, a unitary constellation of child characteristics, could explain variations in antisocial behavior. Consistent with all of these theorists, we posit that the origins of conduct problems cannot be understood without a consideration of individual differences. In addition, although antisocial propensity is often inferred from conduct problems, it must be defined and measured independently to avoid circularity. We thus draw on the work of Gottfredson and Hirschi (1990) and Farrington (1991, 1995) and define antisocial propensity in terms of early developing dispositional dimensions and cognitive ability. Furthermore, drawing on work in developmental psychopathology (e.g., Keenan & Shaw, 2003; Rutter, 1988; Olson, Bates, Sandy, & Lanthier, 2000; Sanson & Prior, 1999), developmental epidemiology (Rutter, 1997), and behavior genetics (Plomin, DeFries, & Loehlin, 1977; Rutter et al., 1997), our model yields hypotheses regarding the genetic and environmental influences underlying antisocial propensity. We also construe an "epigenetic" developmental process, in that relatively undifferentiated dispositional dimensions (with substantial underlying genetic influences) develop into more complex behaviors (e.g., conduct problems) through transactions with the environment. In addition, these dispositional dimensions may moderate the social learning environment and thus influence the child's reactions to it, altering the likelihood that the child will develop conduct problems.

The Ontogeny of Conduct Problems

The developmental trajectory of antisocial behavior is not unitary; that is, youths traverse different conduct problem developmental pathways (Farrington, 1991; Loeber, 1988). Like others, we propose that variations in developmental trajectories are crucial to understanding the etiology of antisocial behavior (Hinshaw, Lahey, & Hart, 1993; Moffitt, 1993; Patterson, Reid, & Dishion, 1992). Moffitt (1993) has proposed a developmental taxonomy of antisocial behavior in which there are two qualitatively distinct forms of conduct problems with distinct developmental trajectories. Contrary to this view, we propose that there is a continuum of developmental trajectories that result from individual differences in the components of antisocial propensity and social influence.

In order to summarize variability in developmental trajectories, we make a similar distinction to that of Moffitt (1993) between *developmentally early* and *developmentally late* conduct problems. Developmentally early conduct problems (e.g., lying, minor aggression) are highly prevalent in children at the time of school entry but become less prevalent in most youths with increasing age. In contrast, developmentally late conduct problems such as status and property offenses (e.g., stealing, running away from home, truancy, breaking and entering) and more severe forms of aggression (e.g., robbery, use of a weapon, and forced sex), while very uncommon in early childhood, increase with age, reaching a peak during adolescence.

For many theorists, the age of onset of antisocial behavior has been a key factor in differentiating developmental trajectories. Whereas it may be meaningful to identify the age of a first criminal conviction or the age of onset of developmentally late conduct problems that *never* occur in very young children (e.g., automobile theft), as Tremblay et al. (1996, 1999) have noted, measuring the age of onset of developmentally early conduct problems is problematic. Tremblay et al. (1996, 1999) have shown that ~50% of toddlers engage in developmentally early conduct problem behaviors such as hitting, kicking, intentionally breaking things, taking other children's toys, stating untruths, and resisting the authority of adults. As children develop, most become less likely to exhibit these behaviors, but others continue to do so. Thus, although it may be valid to view some behaviors, such as drug sales or theft, as newly emerging in late childhood or early adolescence, it may also be accurate to view children as sometimes failing to *unlearn* developmentally early behaviors (Tremblay, 2000). Based on this, it seems plausible that there may be different causal influences on developmentally early and developmentally late conduct problems. Hypotheses regarding these differences will be offered below.

Across development, children with high initial levels of developmentally early conduct problems that persist are at increased risk of developmentally late, often more severe and violent, conduct problems by adolescence (Brame, Nagin, & Tremblay, 2001; Sampson & Laub, 1992; Haemaelaeinen & Pulkkinen, 1996). In addition, some children with initially low levels of developmentally early conduct problems will add developmentally late conduct problems to their behavioral repertoires, though these are typically less serious nonviolent, offenses (e.g., truancy, theft) (Brame et al., 2001). A comprehensive model of conduct problems must account for both the causes of initial levels of conduct problems as well as the causes of their persistence, worsening, or improvement.

Components of Antisocial Propensity

The individual elements of antisocial propensity are critical to our model and include three dispositional dimensions in addition to cognitive abilities. We first present a description of these dispositional dimensions, followed by hypotheses regarding how they contribute causally to the development of conduct problems.

Dispositional Dimensions

Like others' definitions of temperament (Allport, 1937; Buss & Plomin, 1984; Goldsmith, Losoya, Bradshaw, & Campos, 1994), we operationalize dispositions as broad aspects of socioemotional functioning that emerge early in life, are relatively stable, and constitute the foundation for many adult personality traits (Caspi, 1998, 2000; Clark & Watson, 1999; Rothbart & Ahadi, 1994; Rutter, 1987). We describe three independent dispositional dimensions as well as hypotheses regarding their contribution to antisocial propensity and to the risk of developing conduct problems.

The boundary between dispositions and psychopathology is often fuzzy in that there are overlapping items included in measures of both construct domains, which blurs the distinction between them. Our model addresses this issue in two ways. First, through a review of the extant literature on temperament–conduct problem associations, we developed a new measure of dispositional dimensions, the Child and Adolescent Dispositions Scale (CADS; Lahey et al., 2003), which was designed in part to examine relations between dispositions and conduct problems. Second, we were careful to exclude from the CADS contaminating items (i.e., synonyms and antonyms of CD or other disorders). This is important because it prevents the possibility that correlations between temperament dimensions and symptoms of CD or other disorders actually reflect item overlap between measures (Sanson, Prior, & Kyrios, 1990). This differentiates our measure from all other existing personality scales, which contain items such as "angry," "aggressive," "anxious," "nervous," and "fearful." It is important to recognize that we have addressed the issue of overlap at a measurement level by eliminating items that are synonyms or antonyms, rather than at the construct level. In our view, the issue of whether or to what extent dispositions and psychopathological entities represent similar or distinct constructs is an empirical matter to be addressed by future research, rather than being decided a priori by fiat. Several researchers have examined the effect of overlapping items on temperament–psychopathology relations by using "purified" temperament measures that eliminated items common to both temperament and psychopathology measures (Lengua, West, & Sandler, 1998; Lemery, Essex, & Smider, 2002). These studies suggest that not all of the temperament–conduct problem association is due to overlapping item content. Nonetheless, they support the decision to develop a measure that does not include such overlapping items. The CADS was developed through exploratory factor analysis and validated using confirmatory factor analysis in an independent sample (Lahey et al., 2003). Three dispositional dimensions emerged from factor analyses: negative emotionality, prosociality, and daring.

Negative Emotionality. Frequent, intense, and disproportionate expression of negative emotions is characteristic of children with high ratings of negative emotionality (NE). Items loading on this scale refer generally to negative emotions rather than to specific emotions. Due to the nonspecific nature of this dimension, we contend that it reflects a general tendency to react negatively, similar to the "fight-or-flight" system proposed by Gray and McNaughton (1996). All major temperament and personality measures include an NE dimension, although it is sometimes labeled neuroticism (Bouchard & Loehlin, 2001; Digman, 1989; Digman & Inouye, 1986; Eysench, 1947; Goldberg, 1993) or negative affectivity (Rothbart, Ahadi, Hershey, & Fisher, 2001; Watson, Clark, & Tellegen, 1988; Zuckerman, Kuhlman, Joireman, Teta, & Kraft, 1993).

Consistent with our view of NE as a nonspecific tendency to react negatively, NE is associated with a wide range of psychopathology, including both internalizing (depression and anxiety) and externalizing (antisocial behavior) problems in childhood, adolescence, and adulthood (Anthony, Lonigan, Hooe, & Phillips, 2002; Barlow, 2000; Caspi et al., 1994; Depue,

1995; Eysenck & Eysenck, 1970; Farmer et al., 2002; Gershuny & Sher, 1998; Gjone & Stevenson, 1997; Goma-I-Freixnet, 1995; Goodyer, Ashby, Altham, Vize, & Cooper, 1993; Krueger, 1999; Moffitt, Caspi, Dickson, Silva, & Stanton, 1996; Roberts, & Kendler, 1999; Shiner, Masten, & Tellegen, 2002). Overall, the extant data suggest a significant positive association between NE and externalizing behavior including conduct problems. It should be noted, however, that some studies have found no association between NE and conduct problems (e.g., Heaven, 1996; John, Caspi, Robins, Moffitt, & Stouthamer-Loeber, 1994; Powell & Stewart, 1983; Tranah, Harnett, & Yule, 1998). These nonsignificant findings may be due to relatively small sample sizes and newly developed measures of NE with uncertain psychometric properties. For example, the results of Tranah et al. (1998) were based on a sample of just 20 children with conduct disorder and 20 control participants. Furthermore, although their results did not reach statistical significance, the association was in the predicted direction. John et al. (1994) used a newly developed measure of the five-factor model of personality for adolescents. Further study is necessary to determine whether the construct of NE measured by this instrument is equivalent to NE as measured by more commonly used measures.

Prosociality. Our conceptualization of prosociality is based largely on Eisenberg and Mussen's (1991) construct of "dispositional sympathy" and is characterized by frequent manifestations of concern for others' feelings. Prosociality is similar to the Agreeableness factor in the five-factor model of personality, which includes characteristics such as behaving in a giving way, being considerate, trustfulness, and compassion (McCrae & Costa, 1987). Evidence that sympathy, concern for others, and agreeableness are inversely correlated with conduct problems has emerged from both concurrent and longitudinal studies (e.g., Cohen & Strayer, 1996; Eisenberg, Fabes, Murphy, et al., 1996; Graziano, 1994; Graziano & Ward, 1992; Haemaelaeinen & Pulkkinen, 1996; Hastings, Zahn-Waxler, Robinson, Usher, & Bridges, 2000; Hughes, White, Sharpen, & Dunn, 2000; John et al., 1994; Luengo, Otero, Carrillo-de-la-Pena, & Miron, 1994).

Daring. Daring is characterized by adventurousness and enjoyment of loud, rough, and risky activities (Lahey & Waldman, 2003). The label for this dimension was inspired by Farrington and West's (1993) finding that children rated high on a single item of "daring" were at greater risk for chronic criminal offenses later in adolescence and adulthood. This dimension resembles several personality traits in the adult literature that have been found to be positively correlated with conduct problems (Arnett, 1996; Daderman, 1999; Daderman, Wirsen, & Hallman, 2001; Goma-I-Freixnet, 1995; Greene, Krcmar, Walters, Rubin, & Hale, 2000; Luengo et al., 1994; Newcomb & McGee, 1991; Schmeck & Poustka, 2001). These traits have been termed "sensation seeking" (Zuckerman, 1996) and "novelty seeking" (Cloninger, 1987).

It seems likely that *daring* represents a characteristic similar to the inverse of behavioral inhibition (Kagan, Reznick, & Snidman, 1988), a prominent construct in the child psychopathology literature. Children classified as "behaviorally inhibited" are typically fretful, slow to respond to persons and objects, and slow to vocalize when exposed to challenging laboratory situations (Garcia-Coll, Kagan, & Reznick, 1984; Kagan, Reznick, Snidman, Gibbons, & Johnson, 1988; Schwartz, Snidman, & Kagan, 1996). Studies suggest that behaviorally inhibited children may be at heightened risk for anxiety disorders (Biederman et al., 2001; Muris, Merckelbach, Schmidt, Gadet, & Bogie, 2001). Children who displayed the opposite behavioral pattern were classified as "behaviorally disinhibited." Several studies indicate that children with high levels of behavioral disinhibition are at increased risk of externalizing behavior problems (Biederman et al., 2001; Hirshfeld et al., 1992; Hirshfeld-Becker et al., in press; Kerr, Tremblay, Pagani-Kurtz, & Vitaro, 1997; Raine, Reynolds, Venables, Mednick, & Farrington, 1998; Schwartz et al., 1996). An important caveat to the parallels between behavioral disinhibition and daring is that, while the former is conceptualized as categorical in nature, the latter is conceptualized as a continuous trait. Nonetheless, the results of studies of behavioral disinhibition as well as studies of sensation and novelty seeking lead us to hypothesize that *daring* will be positively associated with conduct problems.

Cognitive Abilities

Drawing on studies that have found an inverse relation between cognitive abilities, particularly verbal abilities, and the development of conduct problems (Elkins, Iacono, Doyle, & McGue, 1997; Ge, Donnellan, & Wenk, 2001; Giancola, Martin, Tarter, Pelham, & Moss, 1996; Kratzer & Hodgins, 1999; Lynam, Moffitt, & Stouthamer-Loeber, 1993; Moffitt & Silva, 1988; Seguin, Boulerice, Harden, Tremblay, & Pihl, 1999; Stattin & Klackenberg-Larsson, 1993), we hypothesize that lower cognitive ability and slow language development also represent risk factors for conduct problems. Differences in socioeconomic status, in the probability of more intelligent youths avoiding detection and in the motivation to perform well on cognitive tests, do not appear to account for correlations between cognitive abilities and conduct problems (Lynam et al., 1993; Moffitt & Silva, 1988). Deficits in a wide range of cognitive constructs, including verbal intelligence, language performance, and neuropsychological and executive functions, have been associated with conduct problems, but it is not clear whether one or more of these constructs is more germane than the others.

Despite the importance of cognitive ability to our model, given that the focus of this volume is on personality and psychopathology (rather than on cognitive ability), the remainder of the chapter will focus solely on the association of dispositional dimensions with conduct problems as well as behavior genetic analyses of these traits and of their association. Readers can refer to extant literature reviews regarding the association of conduct problems and cognitive ability and on behavior genetic studies relating to that subject.

ASSOCIATIONS BETWEEN
DISPOSITIONAL DIMENSIONS AND CD

Prosociality

In a review of 15 studies examining the association between empathy and antisocial behavior, Miller and Eisenberg (1988) concluded that there is a significant negative relation. The more recent literature suggests that Sociability, one component of Prosociality, is not associated with externalizing behavior such as CD (Chen, Li, Li, Li, & Liu, 2000; Gjone & Stevenson, 1997; Rende, 1993; Silverman & Ragusa, 1992). In contrast, Guerin, Gottfried, and Thomas (1997) found that among two age groups (7–9 and 10–12) mother ratings yielded significant associations between Sociability and externalizing behavior. Additional studies of prosocial behavior (empathy) further suggest that Prosociality may be related to behavior problems, such as CD. In a study comparing empathic responses of conduct disordered youths to normal comparison youths, Cohen and Strayer (1996) found that adolescents with CD exhibited significantly less empathy. A large representative British sample, using a measure of prosocial behavior among 5- to 15-year-olds yielded a negative association with lying, fighting, stealing, disobedience, and temper tantrums (Goodman, 2001; Lahey & Waldman, 2003). Furthermore, in a 19-year longitudinal study, criminal offenses among 27-year-olds could be predicted by prosocial behavior rated at age 8 (Haemaelaeinen & Pulkkinen, 1996). In a younger sample, a more complex relationship emerged (Hastings et al., 2000). This study suggested that differences in empathic concern for others at age 6–7, but not 4–5, were associated with CD at age 9 (Hastings et al., 2000). In a study of preschoolers, a group of "hard-to-manage" children was characterized by both greater conduct problems and fewer prosocial behaviors/empathic responses than a comparison group of children (Hughes et al., 2000). These studies suggest that there is an association between Prosociality and CD, but developmental considerations should be taken into account, as it is not clear that prosociality is predictive at young ages

Daring

Farrington and West (1993) found that adolescent and adult criminal offenders were more likely characterized as "daring" when they were children. Their conceptualization of daring is similar in many ways to both sensation seeking and novelty seeking (Lahey & Waldman, 2003), and studies of these concepts indicate a relation with CD. For example, in a sample of school-age children Frick, O'Brien, Woulton, and McBurnett (1994) found that sensation seeking was significantly associated with conduct problems. Ang and Woo (2003) similarly found a significant association between sensation seeking and conduct problems in a sample of seventh-grade (mean age of 14) boys.

Negative Emotionality

Studies examining the relation between emotionality and behavior problems generally yield moderate correlations (e.g., Earls & Jung, 1987; Nelson, Martin, Hodge, Havill, & Kamphaus, 1999; Teerikangas, Aronen, Martin, & Huttunen, 1998). With respect to externalizing behavior, the literature suggests a positive association between emotionality and externalizing problems. For example, Rende (1993) examined NE in preschool-age children and externalizing behavior several years later (age 7). Results indicate that there is a significant association, but only for boys, suggesting there may be gender specificity in the association. Other studies find associations for both boys and girls (Lambert, 1988; Schmitz et al., 1999). Nelson et al. (1999) assessed NE in kindergarten and behavior problems 3 years later. Not only was there a significant association with overall externalizing problems, but the magnitude of the association was roughly equivalent across aggression, conduct problem, and hyperactivity domains. Additional studies lend support for an association between NE and more specific dimensions of psychopathology, such as aggression and CD. Rothbart, Ahadi, and Hershey (1994) found a significant correlation of .35 between a dispositional "Negative Affect" factor and later aggression. Further support for this association comes from its consistency across development. Gjone and Stevenson (1997) conducted a longitudinal study using four age cohorts. Participants in this study ranged from 5–6 years to 14–15 years when a number of dispositional characteristics were assessed. Behavior problems were assessed 2 years later for each cohort. The most consistent correlation to emerge from this study was that between NE and aggression, ranging from .41 to .51 across age cohorts.

Alternative Models of Developmental Propensity for Childhood Conduct Problems

While we hypothesize that each of the dispositional dimensions and cognitive ability are important components of the underlying propensity to antisocial behavior and CD, it remains for future studies to determine whether these dimensions combine in an additive or interactive manner. An additive model would imply that each of these dimensions' contributions to risk for antisocial behavior and CD is *independent* of that of each of the other dimensions, and that the risk conferred by each dimension is cumulative in the sense that the risks "sum up" over all of the constituent dimensions. In contrast, an interactive model would imply that each of the dimensions' contributions to risk for antisocial behavior and CD is multiplicative and *contingent* on that of each of the other dimensions, in the sense that the risk conferred by each dimension depends on the child's level on each of the other dimensions. While few studies have heretofore tested whether the contribution of such dimensions to the development of antisocial behavior is additive or interactive in nature, Cloninger's (1986) model of personality posits that the dimensions interact. More specifically, he asserts that high levels in one personality facet depend on the other personality factors. In a longitudinal investigation of the relation of personality dimensions and conduct problems, Tremblay, Pihl, Vitaro, and Dobkin (1994) examined profiles corresponding to Cloninger's model. Although they did not include the personality dimensions in our model, their results support the use of personality profiles in predicting behavioral outcomes. For example, using Cloninger's model (1986), Tremblay et al. (1994) found that a profile of high impulsivity, low anxiety, and low reward dependence was predictive of delinquency. Clearly, more work to determine the additive or interactive nature of personality dimensions in predicting psychopathological outcomes is needed.

Another integral feature of our developmental propensity model for antisocial behavior and CD is that it is a *mediational* model. This means that the dispositional dimensions not only are thought to be related to or to predict antisocial behavior and CD but also are posited to occupy a central place in the etiological pathways underlying antisocial behavior and CD. Specifically, in our model the dispositional dimensions are hypothesized to represent the more proximal effects of the genetic and environmental influences that cause antisocial behavior and CD. As such, we expect that much if not all of the genetic and environmental influences underlying antisocial behavior and CD will be indirect via their influences on the dispositional dimensions, and consequently that the direct effects of the genetic and environmental influences on antisocial behavior and CD will be relatively small once the dispositional dimensions are included in appropriate statistical models. The statistical models required to test our hypotheses regarding the genetic and environmental influences underlying antisocial behavior and CD, and their mediation via the dispositional dimensions, are standard biometric model-fitting analyses that are used with behavior genetic designs, such as the twin studies commonly employed to test etiological hypotheses.

Analyses investigating whether the genetic influences on psychopathological conditions are mediated by dispositional characteristics are appropriate only if several prerequisites are met. First, it must be shown that these dispositional dimensions are, in fact, associated with CD symptoms. Second, it must be demonstrated that there are genetic influences underlying the dispositional dimensions (i.e., Prosociality, Daring, and NE). Third, it must be demonstrated that there are also genetic influences underlying CD symptoms. After briefly reviewing the elements of univariate behavior genetic analytic models, we briefly present the results from behavior genetic studies of dispositional dimensions and of antisocial behavior and CD. We then provide evidence for the relation between antisocial behavior and CD and the focal dispositional dimensions of our theory. We next review the important features of several multivariate behavior genetic models useful for understanding the genetic and environmental influences that contribute to the *covariation* among multiple traits or symptom dimensions, and provide suggestions for which of these models may be best suited to testing mediational models within a behavior genetic framework. Finally, we present the results of the few behavior genetic studies that have examined the etiology of the covariation between dispositional dimensions and antisocial behavior, and conclude with implications for studies of specific candidate genes and specific environmental influences on antisocial behavior and CD.

Drawing Inferences Regarding Genetic and Environmental Influences Using Twin Data

As the reader is no doubt aware, there have been many theoretical approaches posited to explain the etiology of CD and other psychopathological conditions. Unfortunately, in their typical form most of these theories are often more casual than causal (Rogosa, 1987) in that it is hard to envision what data or pattern of results could result in their falsification. This highlights a vital property of rigorous theories, namely, their testability and the possibility that they can be subject to serious challenge and be rejected given particular results that contradict their predictions. This property, unfortunately rare in the social sciences, can be summarized by the position that a theory that cannot be mortally endangered cannot be alive (Meehl, 1978; Popper, 1959). Thus, perhaps the most important feature of behavior genetic designs and their attendant analyses is their testability, particularly their inherent comparison of alternative, a priori etiological hypotheses. The following brief description of the use of data from twins to test alternative hypotheses regarding the genetic and environmental influences underlying a trait or disorder and to estimate these influences may be helpful before presenting more complex behavior genetic models for understanding the covariation among multiple traits and mediation.

BEHAVIOR GENETIC APPROACHES TO THE ETIOLOGY OF DISPOSITIONS AND PSYCHOPATHOLOGY

Behavior geneticists typically are interested in disentangling three sets of influences that may cause individual differences or variation in a given trait. First, heritability, or h^2, refers to the proportion of variance in the trait that is due to genetic differences among individuals in the population. Second, shared environmental influences, or c^2, refer to the proportion of variance in the trait that is due to environmental influences that family members experience in common which increase their similarity for the trait. Third, nonshared environmental influences, or e^2, refer to the proportion of variance in the trait that is due to environmental influences that are experienced uniquely by family members which decrease their similarity for the trait.

In order to estimate these influences, twin studies rely on the fact that monozygotic (MZ) twins are identical genetically whereas fraternal or dizygotic (DZ) twins, just like nontwin siblings, are on average only 50% similar genetically. It also is assumed that MZ twins are no more similar than DZ twins for the *trait-relevant* aspects of the shared environment; i.e., that environmental influences on the trait of interest are shared in common between members of fraternal twin pairs to the same extent as between members of identical twin pairs (this is known as the *equal environments assumption*). It also is assumed that the parents of the twins mate at random with respect to the trait being studied (i.e., that there is no *assortative mating*). Similar to the assumptions underlying other statistical analyses (e.g., normality of the residuals in a regression analysis), these assumptions are unlikely to be completely met, but quantitative genetic analyses are quite robust to minor violations of them. Given these assumptions, the correlation between identical twins comprises heritability and shared environmental influences (i.e., $r_{MZ} = h^2 + c^2$), as these are the two sets of influences that can contribute to identical twins' similarity for the trait. In contrast, the correlation between fraternal twins comprises one-half of heritability and shared environmental influences (i.e., $r_{DZ} = \frac{1}{2}h^2 + c^2$), reflecting the smaller degree of genetic similarity between fraternal twins. Algebraic manipulation of the two equations for twin similarity allows one to estimate h^2, c^2, and e^2 (viz., $h^2 = 2\ [r_{MZ} - r_{DZ}]$; $c^2 = 2r_{DZ} - r_{MZ}$; $e^2 = 1 - r_{MZ}$).

Although estimation of these influences using the twin correlations can be done simply by hand, contemporary behavior geneticists use biometric model-fitting analytic methods that can incorporate additional information on familial relationships (e.g., correlations between nontwin siblings or parents and their children), provide statistical tests of the adequacy of these three influences (viz., h^2, c^2, and e^2) in accounting for the observed familial correlations, and test alternative models for the causal influences underlying the trait (e.g., a model including genetic and nonshared environmental influences vs. a model that also includes shared environmental influences). Especially pertinent to this chapter, these analyses can be extended to examine genetic and environmental influences on the covariation among different traits or symptom dimensions. A recent trend in behavior genetic analyses has been to extend the investigation of genetic and environmental influences on traits considered singly (i.e., univariate behavior genetic analyses) to the case of multiple traits considered conjointly (Neale & Cardon, 1992). Multivariate behavior genetic analyses seek to explain the covariation among different traits by examining the genetic and environmental influences that they share in common. As suggested below, such analyses can shed considerable light on the classification and etiology of psychopathology by permitting tests of mediational hypotheses.

Before showing more complex path models for multivariate behavior genetic analyses pertinent to mediation, we present a comprehensive biometric model for the genetic and environmental influences on a single trait for two twins or siblings in the path diagram in Figure 5.1. Although this path model represents the full set of potential causes on twins' dispositional dimensions or CD symptoms, there is not enough information in the conventional twin study design to estimate all 5 of these parameters simultaneously. As a consequence, contemporary twin studies present and contrast the results of a series of restricted models (i.e., models containing a subset of all potential causes) in order to find the most parsimonious model that fits the data well.

In the path diagram in Figure 5.1, D represents dominance genetic influences, A represents additive genetic influences, C represents shared environmental influences, E represents nonshared environmental influences, and i represents the direct influence of one twin or sibling's dispositions or conduct problems on their cotwin or cosibling's dispositions or conduct problems (or alternatively rater contrast effects). The circles containing these capital letters represent these latent causal genetic and environmental variables, whereas the corresponding lower-case letters (namely, d, a, c, e, and i) represent the magnitude of these influences (i.e., the parameter estimates, which are regression coefficients) on each twin or sibling's dispositions or conduct problems. The square of these parameter estimates (namely, d^2, a^2, c^2, and e^2) represent the variance components corresponding to dominance and additive genetic influences, and shared and non-shared environmental influences. The three correlations in the model—r_d, r_a, and r_c—represent the similarity of particular causal influences between twins or siblings. For example, MZ and DZ twins and nontwin siblings all are correlated 1.0 for shared environmental influences (namely, r_c) consistent with the equal environments assumption. In contrast, MZ twins are correlated 1.0 for both dominance and additive genetic influences (viz., r_d and r_a), whereas DZ twins and non-twin siblings are both correlated .25 and .5 for dominance and additive genetic influences, respectively, consistent with their average level of genetic similarity.

Structural equation modeling programs such as LISREL and MX (Jöreskog & Sörbom, 1993; Neale, 1997) can iteratively fit such models to twin and sibling variances and covariances to provide the best estimates of the parameters, that is, parameter estimates that minimize the difference between the twin and sibling covariances implied by the model and those observed in the data. The fit of the model to the data is summarized by a χ^2 statistic, which allows both the fit of a given model and the comparative fit of alternative models to be tested statistically. This property often results in restricted models—models containing only a subset of the parameters in the full model (e.g., only a and e)—that provide an adequate fit to the data. In addition, although we presented the biometric model as applied to data from twins, the model is equally applicable to adoption study data on biologically related and adoptive siblings, and can be extended to analyze data from biologically related and adoptive parent–offspring pairs.

BEHAVIOR GENETIC STUDIES
OF DISPOSITIONAL DIMENSIONS

Prosociality

The behavior genetic literature on prosociality, as a dispositional characteristic, is limited. Two major adult personality taxonomies, the Big Three (Eysenck, 1947, 1964) and the Big Five (Costa & McCrae, 1992), posit a dimension of Extraversion, which parallels the Sociability component of Prosociality. Studies in the adult literature consistently yield evidence for both genetic and environmental influences underlying the adult Sociability dimension, with heritabilities typically between .29 and .53 (Eid, Riemann, Angleitner, & Borkenau, 1999; Gunderson, Triebwasser, Phillips, & Sullivan, 1999; Heath, Cloninger, & Martin, 1994; Loehlin & Martin, 2001).

Consistent with the adult literature, studies of the etiology of childhood Sociability consistently yield moderate additive genetic influences, moderate nonshared environmental influences, and no shared environmental influences. Saudino et al. (1995) found evidence for substantial genetic

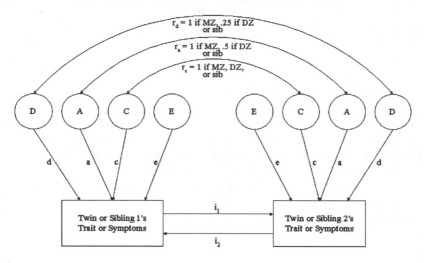

FIGURE 5.1. Path model for univariate behavior-genetic analyses of a trait or symptom dimension.

influences and nonshared environmental influences on parental reports of Sociability, with no evidence for shared environmental influences. Gjone and Stevenson's (1997) study yielded similar results, suggesting substantial genetic and nonshared environmental influences underlying Sociability. Paralleling these studies, a meta-analysis of seven twin studies yielded evidence for substantial additive genetic influences, nonshared environmental influences, and no shared environmental influences on Sociability (Goldsmith, Buss, & Lemery, 1997). In summary, both the adult and child literatures regarding the etiology of Sociability (Extraversion) indicate substantial genetic influences underlying this characteristic.

Twin studies of empathy, another component of Prosociality, also indicate substantial heritability. Adult twin studies have yielded substantial heritabilities for empathic responsiveness (h^2 = .71) (Matthews, Batson, Horn, & Rosenman, 1981) as well as altruism (h^2 = .56) and empathy (h^2 = .68) (Rushton et al., 1986). Studies of empathy in toddlerhood, childhood, and adolescence also suggest genetic underpinnings. In a sample of 14- and 20-month-old twins Zahn-Waxler, Robinson, and Emde (1992) found moderate genetic and nonshared environmental influences on both observational and maternal ratings of empathic concern. Similarly, Emde et al. (1992) found moderate heritability (.32) for observed empathy in a sample of 14-month-old twins. An investigation of the etiological influences underlying empathic concern in a group of high school twins yielded a heritability estimate of .28 for empathic concern in adolescence (Davis, Luce, & Kraus, 1994). Overall, twin studies in adulthood and childhood indicate that there are moderate genetic influences underlying the component dimensions of Prosociality.

Daring

The dispositional characteristic of Daring is conceptually similar to aspects of sensation seeking (Zuckerman, 1996), novelty seeking (Cloninger, 1987), and behavioral disinhibition (Kagan et al., 1988). Twin studies in both adolescent and adult samples indicate that there are genetic influences underlying these characteristics. A literature review concerning the biological correlates of sensation seeking concluded that this personality trait has moderate to strong genetic underpinnings (Zuckerman, Buchsbaum, & Murphy, 1980). Adult samples have yielded heritability estimates of .41–.58 for traits such as sensation seeking, disinhibition, and novelty seeking (e.g., Eysenck, 1990; Heath et al., 1994

It has been suggested that the heritability of a Daring disposition may vary across development. Consistent with the literature, Zuckerman (1971) found substantial heritability for sensation seeking in adults (.58); however, in a subsequent study (Zuckerman, 1974) the heritability estimate was substantially lower (.28) in an adolescent sample. While the magnitude of genetic influences underlying sensation seeking was lower in adolescence, a moderate influence remained. Furthermore, more recent studies have yielded greater heritability estimates in adolescents. In a large sample of adolescent and young adult twins, Koopmans, Boomsma, Heath, and van Doornen (1995) estimated that 48–63% of the variance in sensation seeking is due to underlying genetic influences. Ando et al. (2002) in a twin sample ranging in age from 14 to 28 years old, also found substantial genetic and nonshared environmental influences on novelty seeking. Similar estimates emerged from Miles et al.'s (2001) study with a sample of 7th- to 12th-grade twins. Their univariate analyses of risk-taking indicated that some components of risk taking (risk-taking attitude, riding a motorcycle, taking dangerous dares) were moderately heritable, with estimates ranging from .28 to .55. In a much younger sample of twins (14–24 months old) heritability estimates of disinhibition ranged from .34 at 14 months to .68 at both 20 and 24 months of age (Robinson, Kagan, Reznick, & Corley, 1992).

Negative Emotionality

What we have conceptualized as NE is often referred to Neuroticism (particularly in the adult literature) or simply Emotionality (particularly in the childhood literature). There is a substantial body of literature concerning the etiology of NE, which consistently yields moderate additive genetic influences, moderate nonshared environmental influences, and no shared environmental influences. Studies of adult samples have yielded substantial heritability estimates for NE. For example, Tellegen et al. (1988) and Eysenck (1990) found heritability estimates of .55 and 60, respectively. In a longitudinal study, McGue, Bacon, and Lykken (1993) yielded evidence that the genetic influences on NE may decrease across adult development. Although genetic influences remained moderate at the second wave of data collection, the magnitude of genetic influences underlying NE was substantially lower. Additional studies converge on these finding(s), suggesting moderate to substantial genetic underpinnings (Lake et al., 2000; Macaskill et al., 1994; Pedersen, Plomin, McClearn, & Friberg, 1988).

Twin studies conducted with toddler, school-age, and adolescent twins parallel adult studies. In their meta-analysis, Goldsmith et al. (1997) found substantial additive genetic and nonshared environmental influences but no evidence for shared environmental influences. Gjone and Stevenson's (1997) twin study also yielded genetic influences, with a heritability estimate of .71 for NE. Similarly, Schmitz et al. (1999) found that NE was influenced by genetic and nonshared environmental influences in their twin sample, with little impact of shared environmental influences. Many additional studies have yielded similar results with regard to NE (Cyphers, Phillips, Fulker, & Mrazek, 1990; Emde et al., 1992; Phillips & Matheny, 1997; Saudino, Plomin, & DeFries, 1996). Taken together, twin studies conducted in childhood, adolescence, and adulthood suggest that NE is due to both additive genetic influences and moderate nonshared environmental influences.

BEHAVIOR GENETIC STUDIES OF CD

CD falls under the umbrella of the broader concept of externalizing disorders, which also includes ADHD and ODD (Pennington, 2002). Familiality and heritability has been established in the literature for the broadband externalizing symptom dimension. Behavior genetic studies of externalizing symptoms suggest that both genetic and shared and nonshared environmental influences underlie this dimension. In a twin study using independent samples drawn from Sweden and the United Kingdom, Eley et al. (1999) found evidence of substantial genetic influences and no evidence for shared environmental influences on externalizing behavior, with heritability estimates of .70 and .69 in the Swedish and British samples, respectively. Similar heritability estimates ($h^2 = \sim.50$) emerged at ages 3 and 7 in a Dutch longitudinal study of twins (van der Valk, van den Oord, Verhulst, & Boomsma, 2003). This study also revealed moderate shared environmental ($c^2 = \sim.30$) and nonshared environmental influences ($e^2 = \sim.20$) on externalizing problems. Additional studies converge on these findings, indicating that both genetic and environmental influences underlie external-izing problems (e.g., Krueger et al., 2002).

Looking more specifically at the antisocial behavior components of the externalizing dimension, behavior genetic studies of CD and ODD have yielded evidence for substantial genetic influences. For example, Nadder et al. (1998) found heritability estimates of .65 for boys and .53 for girls. A large twin study ($N = 2,682$ pairs) yielded similar estimates, with genetic influences accounting for 71% of the variance on CD (Slutske et al., 1997). In contrast to Nadder et al. (1998), however, there was no evidence for gender differences in the genetic influences underlying CD. In a large Australian sample of 3- to 15-year-old twins ($N = 2,043$ pairs), both genetic and shared environmental influences were moderate for CD symptoms ($h^2 = .51$ and $c^2 = .34$), with the remaining variance due to nonshared environmental influences ($e^2 = .14$) (Waldman, Rhee, Levy, & Hay, 2001). Lyons et al. (1995) investigated genetic and environmental influences on antisocial behavior in both adolescence and adulthood. Their results indicated that adolescent conduct problems (e.g., truancy, initiating fights, use of weapons, cruelty to animals, and lying) were genetically influenced (h^2 ranged from .21 to .41). Additional adolescent behaviors (running away, cruelty to people, damaging property, starting fires, and stealing without confrontation) did not yield evidence for genetic influences but reflected shared environmental influences. In adulthood nearly all antisocial behaviors were genetically influenced (h^2 ranged from .22 to .52), with no evidence for shared environmental influences. Finally, a recent meta-analysis of behavior genetic studies of antisocial behavior in children, adolescents, and adults found that genetic and nonshared environmental influences were strongest across studies. Across 51 studies the best-fitting model yielded moderate additive genetic influences (.32), nonadditive genetic influences (.09), and both shared (.16) and nonshared (.43) environmental influences (Rhee & Waldman, 2002). Perhaps more importantly, the authors found heterogeneity in the genetic and environmental influences on antisocial behavior due to age, operationalization and assessment method, and zygosity determination method. Consistent with studies that document higher heritability for aggressive than for nonaggressive conduct problems, these findings suggest that antisocial behavior may represent a phenotype whose etiology is highly variable.

Using Twin Data to Estimate Genetic and Environmental Influences on the Covariation among Traits

Multivariate behavior genetic analyses of twin study data, although not a panacea, represent state-of-the-art methods for addressing questions of covariation and of the mediating mechanisms underlying psychopathology (to be described below). Multivariate behavior genetic methods share the advantages of univariate biometric model-fitting methods mentioned above, but possess a number of additional features that make them especially useful for testing hypotheses regarding covariation and mediation. First, such models seek to explain the covariation among two or more traits or symptom dimensions in terms of their common causes by disentangling the genetic and environmental influences that contribute to such covariation. Hence, one can test alternative models for the causes of covariation among different traits or symptom dimensions, or for the mediational role of putative underlying mechanisms, as well as estimate the relative contribution of common genetic and environmental influences to covariation or mediation.

Second, univariate behavior genetic models use estimates of genetic and environmental influences to explain twin correlations (or variances and covariances) for a single trait or symptom dimension. Hence, the data these models attempt to explain are the correlations or covariances between twins for a single trait or symptom dimension. Multivariate behavior genetic models are fit not only to these data but also to the within-twin cross-trait correlations (e.g., twin 1's daring and CD symptoms) and the cross-twin cross-trait correlations (e.g., twin 1's daring and twin 2's CD symptoms). Indeed, it is these cross-twin cross-trait correlations that afford these analyses their ability to discriminate among competing models for the covariation among traits or symptom dimensions because alternative models yield different expectations for the cross-twin cross-trait correlations (see Waldman & Slutske, 2000, for detailed examples). Multivariate behavior genetic models also may facilitate a stronger resolution than univariate models of the causes underlying a single trait or symptom dimension because more information (namely, both within-twin and cross-twin cross-trait correlations) is used in analyses. In the sections below, we describe two alternative multivariate behavior genetic models that may be used to test alternative substantive hypotheses for the causes of the observed covariation between dispositional dimensions and cognitive ability and CD symptoms. In each section below we highlight important characteristics of the models, especially those characteristics that permit the distinction between genetic and environmental contributions to covariation or mediation and which differentiate the alternative models of covariation from one another.

TWO MEDIATIONAL MODELS
OF THE CAUSES UNDERLYING CD SYMPTOMS

In the sections below, we review two mediational models for the etiology of CD symptoms. In the first model, shown in Figure 5.2, one can consider the mediation of the causes underlying CD to occur at the *phenotypic level*,

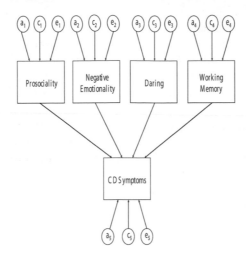

FIGURE 5.2. Path model for direction of causation analyses of temperament, working memory, and CD.

whereas in the alternative model, shown in Figure 5.4, the mediation of the causes underlying CD occurs at the *etiological level*. As shown in Figure 5.2, each of three dispositional dimensions (namely, prosociality, NE, and daring) and working memory have their own etiologies (i.e., genetic and shared and nonshared environmental influences, symbolized by a, c, and e 1–4, respectively) and in turn cause variation in CD symptoms. In addition to the causal influences from the dispositional dimensions and working memory, CD symptoms also have their own genetic and shared and nonshared environmental influences, symbolized by a_5, c_5, and e_5, respectively. There are several aspects of this causal model that are important to note. First, given the fact that mediation is hypothesized to occur at the level of the phenotypes, the genetic and environmental influences on CD symptoms (i.e., a_5, c_5, and e_5) represent genetic and environmental influences on CD residualized on the effects of the dispositional dimensions and working memory, rather than on CD per se. Second, given the nature of the path model shown in Figure 5.2, the genetic and shared and nonshared environmental influences on the three dispositional dimensions and working memory also represent *indirect* genetic and environmental influences on CD symptoms, the effects of which are mediated by those dispositions and cognitive phenotypes.

Third, and perhaps most importantly, the mediational model shown in Figure 5.2 is a substantially simplified version of the full multivariate behavior genetic model that would actually be tested, which would include not only the directional causal paths shown in the figure but also alternative causal paths pointing in the reverse direction, as well as correlations among each of the genetic and shared and nonshared environmental influences underlying the three dispositional dimensions, working memory, and CD symptoms. Given that the inclusion of all of these alternative paths and genetic and environmental correlations in Figure 5.2 would be cumbersome and would result in a path diagram that is difficult to parse and comprehend, in Figure 5.3 we present a reduced version of this diagram that represents the possible etiologies of the covariation between negative emotionality and CD symptoms in one twin. (Although not shown, the model is extended to include the other twin via the appropriate correlations of genetic and environmental influences.) This model encompasses the following alternative hypotheses:

1. Negative emotionality and CD symptoms are correlated because negative emotionality causes CD symptoms.
2. Negative emotionality and CD symptoms are correlated because CD symptoms cause negative emotionality.
3. Negative emotionality and CD symptoms are correlated because the two sets of problems reciprocally influence each other.
4. Negative emotionality and CD symptoms are correlated because they share common causes (i.e., the correlated genetic and environmental influences shown in the figure).

This model is typically referred to as the *direction of causation* model in the behavior genetics literature.

The Direction of Causation Model

Recently, a number of researchers (Duffy & Martin, 1994; Heath et al., 1993; Neale & Cardon, 1992) have proposed and investigated the properties of behavior genetic models for analyzing the direct causal effects of one variable on another, using cross-sectional data from relatives. Although these models lack some of the classical criteria (e.g., temporal ordering of the variables) used to infer causation in epidemiological studies (Goldberg & Ramakrishnan, 1994), under certain circumstances their application to data on relatives may permit valid inferences to be made regarding the causal relation among variables. Although models for the direction of causation between two variables may be tested using data from any type of relatives (Carey, 1994), much greater resolving power is afforded by the use of data on genetically informative relatives such as MZ and DZ twins or adoptive and biologically related siblings. Genetically informative relatives provide much greater information for direction of causation analyses be-

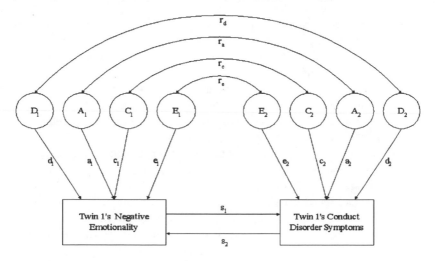

FIGURE 5.3. Full model for direction of causation analyses of NE and CD. D, dominance genetic influences; A, additive genetic influences; C, shared environmental influences; E, nonshared environmental influences; 1, influences on negative emotionality; 2, influences on CD symptoms; r_d, correlation of dominance genetic influences; r_a, correlation of addictive genetic influences; r_c, correlation of shared genetic influences; r_e, correlation of nonshared environmental influences; s_1, the causal effects of negative emotionality on CD symptoms; s_1, the causal effects of CD symptoms on NE.

cause the sources of familial correlations (i.e., genetic and environmental influences) for the traits in the analysis can be disentangled. One consequence of this is that two traits that show similar familial correlations, and hence seem unsuitable for such analyses, may have different causal contributions to those correlations. For example, trait 1 may be correlated in relatives due to additive and dominance genetic influences whereas trait 2 is correlated due to shared environmental influences. Thus, in contrast to the use of familial correlations, the use of data on genetically informative relatives such as twins would permit the testing of alternative models for the direction of causation between the two traits. Important characteristics of the direction of causation model are described in further detail in Waldman and Slutske (2000).

The results of direction-of-causation analyses of real data (Duffy & Martin, 1994; Neale et al., 1994), as well as of power analyses on simulated data (Heath et al., 1993), have led behavior geneticists to propose a number of qualifications to testing direction-of-causation models and distinguishing them from the general bivariate behavior genetic model. These caveats and conditions (Duffy & Martin, 1994; Heath et al., 1993) include:

1. Alternative direction-of-causation models differ mainly in their expectations for the cross-twin cross-trait correlations.
2. The fit of alternative models for direction of causation (i.e., trait 1 → trait 2 vs. trait 2 → trait 1) can be distinguished only if the traits show different patterns of underlying causal influences contributing to their familial correlations (e.g., additive and dominance genetic influences for trait 1 and shared environmental influences for trait 2).
3. If the measurement error of the two traits is not included explicitly in the models, spurious inferences regarding the direction of causation are likely to occur.
4. A model in which the correlation between the two traits is due to common genetic influences will be hard to distinguish from one in which the more heritable trait directly influences the less heritable trait.
5. A model in which the correlation between the two traits is due to common environmental influences will be hard to distinguish from one in which the less heritable trait directly influences the more heritable trait.
6. Rejection of models in which the correlation between the two traits is incorrectly posited to be due to common genetic and/or environmental influences is most likely when the two traits are highly heritable.
7. The impact of these caveats and conditions may be diminished in large samples, but their influence on the discrimination of causal models still will be present.

In conclusion, although direction-of-causation models may represent a useful adjunct to the general bivariate behavior genetic model, and their application to substantive issues of covariation and mediation should be explored further in future applications, these models have seen limited application due to the difficulties in resolving alternative models mentioned above.

The Cholesky Decomposition Model

As stated above, a second mediational model for the etiology of CD symptoms considers the mediation of the causes underlying CD to occur at the *etiological level* rather than at the *phenotypic level*, as in the *direction of causation* model discussed above. This alternative mediational model, referred to as a *Cholesky decomposition model*, is shown in Figure 5.4 and represents a particular method of fully exhausting the information contained in the covariances among the phenotypic variables in the model (shown as the rectangles in the figure). The full Cholesky decomposition model contains as many additive genetic, shared environmental (or dominance genetic), and nonshared environmental latent causal variables (shown as circles in the figure) as there are manifest phenotypic variables in the model. Note that for the purpose of simplicity only additive genetic and nonshared environmental influences are shown in Figure 5.4. The Cholesky decomposition is an interesting structural equation model, as it represents in many ways a hybrid of factor analytic and hierarchical regression analytic approaches. The factor analytic aspect of this model is evidenced by the path coefficients, or "loadings," of each of the phenotypic variables on the genetic, shared environmental, and nonshared environmental latent causal variables, or "factors." These path coefficients represent the magnitude of a particular etiological influence on each of the specific phenotypic variables. The hierarchical regression aspect of this model lies in the fact that the causal influences on the phenotypic variables are considered in a sequential fashion, moving from left to right in the path model, although all of these influences in the model are estimated simultaneously. This sequential aspect of the Cholesky decomposition model means that the left-most variable, the one associated with the first genetic (or shared or nonshared environmental) factor, is considered to be causally prior to the others in the sense that the genetic (or shared or nonshared environmental) influences that each of the subsequent variables shares in common with it are characterized first. After these genetic (or shared or nonshared environmental) influences have been "partialled out," as it were, the second variable and its genetic (or shared or nonshared environmental) factor are similarly considered in the sense that the residual genetic (or shared or nonshared environmental) influences that each of the subsequent variables shares in common with it are characterized. This process continues until the influences due to all of the genetic (or shared or nonshared environmental) factors are considered in turn and exhausted. Given that these subsequent genetic (or shared or nonshared environmental) factors are explaining residual genetic (or shared or nonshared environmental) influences, some of them may not be necessary for explaining all of the covariances among the phenotypic variables in the model and may be dropped, resulting in reduced models that show an adequate and similar fit to the observed data to that of the full Cholesky decomposition model. It is worth noting that, as in a hierarchical regression analysis, while the specific ordering of the variables in the model affects the *relative contribution* of genetic (or shared or nonshared environmental) variance that is attributable to each factor, the *total amount* of genetic (or shared or nonshared environmental) variance explained in any particular phenotypic variable will be the same regardless of the order-

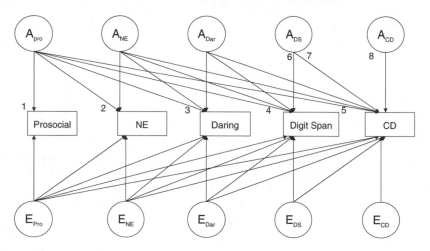

FIGURE 5.4. Cholesky decomposition model for the mediation of genetic and environmental influences on CD.

ing of the variables in the model. Further detail on the properties and characteristics of model fitting and testing using the Cholesky decomposition model can be found in Loehlin (1996) and Neale and Cardon (1992).

Tracing through a specific example illustrated in Figure 5.4 might help to understand these two important statistical aspects of the Cholesky decomposition model. The path coefficients labeled 1–5 represent the loadings of each of the phenotypic variables on the first additive genetic factor, which corresponds to the prosocial dispositional dimension. These loadings represent the additive genetic influences on each of the phenotypic variables that is shared in common with the additive genetic influences on the first phenotypic variable (i.e., prosociality). That is, loadings 2–5 represent the additive genetic influences on negative emotionality, daring, working memory, and CD that are shared in common with the additive genetic influences on prosociality. The loadings on each of the subsequent additive genetic latent variables represent the additive genetic contribution to each of the phenotypic variables *after partialing out* the contribution of the first additive genetic factor (i.e., the prosocial additive genetic factor), and thus may be considered as *residual* additive genetic influences. The same will hold true for the latent variables representing the contributions of each of the sets of shared and nonshared environmental influences. Thus, loading 7 represents the *residual* additive genetic influences on CD that are shared with the additive genetic influences on working memory (i.e., loading 6) after accounting for the additive genetic influences on both variables that are shared in common with prosociality, negative emotionality, and daring. Finally, loading 8 represents the *residual* additive genetic influences on CD after accounting for the additive genetic influences on CD that are shared in common with prosociality, negative emotionality, daring, and working memory. The relative contributions of these additive genetic influences indicate the extent to which the genetic influences on CD are direct versus mediated through their effects on the dispositional dimensions and on working memory. We will be testing exactly these alternative hypotheses using the Cholesky decomposition model in future twin study analyses.

STUDIES OF MEDIATION OF GENETIC AND ENVIRONMENTAL INFLUENCES ON CD VIA DISPOSITIONAL DIMENSIONS

Three prerequisites for examining dispositional mediation of the genetic influences on CD were laid out above. Brief reviews of behavior genetic studies of the three relevant dispositional dimensions, behavior genetic studies of CD, and associations between each of the dispositional dimensions and CD indicate that these prerequisites have been met. The extant literature suggests that not only are both the dispositional dimensions and CD genetically influenced, but also that there are significant associations between them. A few researchers have thus tested mediational models of genetic and environmental influences, and the results have been mixed.

Two studies suggest that a very large portion of the association between dispositional characteristics and psychopathology is due to genetic influences common to both variables (Schmitz et al., 1999; Lemery et al., 2002). Schmitz et al. (1999) examined NE several times from age 14 months to 36 months and behavior problems at 48 months of age. While the authors did not examine CD specifically, they did investigate the broader dimension of CBCL externalizing problems, which is composed of oppositional behavior as well as aggressive and nonaggressive conduct problems. Their results indicated that nearly all (96%) of the association between NE and externalizing was due to genetic influences common to both variables. In a similar study, Lemery et al. (2002) found that the genetic influences on age 7 conduct problems were substantially mediated by dispositional characteristics (including Negative Affect and Surgency, a variable similar to Daring) at age 5. A third study (Gjone & Stevenson, 1997) yielded mixed results. While common genetic influences accounted in part for a prospective association between NE and Aggression, common genetic influences were not implicated in the association between NE and Delinquency.

The Role of Dispositions in the Search for Candidate Genes and Environments for CD

In well-designed candidate gene studies, an understanding of the underlying biology of the trait or disorder is used to choose genes based on the suspected involvement of their gene product in the etiology of the trait or disorder (i.e., its pathophysiological function and etiological relevance). Genes underlying various aspects of the dopaminergic and serotonergic neurotransmitter pathways may be conjectured to be involved in the etiology of antisocial behavior and CD, based on converging evidence that suggests that these neurotransmitter systems play a role in their etiology and pathophysiology. For example, there is considerable overlap between ADHD and childhood antisocial behavior (i.e., ODD and CD) both at the phenotypic level (e.g., Lilienfeld & Waldman, 1990) and genotypic level (Waldman et al., 2001); thus, candidate genes for ADHD may also be relevant candidates for antisocial behavior and CD. Dopamine genes are plausible candidates for ADHD, based on the fact that the stimulant medications that are frequently and effectively used to treat ADHD appear to act primarily by regulating dopamine levels in the brain (Seeman & Madras, 1998; Solanto, 1984), although these medications also appear to affect noradrenergic and serotonergic function (Solanto, 1998). In addition, studies in which the behavioral effects of the deactivation of specific genes are examined in mice (i.e., "knock-out" gene studies) have further demonstrated the putative relevance of genes within these neurotransmitter systems. Results of such studies have supported the consideration of genes within the dopaminergic system—and to a lesser extent the serotonergic and noradrenergic systems—as candidate genes for ADHD. There are several genes within the dopamine system that appear to be risk factors for ADHD (see Waldman & Gizer, in press, for a recent review), including the dopamine transporter gene (*DAT1*; Giros, Jaber, Jones, Wightman, & Caron, 1996) and the dopamine receptor D3, D4, and D5 genes (*DRD3*, *DRD4*, and *DRD4*; Accili et al., 1996; Dulawa, Grandy, Low, Paulus, & Geyer, 1999; Lowe et al., 2004; Rubinstein et al., 1997; Tahir et al., 2000). In addition, genes within the serotonergic system, such as the serotonin 1ß receptor gene (*HTR1ß*; Saudou et al., 1994) and serotonin transporter gene (*5-HTT*; Lesch et al., 1996), also are plausible candidates for ADHD and for antisocial behavior and CD in particular, given the demonstrated relations between serotonergic function and impulsivity, aggression, and violence (Berman, Kavoussi, & Coccaro, 1997).

Candidate genes for neurotransmitter systems may include (1) *precursor genes* that control the rate at which neurotransmitters are converted from precursor amino acids (e.g., tyrosine hydroxylase for dopamine, tryptophan hydroxylase for serotonin); (2) *receptor genes* that code for the production or sensitivity of the receptors important for receiving neuro-transmitter signals (e.g., genes corresponding to the five dopamine receptors [*DRD1, D2, D3, D4*, and *D5*] and to the serotonin receptors [e.g., *HTR1ß* and *HTR2A*]); (3) *transporter genes* that code for the mechanisms involved in the reuptake of neurotransmitters from the synapse back into the presynaptic terminal (e.g., the dopamine and serotonin transporter genes [*DAT1* and *5-HTT*]); (4) genes that are responsible for the metabolism or degradation of neurotransmitters (e.g., the genes for catechol-O-methyltransferase [*COMT*] and for monoamine oxidase A and B [*MAOA* and *MAOB*]); and (5) genes that are involved in the *conversion* of one neurotransmitter into another (e.g., dopamine beta-hydroxylase [*DßH*], which converts dopamine into norepinephrine).

Dispositional dimensions such as prosociality, negative emotionality, and daring can aid in the identification of candidate genes for antisocial behavior and CD in several ways. First, to the extent that the Cholesky decomposition analyses described above reveal that a substantial proportion of the genetic influences on CD are shared in common with the genetic influences on the dispositional dimensions, and to the extent that the latter are of greater magnitude than the former, it may be more profitable to examine associations of the candidate genes with the dispositional dimensions rather than with CD itself. Second, insofar as CD shares genetic influences in common with the dispositional dimensions, novel candidate genes may be suggested for CD based on their hypothesized role in the dispositional dimensions themselves. Finally, it is possible that stronger associations with candidate genes may be revealed by moderator analyses in which high levels of CD symptoms are accompanied by elevations on one or more of the dispositional dimensions.

There are many environmental variables that have been posited as risk factors for antisocial behavior and CD. Relevant environmental domains may include pre- and perinatal influences, such as maternal drinking and smoking and obstetrical complications; aspects of parenting such as warmth and control, harsh discipline, and supervision and monitoring; family background variables, such as living in poverty, family size, disruption, divorce, and single- versus dual-parent status; the influences of siblings or peers, such as levels of aggression and antisocial behavior, substance use or abuse, and academic achievement and aspirations; and characteristics of neighborhoods such as economic inequality, crime rates, and cohesion and collective efficacy. It is unfortunately difficult to interpret much of the literature on the relation between environmental variables and antisocial behavior and CD because the environmental influences that putatively underlie such relations are confounded with genetic influences that also may be involved in their etiology. For example, the apparent effects of parental supervision and monitoring on children's antisocial behavior could be due to a direct environmental influence, to background environmental influences such as socioeconomic status, or to shared genetic influences, in which the same genes that underlie parents' tendencies to carefully or laxly monitor their children's activities also underlie their children's antisocial behavior. Given these confounds, the candidate environmental influences on antisocial behavior mentioned above can be considered putative at best, and must be studied in genetically informative designs to validate their mechanism of effect as truly environmental.

Fortunately, behavior genetic designs and analyses that are able to discriminate among these causal possibilities have recently been developed (e.g., D'Onofrio et al., 2002), and researchers are beginning to investigate the relations of environmental variables with antisocial behavior in such genetically informative designs. For example, a recent study (Jaffee, Caspi, Moffitt, & Taylor, 2004) assessed the environmental effects of physical maltreatment on children's antisocial behavior within the context of a twin study design. Although physical maltreatment was significantly and substantially related to parental antisocial behavior, and the heritability of child antisocial behavior was appreciable (h^2 = .67), the direct environmental effects of physical maltreatment on children's antisocial behavior remained after controlling for the genetic influences on their antisocial behavior (which accounted for 56% of the effects of physical maltreatment).

Similar to the search for candidate genes for CD described above, dispositional dimensions such as prosociality, negative emotionality, and daring can aid in the identification of "candidate environments" for antisocial behavior and CD in several ways that parallel those described above. It is worth noting that such candidate environments are likely to constitute nonshared environmental influences, given the behavior genetic literature on the dispositional dimensions reviewed above. First, to the extent that the Cholesky decomposition analyses described above reveal that a substantial proportion of the environmental influences on CD are shared in common with the environmental influences on the dispositional dimensions, and to the extent that the latter are of greater magnitude than the former, it may be more profitable to examine associations of putative specific environmental influences (e.g., parental supervision and monitoring) with the dispositional dimensions rather than with CD itself. Second, insofar as CD shows common environmental influences with the dispositional dimensions, novel environmental influences may be suggested for CD based on their hypothesized etiological role in the dispositional dimensions themselves. Finally, stronger associations with environmental influences may emerge from moderator analyses in which high levels of CD symptoms are accompanied by elevations on one or more of the dispositional dimensions.

REFERENCES

Accili, D., Fishburn, C. S., Drago, J., Steiner, H., Lachowicz, J. E., Park, B. H., et al. (1996). A targeted mutation of the D3 dopamine receptor gene is associated with hyperactivity in mice. *Proceedings of the National Academy of Sciences of the United States of America, 93,* 1945–1949.

Allport, G. W. (1937) *Personality: A psychological interpretation.* Oxford, UK: Holt.

American Psychiatric Association. (1994). *Diagnostic and statistical manual of mental disorders* (4th ed.). Washington, DC: Author.

Ando, J., Ono, Y., Yoshimura, K., Onoda, N., Shinohara, M., Kanba, S., et al. (2002). The genetic structure of Cloninger's seven-factor model of temperament and character in a Japanese sample. *Journal of Personality, 70,* 583–609.

Ang, R. P., & Woo, A. (2003). Influence of sensation seeking on boys' psychosocial adjustment. *North American Journal of Psychology, 5,* 121–136.

Anthony, J. L., Lonigan, C. J., Hooe, E. S., & Phillips, B. M. (2002). An affect-based, hierarchical model of temperament and its relations with internalizing symptomatology. *Journal of Clinical Child and Adolescent Psychology, 31,* 480–490.

Arnett, J. J. (1996). Sensation seeking, aggressiveness, and adolescent reckless behavior. *Personality and Individual Differences, 20,* 693–702.

Barlow, D. H. (2000). Unraveling the mysteries of anxiety and its disorders from the perspective of emotion theory. *American Psychologist, 55,* 1247–1263.

Berman, M. E., Kavoussi, R. J., & Coccaro, E. F. (1997). Neurotransmitter correlates of human aggression. In D. M. Stoff, J. Breiling, & J. D. Masur (Eds.), *Handbook of antisocial behavior* (pp. 305–313). New York: Wiley.

Biederman, J., Hirshfeld-Becker, D. R., Rosenbaum, J. F., Herot, C., Friedman, D., Snidman, N., et al. (2001). Further evidence of association between behavioral inhibition and social anxiety in children. *American Journal of Psychiatry, 158,* 1673–1679.

Bouchard, T. J., & Loehlin, J. C. (2001). Genes, evolution, and personality. *Behavior Genetics, 31,* 243–273.

Brame, B., Nagin, D. S., & Tremblay, R. E. (2001). Developmental trajectories of physical aggression from school entry to late adolescence. *Journal of Child Psychology and Psychiatry, 42,* 503–512.

Buss, A. H., & Plomin, R. (1984). *Temperament: Early developing personality traits.* Hillsdale, NJ: Erlbaum.

Carey, G. (1994). Direction of causality: A comment. *Genetic Epidemiology, 11,* 473–476.

Caspi, A. (1998). Personality development across the life course. In N. Eisenberg (Ed.), *Handbook of child psychology* (5th ed., Vol. 3, pp. 311–388). New York: Wiley.

Caspi, A. (2000). The child is father of the man: Personality continuities from childhood to adulthood. *Journal of Personality and Social Psychology, 78,* 158–172.

Caspi, A., Moffitt, T. E., Silva, P. A., Stouthamer-Loeber, M., Schmutte, P. S., & Krueger, R. (1994). Are some people crime-prone? Replications of the personality-crime relation across nation, gender, race and method. *Criminology, 32,* 301–333.

Chen, X., Li, D., Li, Z., Li, B., & Liu, M. (2000). Sociable and prosocial dimensions of social competence in Chinese children: Common and unique contributions to social, academic, and psychological adjustment. *Developmental Psychology, 36,* 302–314.

Clark, L. A., & Watson, D. (1999) Temperament: A new paradigm for trait psychology. In L. A. Pervin & O. P. John (Eds.), *Handbook of personality: Theory and research* (2nd ed., pp. 399–423). New York: Guilford Press.

Cloninger, C. R. (1986). A unified biosocial theory of personality and its role in the development of anxiety states. *Psychiatric Development, 3,* 167–226.

Cloninger, C. R. (1987). A systematic method for clinical description and classification of personality variants: A proposal. *Archives of General Psychiatry, 44,* 573–588.

Cohen, D. C., & Strayer, J. (1996). Empathy in conduct-disordered and comparison youth. *Developmental Psychology, 32,* 988–998.

Costa, P. T., & McCrae, R. R. (1992) The five-factor model of personality and its relevance to personality disorders. *Journal of Personality Disorders, 6,* 343–359.

Costa, P. T., & McCrae, R. R. (1995). Primary traits of Eysenck's P-E-N system: Three- and five-factor solutions. *Journal of Personality and Social Psychology, 69,* 308–317.

Cyphers, L. H., Phillips, K., Fulker, D. W., & Mrazek, D. A. (1990). Twin temperament during the transition from infancy to early childhood. *Journal of the American Academy of Child and Adolescent Psychiatry, 29,* 392–397.

Daderman, A. M. (1999). Differences between severely conduct-disordered juvenile males and normal juvenile males: The study of personality traits. *Personality and Individual Differences, 26,* 827–845.

Daderman, A. M., Wirsen, M. A., & Hallman, J. (2001). Different personality patterns in non-socialized (juvenile delinquents) and socialized (air force pilot recruits) sensation seekers. *European Journal of Personality, 15,* 239–252.

Davis, M. H., Luce, C., & Kraus, S. J. (1994). The heritability of characteristics associated with dispositional empathy. *Journal of Personality, 62,* 369–391.

Depue, R. A. (1995). Neurobiological factors in personality and depression. *European Journal of Personality, 9,* 413–439.

Digman, J. M. (1989). Five robust trait dimensions: Development, stability, and utility. *Journal of Personality, 57,* 195–214.

Digman, J. M., & Inouye, J. (1986). Further specification of the five robust factors of personality. *Journal of Personality and Social Psychology, 50,* 116–123.

D'Onofrio, B. M., Turkheimer, E., Eaves, L. J., Corey, L. A., Berg, K., Solaas, M. H., et al. (2003). The role of the Children of Twins design in elucidating causal relations between parent characteristics and child outcomes. *Journal of Child Psychology and Psychiatry, 44,* 1130–1144.

Duffy, D. L., & Martin, N. G. (1994). Inferring the direction of causation in cross-sectional twin data: Theoretical and empirical considerations. *Genetic Epidemiology, 11,* 483–502.

Dulawa, S. C., Grandy, D. K., Low, M. J., Paulus, M. P., & Geyer, M. A. (1999). Dopamine D4 receptor-knock-out mice exhibit reduced exploration of novel stimuli. *Journal of Neuroscience, 19,* 9550–9556.

Earls, F. E., & Jung, K. G. (1987). Temperament and home environment characteristics as causal factors in the early development of childhood psychopathology. *Journal of American Academy of Child and Adolescent Psychiatry, 26,* 491–498.

Eid, M., Riemann, R., Angleitner, A., & Borkenau, P. (2003). Sociability and positive emotionality: Genetic and environmental contributions to the covariation between different facets of extraversion. *Journal of Personality, 71,* 319–346.

Eisenberg, N., Fabes, R. A., Murphy, B., Karbon, M., Smith, M., & Maszk, P. (1996). The relations of children's dispositional empathy-related responding to their emotionality, regulation, and social functioning. *Developmental Psychology, 32,* 195–209.

Eisenberg, N., & Mussen, P. H. (1991). *The roots of pro social behavior in children.* New York: Cambridge University Press.

Eley, T. C., Lichtenstein, P., & Stevenson, J. (1999). Sex differences in the etiology of aggressive and nonaggressive antisocial behavior: Results from two twin studies. *Child Development, 70,* 155–168.

Elkins, I., Iacono, W., Doyle, A., & McGue, M. (1997). Characteristics associated with the persistence of antisocial behavior: Results from recent longitudinal research. *Aggression and Violent Behavior, 2,* 101–124.

Emde, R. N., Plomin, R., Robinson, J., Corley, R., DeFries, J., Fulker, D. W., et al. (1992). Temperament, emotion, and cognition at fourteen months: The MacArthur Longitudinal Twin Study. *Child Development, 63,* 1437–1455.

Eysenck, H. J. (1947). *Dimensions of personality.* New York: Praeger.

Eysenck, H. J. (1964). *Crime and personality.* New York: Houghton Mifflin.

Eysenck, H. J. (1990). Genetic and environmental contributions to individual differences: The three major dimensions of personality. *Journal of Personality, 58,* 245–261.

Eysenck, S. G., & Eysenck, H. J. (1970). Crime and personality: An empirical study of the three-factor theory. *British Journal of Criminology, 10,* 225–239.

Farmer, A., Redman, K., Harris, T., Mahmood, A., Sadler, S., Pickering, A., et al. (2002). Neuroticism, extraversion, life events and depression: The Cardiff Depression Study. *British Journal of Psychiatry, 181,* 118–122.

Farrington, D. P. (1991). Antisocial personality from childhood to adulthood. *The Psychologist, 4,* 389–394.

Farrington, D. P. (1995). The development of offending and antisocial behaviour from childhood: Key findings from the Cambridge Study in Delinquent Development. *Journal of Child Psychology and Psychiatry, 6,* 929–964.

Farrington, D. P., & West, D. J. (1993). Criminal, penal and life histories of chronic offenders: Risk and protective factors and early identification. *Criminal Behaviour and Mental Health, 3,* 492–523.

Frick, P. J., O'Brien, B. S., Wootton, J. M., & McBurnett, K. (1994). Psychopathy and conduct problems in children. *Journal of Abnormal Psychology, 103,* 700–707.

Garcia-Coll, C., Kagan, J., & Reznick, J. S. (1984). Behavioral inhibition in young children. *Child Development, 55,* 1005–1019.

Ge, X., Donnellan, M. B., & Wenk, E. (2001). The development of persistent criminal offending in males. *Criminal Justice and Behavior, 26,* 731–755.

Gershuny, B. S., & Sher, K. J. (1998). The relation between personality and anxiety: Findings from a 3-year prospective study. *Journal of Abnormal Psychology, 107,* 252–262.

Giancalo, P. R., Martin, C. S., Tarter, R. E., Pelham, W. E., & Moss, H. B. (1996). Executive cognitive functioning and aggressive behavior in preadolescent boys at high risk for substance abuse/dependence. *Journal of Studies on Alcohol, 57*, 352–359.

Giros, B., Jaber, M., Jones, S. R., Wightman, R. M., & Caron, M. G. (1996). Hyperlocomotion and indifference to cocaine and amphetamine in mice lacking the dopamine transporter. *Nature, 379*, 606–612.

Gjone, H., & Stevenson, J. (1997). A longitudinal twin study of temperament and behavior problems: Common genetic or environmental influences? *Journal of American Academy of Child and Adolescent Psychiatry, 36*, 1448–1456.

Goldberg, J., & Ramakrishnan, V. (1994). Commentary: Direction of causation models. *Genetic Epidemiology, 11*, 457–462.

Goldberg, L. R. (1993). The structure of phenotypic personality traits. *American Psychologist, 48*, 26–34.

Goldsmith, H. H., Buss, K. A., & Lemery, K. S. (1997). Toddler and childhood temperament: Expanded content, stronger genetic evidence, new evidence for the importance of environment. *Developmental Psychology, 33*, 891–905.

Goldsmith, H. H., Losoya, S. H., Bradshaw, D. L., & Campos, J. J. (1994). Genetics of personality: A twin study of the five-factor model and parent-offspring analyses. In C. F. Halverson, Jr., & G. A. Kohnstamm (Eds.), *The developing structure of temperament and personality from infancy to adulthood.* Hillsdale, NJ: Erlbaum.

Goma-I-Freixnet, M. (1995). Prosocial and antisocial aspects of personality. *Personality and Individual Differences, 19*, 125–134.

Goodman, R. (2001). Psychometric properties of the Strengths and Difficulties Questionnaire. *Journal of the American Academy of Child and Adolescent Psychiatry, 40*, 1337–1345.

Goodyer, I. M., Ashby, L., Altham, P. M., Vize, C., & Cooper, P. J. (1993). Temperament and major depression in 11 to 16 year olds. *Journal of Child Psychology and Psychiatry and Allied Disciplines, 34*, 1409–1423.

Gottfredson, M. R., & Hirschi, T. (1990). *A general theory of crime.* Stanford, CA: Stanford University Press.

Gray, J. A., & McNaughton, N. (1996). The neuropsychology of anxiety: Reprise. In D. A. Hope (Ed.), *Perspectives on anxiety, panic, and fear: Nebraska Symposium on Motivation* (Vol. 43, pp. 61–134). Lincoln: University of Nebraska Press.

Graziano, W. G. (1994). The development of agreeableness as a dimension of personality. In C. F. Halverson, G. A. Kohnstamm, & R. P. Martin (Eds.), *The developing structure of temperament and personality from infancy to adulthood* (pp. 339–354). Hillsdale, NJ: Erlbaum.

Graziano, W. G., & Ward, D. (1992). Probing the Big Five in adolescence: Personality and adjustment during a developmental transition. *Journal of Personality, 60*, 425–439.

Greene, K., Krcmar, M., Walters, L. H., Rubin, D. L., & Hale, J. L. (2000). Targeting adolescent risk-taking behaviors: The contribution of egocentrism and sensation-seeking. *Journal of Adolescence, 23*, 439–461.

Guerin, D. W., Gottfried, A. W., & Thomas, C. W. (1997). Difficult temperament and behaviour problems: A longitudinal study from 1. 5 to 12 years. *International Journal of Behavioral Development, 21*, 71–90.

Gunderson, F. G., Triebwasser, J., Phillips, K. A., & Sullivan, C. N. (1999). Personality and vulnerability to affective disorders. In C. R. Cloninger (Ed.), *Personality and psychopathology* (pp. 3–32). Washington, DC: American Psychopathological Association.

Haemaelaeinen, M., & Pulkkinen, L. (1996). Problem behavior as a precursor of male criminality. *Development and Psychopathology, 8*, 443–455.

Hastings, P. D., Zahn-Waxler, C., Robinson, J., Usher, B., & Bridges, D. (2000). The development of concern for others in children with behavior problems. *Developmental Psychology, 36*, 531–546.

Heath, A. C., Cloninger, C. R., & Martin, N. G. (1994). Testing a model for the genetic structure of personality: A comparison of the personality systems of Cloninger and Eysenck. *Journal of Personality and Social Psychology, 66*, 762–775.

Heath, A. C., Kessler, R. C., Neale, M. C., Hewitt, J. K., Eaves, L. J., & Kendler, K. S. (1993). Testing hypotheses about direction of causation using cross-sectional family data. *Behavior Genetics, 23*, 29–50.

Heaven, P. C. L. (1996). Personality and self-reported delinquency: A longitudinal analysis. *Journal of Child Psychology and Psychiatry, 37*, 747–751.

Hinshaw, S. P., Lahey, B. B., & Hart, E. L. (1993). Issues of taxonomy and comorbidity in the development of conduct disorder. *Development and Psychopathology, 5*, 31–50.

Hirshfeld, D. R., Rosenbaum, J. F., Biederman, J., Bolduc, E. A., Faraone, S. V., Snidman, N., et al. (1992). Stable behavioral inhibition and its association with anxiety disorder. *Journal of the American Academy of Child and Adolescent Psychiatry, 31*, 103–111.

Hirshfeld-Becker, D. R., Biederman, J., Faraone, S. V., Violette, H., Wrightsman, J., & Rosenbaum, J. F. (2002). Temperamental correlates of disruptive behavior disorders in young children: Preliminary findings. *Biological Psychiatry, 51*, 563–574.

Hughes, C., White, A., Sharpen, J., & Dunn, J. (2000). Antisocial, angry, and unsympathetic: "Hard-to-manage" preschoolers' peer problems and possible cognitive influences. *Journal of Child Psychology and Psychiatry, 41*, 169–179.

Jaffee, S. R., Caspi, A., Moffitt, T. E., & Taylor, A. (2004). Physical maltreatment victim to antisocial child: Evidence of an environmentally mediated process. *Journal of Abnormal Psychology, 113*, 44–55.

John, O. P., Caspi, A., Robins, R. W., Moffitt, T. E., & Stouthamer-Loeber, M. (1994). The "little five": Exploring the nomological network of the five-factor model of personality in adolescent boys. *Child Development, 65*, 160–178.

Jöreskog, K. G., & Sörbom, D. (1993). *LISREL VIII: User's guide*. Chicago: Scientific Software.

Kagan, J., Reznick, J. S., & Snidman, N. (1988). Biological bases of childhood shyness. *Science, 240*, 167–171.

Kagan, J., Reznick, J. S., Snidman, N., Gibbons, J., & Johnson, M. O. (1988). Childhood derivatives of inhibition and lack of inhibition to the unfamiliar. *Child Development, 59*, 1580–1589.

Keenan, K., & Shaw, D. (2003). Starting at the beginning: Exploring etiological factors of later antisocial behavior in the first years of life. In B. B. Lahey, T. E.

Moffitt, & A. Caspi (Eds.), *Causes of conduct disorder and juvenile delinquency* (pp. 153–181). New York: Guilford Press.

Kerr, M., Tremblay, R. E., Pagani-Kurtz, L., & Vitaro, F. (1997). Boys' behavioral inhibition and the risk of later delinquency. *Archives of General Psychiatry, 54,* 809–816.

Koopmans, J. R., Boomsma, D. I., Heath, A. C., & van Doornen, L. J. P. (1995). A multivariate genetic analysis of sensation seeking. *Behavior Genetics, 25,* 349–356.

Kratzer, L., & Hodgins, S. (1999). A typology of offenders: A test of Moffitt's theory among males and females from childhood to age 30. *Criminal Behaviour and Mental Health, 9,* 57–73.

Krueger, R. F. (1999). Personality traits in late adolescence predict mental disorders in early adulthood: A prospective–epidemiologic study. *Journal of Personality, 67,* 39–65.

Krueger, R. F., Hicks, B. M., Patrick, C. J., Carlson, S. R., Iacono, W. G., & McGue, M. (2002). Etiologic connections among substance dependence, antisocial behavior and personality: Modeling the externalizing spectrum. *Journal of Abnormal Psychology, 111,* 411–424.

Lahey, B. B., & Waldman, I. D. (2003). A developmental propensity model of the origins of conduct problems during childhood and adolescence. In B. B. Lahey, T. E. Moffitt, & A. Caspi (Eds.), *Causes of conduct disorder and juvenile delinquency* (pp. 76–117). New York: Guilford Press.

Lahey, B. B., Waldman, I. D., Applegate, B., Rowe, D. C., Urbano, R. C., & Chapman, D. A. (2003). *Dimensions of child and adolescent dispositions relevant to psychopathology.* Manuscript under editorial review.

Lake, R. I. E., Eaves, L. J., Maes, H. H. M., Heath, A. C., & Martin, N. G. (2000). Further evidence against the environmental transmission of individual differences in neuroticism from a collaborative study of 45,850 twins and relatives on two continents. *Behavior Genetics, 30,* 223–233.

Lambert, N. M. (1988). Adolescent outcomes for hyperactive children: Perspectives on general and specific patterns of childhood risk for adolescent educational, social, and mental health problems. *American Psychologist, 43,* 786–799.

Lemery, K. S., Essex, M. J., & Smider, N. A. (2002). Revealing the relations between temperament and behavior problem symptoms by eliminating measurement confounding: Expert ratings and factor analyses. *Child Development, 73,* 867–882.

Lengua, L. J., West, S. G., & Sandler, I. N. (1998). Temperament as a predictor of symptomatology in children: Addressing contamination of measures. *Child Development, 69,* 164–181.

Lilienfeld, S. O., & Waldman, I. D. (1990). The relation between childhood Attention-Deficit Hyperactivity Disorder and adult antisocial behavior reexamined: The problem of heterogeneity. *Clinical Psychology Review, 10,* 699–725.

Loeber, R. (1988). Natural histories of conduct problems, delinquency, and associated substance abuse: Evidence for developmental progressions. In B. B. Lahey & A. E. Kazdin (Eds.), *Advances in clinical child psychology* (Vol. 11, pp. 73–124). New York: Plenum.

Loeber, R., & LeBlanc, M. (1990). Toward a developmental criminology. In M. Tonry

& N. Morris (Eds.), *Crime and justice* (Vol. 12, pp. 375–473). Chicago: University of Chicago Press.

Loehlin, J. C. (1996). The Cholesky approach: A cautionary note. *Behavior Genetics, 26, 65–69.*

Loehlin, J. C., & Martin, N. G. (2001). Age changes in personality traits and their heritabilities during the adult years: Evidence from Australian twin registry samples. *Personality and Individual Differences, 30,* 1147–1160.

Lowe, N., Kirley, A., Hawi, Z., Sham, P., Wickham, H., Kratochvil, C. J., et al. (2004). Joint analysis of the DRD5 marker concludes association with Attention-Deficit/ Hyperactivity Disorder confined to the Predominantly Inattentive and Combined subtypes. *American Journal of Human Genetics, 74,* 348–356.

Luengo, M. A., Otero, J. M., Carrillo-de-la-Pena, M. T., & Miron, L. (1994). Dimensions of antisocial behaviour in juvenile delinquency: A study of personality variables. *Psychology Crime and Law, 1,* 27–37.

Lynam, D., Moffitt, T., & Stouthamer-Loeber, M. (1993). Explaining the relation between IQ and delinquency: Class, race, test motivation, school failure or self-control? *Journal of Abnormal Psychology, 102,* 187–196.

Lyons, M. J., True, W., Eisen, S., Goldberg, J., Meyer, J., Faraone, S. V., et al. (1995). Differential heritability of adult and juvenile antisocial traits. *Archives of General Psychiatry, 52,* 906–915.

Macaskill, G. T., Hopper, J. L., White, V., & Hill, D. J. (1994). Genetic and environmental variation in Eysenck Personality Questionnaire scales measured on Australian adolescent twins. *Behavior Genetics, 24,* 481–491.

Matthews, K. A., Batson, C. D., Horn, J., & Rosenman, R. H. (1981). "Principles in his nature which interest him in the fortune of others . . . ": The heritability of empathic concern for others. *Journal of Personality, 49,* 237–247.

McGue, M., Bacon, S., & Lykken, D. T. (1993). Personality stability and change in early adulthood: A behavioral genetic analysis. *Developmental Psychology, 29,* 96–109.

McRae, R. R., & Costa, P. T. (1987). Validation of the five-factor model of personality across instruments and observers. *Journal of Personality and Social Psychology, 52,* 81–90.

Meehl, P. E. (1978). Theoretical risks and tabular asterisks: Sir Karl, Sir Ronald, and the slow progress of soft psychology. *Journal of Consulting and Clinical Psychology, 46,* 806–834.

Miles, D. R., van den Bree, M. B. M., Gupman, A. E., Newlin, D. B., Glantz, M. D., Pickens, R. W. (2001). A twin study on sensation seeking, risk taking behavior and marijuana use. *Drug and Alcohol Dependence, 62,* 57–68.

Miller, P. A., & Eisenberg, N. (1988). The relation of empathy to aggressive and externalizing/antisocial behavior. *Psychological Bulletin, 103,* 324–344.

Moffitt, T. E. (1993). Adolescence-limited and life-course-persistent antisocial behavior: A developmental taxonomy. *Psychological Review, 100,* 674–701.

Moffitt, T. E., Caspi, A., Dickson, N., Silva, P., & Stanton, W. (1996). Childhood-onset versus adolescent-onset antisocial conduct problems in males: Natural history from ages 3 to 18 years. *Development and Psychopathology, 8,* 399–424.

Moffitt, T. E., & Silva, P. A. (1988). IQ and delinquency: A direct test of the differential detection hypothesis. *Journal of Abnormal Psychology, 97*, 330–333.

Muris, P., Merckelbach, H., Schmidt, H., Gadet, B., & Bogie, N. (2001). Anxiety and depression as colTelates of self-reported behavioura1 inhibition in normal adolescents. *Behaviour Research and Therapy, 39*, 1051–1061.

Nadder, T. S., Silberg, J. L., Eaves, L. J., Maes, H. H., & Meyer, J. M. (1998). Genetic effects on ADHD symptomatology: Results from a telephone survey. *Behavior Genetics, 28*(2), 83–99.

Nagin, D., & Tremblay, R. E. (1999). Trajectories of boys' physical aggression, opposition, and hyperactivity on the path to physically violent and non-violent delinquency. *Child Development, 70*, 1181–1196.

Neale, M. C. (1997). *Mx: Statistical modeling* (4th ed.). Richmond, VA: Department of Psychiatry, Medical College of Virginia, Virginia Commonwealth University.

Neale, M. C., & Cardon, L. R. (1992). *Methodology for genetic studies of twins and families*. Dordrecht, Netherlands: Kluwer Academic.

Neale, M. C., Walters, E., Heath, A. C., Kessler, R. C., Perusse, D., Eaves, L. J., et al. (1994). Depression and parental bonding: Cause, consequence, or genetic covariance? *Genetic Epidemiology, 11*, 503–522.

Nelson, B., Martin, R. P., Hodge, S., Havill, V., & Kamphaus, R. (1999). Modeling the prediction of elementary school adjustment from preschool temperament. *Personality and Individual Differences, 26*, 687–700.

Newcomb, M. D., & McGee, L. (1991). Influence of sensation seeking on general deviance and specific problem behaviors from adolescence to young adulthood. *Journal of Personality and Social Psychology, 61*, 614–628.

Olson, S. L., Bates, J. E., Sandy, J. M., & Lanthier, R. (2000). Early developmental precursors of externalizing behavior in middle childhood and adolescence. *Journal of Abnormal Child Psychology, 28*, 119–133.

Patterson, G. R. (1982). *Coercive family interactions*. Eugene, OR: Castalia.

Patterson, G. R., Reid, J. B., & Dishion, T. J. (1992). *Antisocial boys*. Eugene, OR: Castalia.

Pedersen, N. L., Plomin, R., McClearn, G. E., & Friberg, L. (1988). Neuroticism, extraversion, and related traits in adult twins reared apart and reared together. *Journal of Personality and Social Psychology, 55*, 950–957.

Pennington, B. F. (2002). *The development of psychopathology: Nature and nurture*. New York: Guilford Press.

Phillips, K., & Matheny, A. P. (1997). Evidence for genetic influence on both cross-situation and situation-specific components of behavior. *Journal of Personality and Social Psychology, 73*, 129–138.

Plomin, R., DeFries, J. C., & Loehlin, J. C. (1977). Genotype–environment interaction and correlation in the analysis of human behavior. *Psychological Bulletin, 84*, 309–322.

Popper, K. R. (1959). *The logic of scientific discovery*. New York: Basic Books.

Powell, G. E., & Stewart, R. A. (1983). The relationship of personality to antisocial and neurotic behaviours as observed by teachers. *Personality and Individual Differences, 4*, 97–100.

Raine, A., Reynolds, C., Venables, P. H., Mednick, S. A., & Farrington, D. P. (1998). Fearlessness, stimulation-seeking, and large body size at age 3 years as early predispositions to childhood aggression at age 11 years. *Archives of General Psychiatry, 55,* 745–751.

Rende, R. D. (1993). Longitudinal relations between temperament traits and behavioral syndromes in middle childhood. *Journal of American Academy of Child and Adolescent Psychiatry, 32,* 287–290.

Rhee, S. H., & Waldman, I. D. (2002). Genetic and environmental influences on antisocial behavior: A meta-analysis of twin and adoption studies. *Psychological Bulletin, 128,* 490–529.

Roberts, S., & Kendler, K. S. (1999). Neuroticism and self-esteem as indices of the vulnerability to major depression in women. *Psychological Medicine, 29,* 1101–1109.

Robinson, J. L., Kagan, J., Reznick, J. S., & Corley, R. (1992). The heritability of inhibited and unihibited behavior: A twin study. *Developmental Psychology, 28,* 1030–1037.

Rogosa, D. (1987). Casual models do not support scientific conclusions—A comment. *Journal of Educational Statistics, 12,* 185–195.

Rothbart, M. K. (1981). Measurement of temperament in infancy. *Child Development, 52,* 569–578.

Rothbart, M. K., & Ahadi, S. A. (1994). Temperament and the development of personality. *Journal of Abnormal Psychology, 103,* 55–66.

Rothbart, M. K., Ahadi, S. A., & Hershey, K. L. (1994). Temperament and social behavior in childhood. *Merrill-Palmer Quarterly, 40,* 21–39.

Rothbart, M. K., Ahadi, S. A., Hershey, K. L., & Fisher, P. (2001). Investigations of temperament at three to seven years: The Children's Behavior Questionnaire. *Child Development, 72,* 1394–1408.

Rubinstein, M., Phillips, T. J., Bunzow, J. R., Falzone, T. L., Dziewczapolski, G., Zhang, G., et al. (1997). Mice lacking dopamine D4 receptors are supersensitive to ethanol, cocaine, and methamphetamine. *Cell, 90,* 991–1001.

Rushton, J. P., Fulker, D. W., Neale, M. C., Nias, D. K. B., & Eysenck, H. J. (1986). Altruism and aggression: The heritability of individual differences. *Journal of Personality and Social Psychology, 50,* 1192–1198.

Rutter, M. (1987). Temperament, personality, and personality disorder. *British Journal of Psychiatry, 150,* 443–458.

Rutter, M. (1988). Epidemiological approaches to developmental psychopathology. *Archives of General Psychiatry, 45,* 486–495.

Rutter, M., Dunn, J., Plomin, R., Siminoff, E., Pickles, A., Maughan, B., et al. (1997). Integrating nature and nurture: Implications of person–environment correlations and interactions for developmental psychopathology. *Development and Psychopathology, 9,* 335–364.

Sampson, R. J., & Laub, J. H. (1992). Crime and deviance. *Annual Review of Sociology, 18,* 63–84.

Sanson, A., & Prior, M. (1999). Temperament and behavioral precursors to oppositional defiant disorder and conduct disorder. In H. Quay & A. Hogan (Eds.), *Handbook of the disruptive behavior disorders.* (pp. 397–417). New York: Kluwer Academic/Plenum.

Sanson, A., Prior, M., & Kyrios, M. (1990). Contamination of measures in temperament research. *Merrill-Palmer Quarterly, 36,* 179–192.

Saudino, K. J., McGuire, S., Hetherington, E. M., Reiss, D., & Plomin, R. (1995). Parent ratings of EAS temperaments in twins, full siblings, half siblings, and step siblings. *Journal of Personality and Social Psychology, 68*, 723–733.

Saudino, K. J., Plomin, R., & DeFries, J. C. (1996). Tester-rated temperament at 14, 20 and 24 months: Environmental change and genetic continuity. *British Journal of Developmental Psychology, 14*, 129–144.

Saudou, F., Amara, D. A., Dierich, A., LeMeur, M., Ramboz, S., Segu, L., et al. (1994). Enhanced aggressive behavior in mice lacking 5-HT1B receptor. *Science, 265*, 1875–1878.

Schmeck, K., & Poustka, F. (2001). Temperament and disruptive behavior disorders. *Psychopathology, 4*, 159–163.

Schmitz, S., Fulker, D. W., Plomin, R., Zahn-Waxler, C., Emde, R. N., & DeFries, J. C. (1999). Temperament and problem behaviour during early childhood. *International Journal of Behavioral Development, 23*, 333–355.

Schwartz, C. E., Snidman, N., & Kagan, J. (1996). Early childhood temperament as a determinant of externalizing behavior in adolescence. *Developmental Psychopathology, 8*, 527–537.

Seeman, P., & Madras, B. K. (1998). Anti-hyperactivity medication: Methylphenidate and amphetamine. *Molecular Psychiatry, 3*, 386–396.

Seguin, J. R., Boulerice, B., Harden, P. W., Tremblay, R. E., & Pihl, R. O. (1999). Executive functions and physical aggression after controlling for attention deficit hyperactivity disorder, general memory and IQ. *Journal of Child Psychology and Psychiatry, 40*, 1197–1208.

Shiner, R. L., Masten, A. S., & Tellegen, A. (2002). A developmental perspective on personality in emerging adulthood: Childhood antecedents and concurrent adaptation. *Journal of Personality and Social Psychology, 83*, 1165–1177.

Silverman, I. W., & Ragusa, D. M. (1992). A short-term longitudinal study of the early development of self-regulation. *Journal of Abnormal Child Psychology, 20*, 415–435.

Slutske, W. S., Heath, A. C., Dinwiddie, S. H., Madden, P. A. F., Bucholz, K. K., Dunne, M. P., et al. (1997). Modeling genetic and environmental influences in the etiology of conduct disorder: A study of 2682 adult twin pairs. *Journal of Abnormal Psychology, 106*, 266–279.

Solanto, M. V. (1984). Neuropharmacological basis of stimulant drug action in attention deficit disorder with hyperactivity: A review and synthesis. *Psychological Bulletin, 95*, 387–409.

Solanto, M. V. (1998). Neuropsychopharmacological mechanisms of stimulant drug action in attention-deficit hyperactivity disorder: A review and integration. *Behavioural Brain Research, 94*, 127–152.

Stattin, H., & Klackenberg-Larsson, I. (1993). Early language and intelligence development and their relationship to future criminal behavior. *Journal of Abnormal Psychology, 102*, 369–378.

Tahir, E., Yazgan, Y., Cirakoglu, B., Ozbay, F., Waldman, I., & Asherson, P. J. (2000). Association and linkage of DRD4 and DRD5 with attention deficit hyperactivity disorder (ADHD) in a sample of Turkish children. *Molecular Psychiatry, 5*, 396–404.

Teerikangas, O. M., Aronen, E. T., Martin, R. P., & Huttunen, M. O. (1998). Effects of infant temperament and early intervention on the psychiatric symptoms of adolescents. *Journal of American Academy of Child and Adolescent Psychiatry, 37,* 1070–1076.

Tellegen, A., Lykken, D. T., Bouchard, T. J., Wilcox, K. J., Segal, N. L., & Rich, S. (1988). Personality similarity in twins reared apart and together. *Journal of Personality and Social Psychology, 54,* 1031–1039.

Tranah, T., Harnett, P., & Yule, W. (1998). Conduct disorder and personality. *Personality and Individual Differences, 24,* 741–745.

Tremblay, R. E. (2000). The development of aggressive behaviour during childhood: What have we learned in the past century? *International Journal of Behavioral Development, 24,* 129–141.

Tremblay, R. E., Boulerice, B., Harden, P. W., McDuff, P., Perusse, D., Pihl, R. O., et al. (1996). Do children in Canada become more aggressive as they approach adolescence? In M. Cappe & I. Fellegi (Eds.), *Growing up in Canada* (pp. 127–136). Ottawa: Statistics Canada.

Tremblay, R. E., Japel, C., Perusse, D., McDuff, P., Boivin, M., Zoccolillo, M., et al. (1999). The search for the age of 'onset' of physical aggression: Rousseau and Bandura revisited. *Criminal Behaviour and Mental Health, 9,* 8–23.

Tremblay, R. E., Pihl, R. O., Vitaro, F., & Dobkin, P. L. (1994). Predicting early onset of male antisocial behavior from preschool behavior. *Archives of General Psychiatry, 51,* 732–739.

van der Valk, J. C., van den Oord, E. J. C. G., Verhulst, F. C., & Boomsma, D. I. (2003). Genetic and environmental contributions to stability and change in children's internalizing and externalizing problems. *Journal of the American Academy of Child Adolescent Psychiatry, 42,* 1212–1220.

Waldman, I. D., & Gizer, I. (in press). The genetics of ADHD. *Clinical Psychology Review.*

Waldman, I. D., Rhee, S. H., Levy, F., & Hay, D. A. (2001). Genetic and environmental influences on the covariation among symptoms of attention deficit hyperactivity disorder, oppositional defiant disorder, and conduct disorder. In D. A. Hay & F. Levy (Eds.), *Attention, genes and ADHD* (pp. 115–138). East Sussex, UK: Brunner-Routledge.

Waldman, I. D., & Slutske, W. S. (2000). Antisocial behavior and alcoholism: A behavioral genetic perspective on comorbidity. *Clinical Psychology Review, 20,* 255–287.

Watson, D., Clark, L. A., & Tellegen, A. (1988). Development and validation of brief measures of positive and negative affect: The PANAS scales. *Journal of Personality and Social Psychology, 54,* 1063–1070.

Young, S. B., Smolen, A., Corley, R. P., Krauter, K. S., DeFries, J. C., Crowley, T. J., & Hewitt, J. K. (2002). Dopamine transporter polymorphism associated with externalizing behavior problems in children. *American Journal of Medical Genetics, 114,* 144–149.

Zahn-Waxler, C., Robinson, J. L., & Emde, R. N. (1992). The development of empathy in twins. *Developmental Psychology, 28,* 1038–1047.

Zuckerman, M. (1971) Dimensions of sensation seeking. *Journal of Consulting Clinical Psychology, 36,* 45–52.

Zuckerman, M. (1974). The sensation seeking motive. In B. Maher (Ed.), *Progress in experimental personality research* (pp. 79–148). New York: Academic Press.

Zuckerman, M. (1996). The psychobiological model for impulsive unsocialized sensation seeking: A comparative approach. *Neuropsychobiology, 34,* 125–129.

Zuckerman, M., Buchsbaum, M. S., & Murphy, D. L. (1980). Sensation seeking and its biological correlates. *Psychological Bulletin, 88,* 187–214.

Zuckerman, M., Kuhlman, D. M., Joireman, J., Teta, P., & Kraft, M. (1993). A comparison of three structural models for personality: The big three, the big five, and the alternative five. *Journal of Personality and Social Psychology, 65,* 757–768.

Chapter 6

What Is the Role of Personality in Psychopathology?

A View from Behavior Genetics

KERRY L. JANG
HEIKE WOLF
ROSEANN LARSTONE

Time and time again, empirical studies of psychiatric comorbidity consistently find that personality features are correlated with virtually all forms of common psychopathology. These relationships are found with broad traits such as neuroticism as well as with more specific facet traits defining domains such as anxiety, warmth, rigidity or compliance. For example, clinical research has shown that individuals with depression frequently report being anxious (Zimmerman, Chelminski, & McDermut, 2002; Kendler, 1996) and that higher measured levels of neuroticism were related to increased levels of emotional discomfort among schizophrenics (Lysaker, Bell, Kaplan, Greig, & Bryson, 1999). Moreover, the importance of personality for many forms of psychopathology is highlighted by the fact that many personality features serve as diagnostic criteria. For example, the diagnostic criteria for DSM-IV major depressive episode (American Psychiatric Association, 1994) includes "feelings of guilt and worthlessness," item content typically found in measures of trait neuroticism.

Despite the recognition that personality features form part of the presentation of many disorders, there has been little research that has examined (1) *why* personality and psychopathology are comorbid and (2) what role personality actually plays in the development and expression of another disorder. What are some of the possibilities? First of all, it could be argued that personality plays no significant role because any observed comorbidity is due to the problem of *criterion overlap*. Criterion overlap occurs when similar descriptive categories are used to define personality dimensions and used to diagnose another disorder. This occurs when the definitions used to define each domain are overly broad or inclusive, or the behavioral exemplars are vague or indistinct. For example, it could be argued that, because not all depressed patients display "feelings of guilt and worthlessness," these behaviors should not be used as indicators of depression and should be considered part of personality. Similar questions swirl around the content of personality scales. One of the primary facet scales of neuroticism in the revised Neuroticism Extraversion Openness Personality Inventory (NEO-PI-R: Costa & McCrae, 1992) is "depression." Does this scale really fit in this domain along with the other facets of anxiety, hostility, self-consciousness, impulsiveness, and vulnerability? Thus, the fact that both the diagnostic criteria for depression and trait neuroticism assess the same content increases the correlation between these domains. On the other hand, it is possible that current definitions do validly reflect the nature of each and that the measured relationship between them reflects a true state of nature. The central issue is to distinguish between these two possibilities.

One approach is to conduct rigorous psychometric studies to determine whether the behaviors used to define neuroticism are more appropriately considered an aspect of personality or an aspect of depression. The focus of this chapter is a complementary approach that tests whether personality is an integral aspect of psychopathology by determining whether the two domains share a common etiological basis and by delineating the pathogenic role of personality.

WHAT DOES PERSONALITY DO?

The literature suggests that personality has been thought to impact psychopathology in three basic ways. A great deal of this theoretical work comes from the temperament literature, and many recent treatments of the subject (e.g., the "pathoplasty model" by Krueger & Tackett, 2003) are variations on these fundamental ideas. The first hypothesizes that personality factors increase the risk for developing psychiatric disorder—the *risk model*. In this model, both temperament and psychopathology are qualitatively distinct entities—but certain temperament dimensions alone or in combination with others increase the likelihood of developing a psychiatric disorder. For example, a child's level of positive or negative emotionality weights the effect of negative parenting on child adjustment (e.g., Rothbart, 2004). The second hypothesis is that personality and psychopathology occupy a single domain and psychopathology is simply a display of the extremes of normal personality function (the *spectrum model*). For example, conduct disorder (CD) is conceptualized as pathological disinhibition. In contrast, the *scar model* hypothesizes that psychopathology influences personality. Under this model, personality variables are hypothesized to play minor roles in the development of the disorder, and changes in observed personality are simply the *result* of the disorder. For example, although minor personality changes are frequently observed before the full-fledged onset of Alzheimer's disease, the major personality changes occur after onset of the core symptoms (Lewinsohn, Steinmetz, Larson, & Franklin, 1981).

The next question is: How would one determine which role any specific personality variable plays in a disorder? Do variations in trait anxiety increase the vulnerability to depression (risk model), or are changes in anxiety simply a consequence of depression (scar model)? How does one test whether depression is the negative extreme of sociability or trait extraversion, as predicted by the spectrum model? Behavior-genetic methods provide one avenue into exploring these alternatives by delineating how the observed relationships between personality and psychopathology have biological bases.

THE BEHAVIOR-GENETIC APPROACH

The purpose of behavior-genetic research is to estimate the extent to which variability in any measured behavior is due to genetic and environmental differences between people. These methods simultaneously estimate the degree to which the observed relationship—covariation or comorbidity—between two or more observed behaviors is attributable to a set of genetic and environmental factors common to both, illustrated by the following equation:

$$r_{X.Y} = (h_X \cdot h_Y \cdot r_G) + (e_X \cdot e_Y \cdot r_E) \qquad \text{Eq. 1}$$

This expression states that the *phenotypic* relationship between two measured variables, X and Y, indexed by the correlation coefficient, $r_{X.Y}$, is a direct function of the degree to which genetic factors, symbolized by h (h_X, h_Y), and environmental factors, symbolized by e (e_X, e_Y) influence X and Y, respectively, weighted by the degree to which the genetic and environmental influences on X and Y stem from a common source, indexed by the genetic and environmental correlation coefficients r_G and r_E, respectively.

The terms in Equation 1 are estimated by comparing the magnitude of the similarities and differences between relatives who share genes to different degrees. The most common classes of designs are (1) family studies, (2) adoption studies, and (3) twin studies. One version of the family study compares the similarities of biological siblings, and another compares parents to their offspring. In general, family study designs are the least powerful because they confound genetic and environmental effects. Siblings, for example, share both genes (50%) and the environments (100%) in which they were raised. These studies are useful to identify which disorders "run in families." However, genetic and environmental influences are easily separated in family study designs when the object is to compare actual DNA polymorphisms extracted from the blood of relatives.

The influence of genetic and environmental factors is readily separated in adoption study designs. One version of this design compares the similarities of adopted-away children and their biological parents. Because adopted-away children were raised apart from their biological parents, any similarities between them indexed by a correlation coefficient can only be due to shared genes. Comparing raised-together monozygotic (MZ) pairs to dizygotic (DZ) twin pairs is one of the most commonly used designs. In this design, a higher within-pair MZ correlation ($r_{MZ\ TWIN1.TWIN2}$) compared to a within-pair DZ correlation ($r_{DZ\ TWIN1.TWIN2}$) suggests that genetic influences are implicated because MZ twins share all of their genes whereas DZ twins share approximately half. When $r_{MZ\ TWIN1.TWIN2} = r_{DZ\ TWIN1.TWIN2}$, no genetic influences are inferred because, despite the two-fold greater genetic similarity of MZ twins, their observed similarity is that of DZ twins.

These correlations (or covariances) are used as the raw data to estimate the heritability coefficient (h^2) that estimates the proportion (%) of the observed variability in any behavioral measure that is directly attributable to genetic differences between people. The actual procedures used to estimate the quantities in Equation 1 are explained in detail in many behavior-genetic textbooks (e.g., Neale & Cardon, 1992; Plomin, DeFries, McClearn, & Rutter, 1997; Jang, 2005), and the details need not be reiterated here.

Just as genetic effects can be estimated, twin data also allow the direct estimation of environmental effects. Two environmental influences are distinguished. The first is the family environment that affects all family members the same way on a measured behavior (c^2) or has the same influence on two variables (r_C). A frequently used example of c^2 is socioeconomic status because it is thought to apply to and affect each person within the family equally while differentiating families. The second major environmental effect is the nonshared family environment (e^2 and r_E). Nonshared environmental influences are defined as any experience, milieu, or circumstance— virtually anything that causes children from the same family to be different from one another, including experiences that systematically differentiate people from one another, such as parental favoritism (see Hetherington, Reiss, & Plomin, 1994) and measurement error.

The point here is not how these quantities are assessed but rather how they can be used to test the veracity of the risk, spectrum, and scar models as explanatory mechanisms for the relationship between personality and psychopathology. The following sections discuss some of these possibilities and illustrate them with some examples drawn from the literature. The following discussions are meant to encourage thinking of how to bridge personality and psychopathology using behavior genetics. They are, to borrow from Rudyard Kipling, "just so stories," and it is not our claim that our interpretations are necessarily correct or the only ones possible. They are provided as concrete examples of how this fascinating problem might be approached.

PERSONALITY AS A RISK FACTOR

How does personality act as a risk factor? There are two mechanisms discussed by behavior geneticists that might be helpful in explaining just how personality increases the risk for the onset of another disorder. These two mechanisms are *gene–environment correlation*, broadly defined as genetic influence on exposure to environments, and *gene–environment interaction* that describes environmental modulation of genetic effects. We propose as a starting point for discussion that personality works via these two phenomena to increase risk for the development of another disorder. The validity of a personality-as-risk-factor model rests on demonstrating comorbidity and that the observed covariance is not merely coincident, but shares a real relationship, such as one due to a shared etiology. Second, validity depends on some form of gene–environment correlation—that is, genetically based personality traits help create or modify environments thought to increase the risk for a particular psychopathology. The third step is to show that the environment that personality helped shape "triggers" the onset of another genetically based disease. For example, people high on the genetically based personality trait of sensation seeking prefer an urban (as opposed to rural) lifestyle where alcohol and other substances are readily available. The accessibility of alcohol could trigger the onset of genetically based alcoholism via the mechanism of gene–environment interaction.

To our knowledge, there is no single study that demonstrates all three processes at this time, partly due to limitations in the methods used by researchers to actually test for gene–environment interaction or correlation. Presently, the behavior-genetic literature contains several smaller studies that illustrate one or two steps in the process. A case in point is *posttrau-*

matic stress disorder (PTSD), where there is some evidence for genetically based aspects of personality influencing the environments (gene–environment correlation) important to the onset of PTSD.

Gene–Environment Correlation

The PTSD literature has recently emerged as a good place to find evidence— clinical studies that could be followed up by behavior-genetic examination— that personality modifies the risk of developing additional psychiatric disorder. For example, Koenen et al. (2002) reported that preexisting conduct disorder in males (considered an early manifestation of antisocial personality) was predictive of both trauma exposure and subsequent PTSD symptoms, using data from veterans of the Vietnam War. From a behavior-genetic perspective, the first step in testing the validity of the personality-as-risk model is to show that PTSD and personality share a common etiological basis. A series of heritability studies of twins who were veterans of the Vietnam War have (e.g., True et al., 1993) shown that like personality, PTSD has a heritable basis. For example, the estimated heritability (h^2) of DSM-III and DSM-III-R PTSD symptoms (e.g., traumatic events are persistently reexperienced, persistent avoidance of stimuli associated with trauma or numbing of general responsiveness, persistent symptoms of increased arousal) ranged from 32 to 45% (True et al., 1993). Moreover, these estimates did not vary when the sample was split into groups of twins who had served in Southeast Asia and those who had not. This suggests that PTSD is not a disorder solely associated with military service (e.g., combat) and that any form of trauma, such as assault, natural disaster, car accident or significant negative life event, can also trigger symptoms.

Stein, Jang, Taylor, Vernon, and Livesley (2002) reported similar findings on a general population sample of 222 MZ and 184 DZ twin pairs recruited in Canada on lifetime exposure to traumatic events and their characteristic responses. The twins were asked to report their experiences on several classes of traumatic events that ranged from sexual assault to car accidents to the death of a close family member or friend. Being a Canadian sample, virtually no twin had been in combat, but 75.4% of the total sample had experienced one or more of the other events. These twins were surveyed on DSM-IV PTSD Cluster B through D symptoms and, as with the study of combat veterans, the h^2 of reexperiencing the event was 36%, avoidance of places associated with the trauma was 28%, feeling numb was 36%, and being hyperaroused was 29%. This study also investigated whether *exposure* to traumatic events has a heritable basis. The types of traumatic events surveyed were submitted to factor analysis that extracted two factors. The first described "assaultive events" (robbery; held captive;

beat up; sexual assault; other life threat) and the second "nonassaultive events" (sudden family death; motor vehicle accident; fire; and tornado, flood, or earthquake). The heritability of assaultive trauma exposure (using data from all subjects; that is, whether or not any trauma was experienced) was $h^2 = 20.3\%$, $c^2 = 21.3\%$, and $e^2 = 58.4\%$. In contrast, a purely environmental model provided the best explanation of liability to exposure to nonassaultive trauma: $c^2 = 38.6\%$ and $e^2 = 61.5\%$. It was also found that PTSD symptoms and the experience of assaultive trauma were inextricably linked by a common set of genetic factors, as the r_G's between exposure to assaultive trauma and PTSD symptoms ranged from 0.71 to 0.83.

The finding that exposure to events is mediated by genetic factors is not a novel finding. For example, Kendler, Heath, Neale, and Kessler (1993) showed that certain kinds of life events have a genetic basis. Specifically, "personal events" (events that primarily impacted the respondent), not "network events" describing events that had a primary impact on individuals in the respondent's social network (e.g., a death, illness/injury to member of the network), were heritable. For example, for personal events such as experiencing marital difficulties, $h^2 = 14\%$; being robbed/assaulted $= 33\%$; interpersonal difficulties $= 39\%$; having financial problems $= 18\%$ with $c^2 = 21\%$; illness/injury $= 21\%$ and having problems at work $= 18\%$ with $c^2 = 21\%$. In contrast, network events were not heritable, with c^2 effects being accountable for 32% to 45% of the variability and e^2 accounting for the remainder.

The heritability studies have established that (1) PTSD symptoms are heritable; (2) exposure to assaultive events is heritable; and (3) the genes influencing symptoms and exposure share a common genetic basis. This suggests that specific interpersonal events are partially under genetic control, but it is unlikely that the event per se is heritable. Rather, given that the genetic bases of both PTSD and personality are established (and permit the possibility of sharing a common basis), it is now possible to hypothesize that what is more likely to be inherited are *factors that influence the person's risk for placing oneself in, or creating, potentially hazardous situations*. It is here we get to the crux of the risk model of association. Clinical research has shown that personality traits, particularly neuroticism, have been implicated in playing this role in PTSD (e.g., Fauerbach, Lawrence, Schmidt, Munster, & Costa, 2000), whereas other traits, such as sensation seeking, have been associated with increased risk for being a victim of rape (e.g., Kilpatrick, Resnick, Saunders, & Best, 1998).

One of the behavior-genetic mechanisms underlying this phenomenon is called *gene–environment correlation* in which genetically influenced factors (such as personality) influence the probability of exposure to adverse events critical to the development of specific psychopathology. Three general types of genotype–environment correlation have been hypothesized: *passive*, *reactive*, and *active* (Plomin, DeFries, & Loehlin, 1977). Passive genotype–environment correlation occurs because children share heredity and environments with their parents and can thus passively inherit environments correlated with their genetic propensities. Reactive genotype–environment correlation refers to experiences of the child derived from others' reactions to the child's genetic propensities. Active genotype–environment correlation is known as "niche building" or "niche picking" (Plomin, DeFries, & McClearn, 1990, p. 251). This occurs when children actively select or create environments that are commensurate with their underlying genetic propensities.

It is also important to note that the term gene–environment correlation is used in the literature to explain the theoretical situations described immediately above but also to describe findings that many measures of the environment are heritable (see Plomin & Daniels, 1987; Vernon, Jang, Harris, & McCarthy, 1997), and this genetic basis is shared to some extent with other genetically based behavior (see also Jang, 2005). In the case of PTSD, support for such a role for personality was indicated by significant genetic correlations between assaultive trauma and personality variables (Jang et al., 2003)—specifically, the genetic correlations between assaultive trauma and the personality disorder trait scales juvenile antisocial behavior (.22) and self-damaging acts (.24), as well as normal personality trait measures such as the NEO Five Factor Inventory's (Costa & McCrae, 1992) Openness to Experience (.14) and the Revised Eysenck Personality Questionnaire's Psychoticism (EPQ-R; Eysenck & Eysenck, 1992) scale (.36). These findings suggest that personality traits increase the risk for developing PTSD by placing individuals in higher-risk situations.

Other examples include Saudino, Petersen, Lichtenstein, and McClearn's (1997) study that showed that all genetic variance on controllable, desirable, and undesirable life events in women were in common to the genetic influences underlying EPQ-R Neuroticism and Extraversion, and NEO-FFI Openness to Experience. Similarly, Jang, Vernon, and Livesley (2000) showed that perceptions of family environment (assessed using the Family Environment Scale [FES]; Moos & Moos, 1974) and personality dysfunction shared a substantial genetic basis. In particular, inhibitedness was found to share a common heritable basis with perceptions of family cohesiveness ($r_G = -.39$), achievement orientation of the family ($r_G = -.58$), and intellectual-cultural orientation of the family ($r_G = -.38$). Emotional lability influenced family cohesiveness ($r_G = -.45$), and antisocial behavior was related to achievement orientation of the family ($r_G = .38$). In short, the broad phenomenon of gene–environment correlation suggests that genetically based personality factors influence the probability of exposure to adverse events, which increases the risk for the development of a disorder.

Gene–Environment Interaction

Another way personality can increase the risk for disorder is via the mechanism of *gene–environment interaction* (G × E; Plomin, DeFries, & Loehlin, 1977). Briefly, G × E is environmental control or modulation of genetic effects. One way its presence is tested is to demonstrate that estimates of h^2, c^2, and e^2 are shown to vary over different levels of environmental condition. Heath, Eaves, and Martin (1989) tested whether being married (marital status) or being in a marriage-like relationship moderates the genetic basis of drinking habits. The study sample was 1,233 MZ and 751 DZ female adult same-sex twin pairs from Australia who were interviewed on the details of total weekly alcohol consumption. This consisted of reported beer, wine, spirits, or sherry consumption measured in standard drink sizes (7 ounces in the case of beer, 4 ounces of wine, 1 ounce of spirits) for each day of the preceding 7-day week. Current marital status information was obtained (single, widowed, married, living together, divorced, or remarried) and was recoded as unmarried (single, separated, divorced, or widowed) or as married (married and living together). The twins were further subdivided into two age cohorts. The first consisted of younger adults (ages 30 years or less) and the other of older adults (ages 31 years and greater).

To test for gene–environment interaction effects, the magnitude of h^2, c^2, and e^2 conditional upon environmental exposure was estimated— married versus unmarried status. In a model where there are no gene–environment interaction effects, estimates of h^2, c^2 or e^2 should not significantly differ between married and unmarried twins. If gene–environment interaction effects are present, it is expected that estimates of h^2, c^2, or e^2 should vary significantly between married and unmarried twins. The results were clear—marital status does moderate (decreases) genetic influences on alcohol consumption. In the younger adult cohort, $h^2 = 60\%$ for unmarried twins as compared to married twins, where $h^2 = 31\%$. In the older adult cohort, h^2 for unmarried twins was estimated at 76%, whereas in married twins $h^2 = 59\%$. When the older and younger cohorts were combined, $h^2 = 77\%$ for unmarried twins and 59% for the married twins.

G × E effects are also demonstrated by showing that more individuals who possess a specific genetic polymorphism (a particular form of a gene implicated in a particular disorder) *and* have been exposed to specific environmental conditions (e.g., subjected to high levels of parental mistreatment) develop a disorder as compared to individuals who possess just the polymorphism *or* have only been exposed to the salient environmental conditions. One of the most dramatic examples of gene–environment interaction is Caspi, McClay, and Moffitt's (2002) study of the development of antisocial behavior. Clinical research has identified abuse as a child, such as erratic, coercive, and punitive parenting, as one of the major risk factors for the development of antisocial behavior in boys and has concluded that the risk for conduct disorder increases the earlier the abuse begins. However, there is often little 1-to-1 correspondence between environmental conditions and phenotype, so the presence of a genetic liability for the disorder must be involved. In the case of antisocial behavior, the monoamine oxidase A gene (MAOA gene Xp11.23–11.4) was selected because it has been associated with aggressive behavior in mice and in some human studies. This sample consisted of 1,037 children who had been assessed at nine different ages for levels of maltreatment (no maltreatment, probable maltreatment, and severe maltreatment) and MAOA activity (low or high activity). They found that the effect of maltreatment was significantly weaker among males with high MAOA activity than those with low activity. Moreover, the probable and high maltreatment group did not differ in MAOA activity, indicating that the genotype did not influence exposure to maltreatment. These results demonstrate that the MAOA gene modifies the influence of maltreatment.

G × E effects are crucial to the personality-as-risk model because it is possible the environmental condition that personality shaped via gene–environment correlation actually "triggers" or activates the underlying genetic liability for another disorder, such as alcoholism. There is some evidence for each of these processes in the literature. First of all, at the phenotypic level, a huge number of clinical studies show that personality variables, particularly those related to antisocial personality, neuroticism, and extraversion, are related to alcohol initiation, abuse and dependence. For example, Heath et al. (1997) examined the association of personality as measured by the EPQ and TPQ, lifetime DSM-III-R Axis I disorders, and DSM-III-R alcohol dependence risk in females and males. Among women, they found that the risk for alcohol dependence was predicted by history of childhood conduct disorder (odds ratio [OR] = 4.6), lifetime history of major depression (OR = 2.1), and high scores on EPQ Extraversion (OR = 1.6), Neuroticism (OR = 1.6), Cloninger's Tridimensional Personality Questionnaire Novelty Seeking scale (OR = 1.6) and scores on social nonconformity measures (OR = 1.9). For men, the same factors predicted alcohol dependence, differing only in terms of magnitude. For example, among males, the association with a history of childhood conduct disorder is somewhat less (OR = 1.9) but greater on EPQ-R Neuroticism (OR = 1.9) as compared to women.

The next step in testing the personality-as-risk model is to introduce behavior-genetic ideas into the relationship and show that the two domains are linked by a common etiology, verifying that personality plays a significant role in alcohol use problems. For example, Slutske et al. (2002) showed that the genetic influences underlying "behavioral undercontrol" (a composite derived from the TPQ Novelty Seeking, EPQ-R Psychoticism, and reverse-coded EPQ-R Lie scales—a dimension representing antisocial behavior) were shared with alcohol dependence in a large sample of Australian twin pairs. Specifically, among males between behavioral undercontrol and alcohol dependence, r_G = .53 (95% CI = .38–.67) and among females, r_G = .71 (95% confidence interval [CI] = .56–.86). They also found that a history of childhood conduct disorder shared a common basis with later alcohol dependence: among males r_G = .59 (95% CI = .45–.72), and among females r_G = .59 (95% CI = .50–.85). In fact, together behavioral undercontrol and childhood conduct disorder accounted for 85% (95% CI = 54% to 100%) of the variability of alcohol dependence in males and 93% (95% CI = 59–100%) in females.

The third step would be to show that personality (and incidentally other genes that may influence alcohol use as well) direct the selection of environments (gene–environment correlation) that provide the essential conditions and experiences that eventually trigger the genetic liability for alcoholism and subsequent onset of the disorder (gene–environment interaction). There is some evidence of gene–environment correlation for alcohol problems, specifically, that perceptions of the family environment are influenced by genetic influences underlying traits delineating personality disorder (Jang, Vernon, & Livesley, 2000). Perceptions of family cohesiveness are significantly related to alcohol misuse (r_G = –.30) and trait inhibition (r_G = –.39); family achievement orientation was related to both alcohol misuse (r_G = –.56) and antisocial personality (r_G = .38) and trait inhibition (r_G = –.56). Other research has shown that genetic factors underlying alcohol use are associated with some purely environmental factors such as decreases in family moral-religious emphases, family cohesion, task orientation at school, and increases in strictness in the classroom (Jang, Vernon, Livesley, Stein, & Wolf, 2001).

The final step, evidence that those environments would moderate the genetic liability for alcoholism, has also been found for alcohol use problems. In our hypothetical example at the beginning of this section, it was suggested that availability of alcohol may be enough to trigger genetically based alcohol use problems. This general idea has been supported by a number of recent papers. For example, Dick, Rose, Viken, Kaprio, and Koskenvuo (2001) examined regional residency effects on longitudinal influences on alcohol use. In this study, longitudinal data on drinking frequency were obtained from adolescents when they were ages 16, 17, and 18.5 years. Heritability analyses over the three ages showed that genetic factors influencing drinking patterns increased over the 30-month period. At age 16, 17 and 18.5 years, the h^2 for drinking frequency was reported to account for 33%, 49%, and 50% of the total variance; c^2 influences accounted for 37%, 20%, 14%, respectively, with e^2 accounting for 29%, 30%, and 36%.

When the estimates are crossed with area of residency, a clear genotype by environment interaction was detected. Despite the distributions of drinking frequencies in twins residing in urban and rural areas being highly similar, the influences on drinking varied between the two environments. Genetic factors assumed a larger role among adolescents residing in urban areas, while shared environmental influences were more important in rural settings. However, they also found that urban and rural settings appear to moderate genetic and environmental influences on adolescent drinking *without* altering drinking frequencies. They point to the fact that there is no effect of residency on (1) observed abstinence rates and (2) drinking frequency among nonabstinent adolescents, but yet find that urban/rural residency significantly modulates h^2 and c^2 influences on alcohol use. This suggests that environmental effects on mean effects are different from the moderating effect of the environment—urban areas may not necessarily encourage adolescents to initiate drinking earlier, to drink more frequently, or to drink greater quantities, but urban areas provide the opportunities for those who are genetically predisposed to engage in drinking to do so. At the same time, the diversity of the urban environment enables adolescents who abstain from drinking (or drink rarely) to find like-minded and supportive peers. In rural areas, environmental influences tend to cluster between communities and thus between families, which are then detected as c^2 effects. The exact nature of the environmental effects needs to be more closely examined. Area of residence is likely a proxy variable for other effects. It was suggested that the Finnish urban–rural split represents several environmental variables such as ease of access to liquor stores; regional variation in levels of community and familial control of adolescent drinking; availability of extended networks of peers; urban and rural adolescents in Finland experiencing quite different exposure to public drinking and intoxication; and well-documented historical and regional differences in religious values and behavior.

Another moderating effect of genetically based alcohol use is religion. Koopmans et al. (1999) showed that genetic variability to initiation of alcohol use varies with religious involvement. In a large sample of Dutch adolescent twin pairs (MZ males = 327, MZ females = 457, DZ males = 284, DZ females = 356, DZ opposite-sex = 543 pairs) initiation of alcohol use was measured, and also whether the probands were currently active in church or reported they were religious but not active in church. They found that the heritability on risk of alcohol use initiation was higher in families without a religious upbringing than in families with it. They also reported that among religious males the heritability of alcohol use was lower than in nonreligious males: $h^2 = 25\%$, $c^2 = 67\%$, and $e^2 = 7\%$ to $h^2 = 40\%$, $c^2 = 47\%$, and $e^2 = 13\%$. Among religious females $h^2 = 0\%$, $c^2 = 88\%$, and $e^2 = 12\%$, and among nonreligious females $h^2 = 39\%$, $c^2 = 56\%$, and $e^2 = 5\%$.

This study also reported that an important aspect of antisocial personality, "behavioral disinhibition," was significantly correlated with alcohol use ($r = .46$ in males and $r = .41$ in females) and that heritability of behavioral disinhibition was significantly greater among those who reported less religious involvement. Koopmans, Slutske, Van Baal, and Boomsma (1999) conclude that genetic influences for disinhibited behavior (which includes heavier and problematic alcohol use) among more religious individuals are attenuated because one's decision on how to behave is based less on personal choice and more on family circumstances or religious proscriptions (p. 446). Thus, religious upbringing not only reduces the impact of genotype on disinhibited behavior but also reduces genetic influences on initiation.

The preceding discussion is one possible way behavior-genetic concepts might be used to test the veracity of the personality-as-risk model. It should be noted that picking and choosing of research from different studies to find evidence of bivariate heritability, gene–environment correlation and interaction provides circumstantial evidence that personality increases the risk for alcohol use problems. An important next step is to be able to test all of these steps within a single comprehensive study using a single set of variables.

PSYCHOPATHOLOGY AS THE EXTREMES OF PERSONALITY FUNCTION

The *spectrum model* hypothesizes that many psychiatric disorders are best conceptualized as extremes of personality. A body of research supports this idea. For example, Trull, Waudby, and Sher (2004) showed that DSM-IV Cluster B personality disorder symptoms (particularly antisocial and borderline disorder symptoms) were consistently associated with alcohol use disorders in a nonclinical sample of 395 young adults. Most interestingly, however, their analyses showed that Cluster B symptoms were significantly associated with alcohol use disorders *above and beyond* what was accounted for by normal personality traits, suggesting that personality disorder symptoms predict unique variance in substance use disorders that reflects maladaptive aspects of personality. The basic ideas underlying a spectrum model are commonly used to explain the development of many disorders, such as schizophrenia. For example, Meehl (1989) suggested that the concept of *schizotaxia* is a form of a spectrum disorder. In his model, schizotaxia describes a genetically based neural defect that either can manifest itself as abnormal personality under ordinary social learning paradigms *or* can develop into schizophrenia when triggered by some major aversive event, childhood trauma, or adult misfortune (p. 935).

As with the risk model discussed above, a critical starting point of the spectrum model is that personality and the other disorder can be shown to share a common etiological basis. However, one possible way of differentiating between the risk and the spectrum model is the degree to which personality and the other disorder share a common genetic basis and how this shared etiology is structured. This next section examines some basic multivariate behavior-genetic models as a starting point for discussion and research on how spectrum models could be tested and distinguished from risk models of psychopathology. It should be clarified at the outset that currently the distinction between the spectrum and risk models is not all that clear if personality and another disorder share a common genetic basis. However, setting conditions on its structure may provide clues regarding the function of personality in a particular disorder.

Behavior-genetic methods have two basic models to represent the different organization or structure of variables. Figure 6.1 illustrates one organization known as the *common pathways model*. The figure is divided into three sections marked A, B, and C. Focusing attention on section B (labeled the "phenotypic factor model"), the boxes in the diagram contain the actual scores measured on a sample of people. Taking the example of schizotaxia, the three boxes can contain personality trait scales such as Eysenck's neuroticism (N) and psychoticism (PSY) and the presence or absence of schizophrenia (SCHIZ). The most important aspect of this figure from the perspective of the spectrum model is the higher-order construct, P, which mediates 100% of the covariance of N, PSY, and SCHIZ. Note that the existence of P is unmeasured and is inferred by the degree to which the measured variables appear together.

This portion of Figure 6.1 is the same as a contemporary factor analysis model. However, the addition of genetic and environmental influences to P (section A of the diagram labeled "genetic and environmental factors in common to all variables") and N, PSY, SCHIZ (section C labeled "genetic and environmental factors unique to each variable") transforms the construct P into a veridical entity that has a basis in biology. Evidence of an independently heritable P constitutes basic personality liability and would provide additional support for the spectrum model. Section C allows for the possibility that each disorder is also influenced by environmental and genetic factors specific to each, but the main point for the spectrum model is that a central genetically based liability rooted in personality underlies other psychopathology.

In contrast, Figure 6.2 illustrates what behavioral geneticists call the "independent pathways model." Although both models hypothesize that personality and psychopathology share a common genetic basis, the primary difference between the independent and common pathway models is that no independently inherited P is required to explain the covariation be-

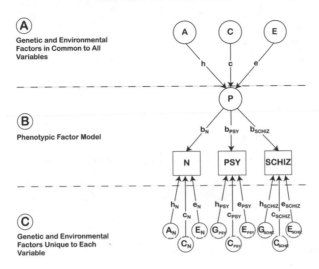

FIGURE 6.1. Common Pathways Model.

tween personality traits and schizophrenia in this example. In fact, the independent pathways model allows for several different genetic factors to influence both personality and other psychopathology, and permits the situation in which the observed covariance between personality and other psychopathology is not necessarily attributable to a common genetic basis at all. It is certainly a less stringent model than the common pathways model that requires that the observed covariance between personality and psychopathology comes from a single etiological source. As such, the ability of a common pathway model to explain the covariance between personality and psychopathology compared to an independent pathway model emerges as better evidence for the validity of a spectrum over a risk model.

Potential evidence for the spectrum model has come from work examining the comorbidity of the major psychiatric disorders. Phenotypically, work by Krueger (1999) has shown that the comorbidity of 10 DSM-III-R common mental disorders can be sorted into two latent higher-order constructs that describe disorders directed inward toward oneself as opposed to disorders that are directed outward. The first latent factor was named "Anxious Misery" because it primarily accounts for the relationship between major depressive episode, dysthymia, and generalized anxiety disorder. The second factor, labeled "Fear," describes the covariation between social phobia, simple phobia, agoraphobia, and panic disorder. The Fear and Anxious-Misery factors are really lower-order factors whose relationship was explained by a higher-order factor labeled "Internalizing" because together they represent disorders that are expressed primarily inward. In

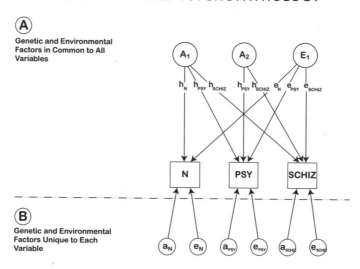

FIGURE 6.2. Independent Pathways Model.

contrast, the covariation between alcohol dependence, drug dependence, and antisocial personality disorder was accounted for by a single factor labeled "Externalizing" because it described maladjustment that is expressed primarily outward as antisocial, disruptive behavior. A path between Internalizing and Externalizing factors was also necessary to account for any comorbidity between all 10 disorders. Vollebergh and colleagues (2001) found a highly similar structure in data from the Netherlands Mental Health Survey and Incidence Study. Moreover, they also found that this three-factor model was stable over a 12-month period.

Do these factors like Internalizing and Externalizing represent genetically homogeneous entities as required by the spectrum model? Krueger et al. (2002) surveyed a sample of twin pairs on DSM-III-R alcohol dependence, drug dependence, adolescent antisocial behavior, and conduct disorder. Antisocial personality was assessed using adolescent antisocial behavior and conduct disorder variables. They fitted a variety of genetic models to the data and found that a one-factor common pathway genetic model (similar in form to Figure 6.1) provided the best explanation for the covariation of these measures, suggesting that the externalizing disorders are inherited as a single genetically based syndrome.

However, despite Krueger et al.'s (2002) report that the fit of the one-factor common pathways model provided a superior fit to any of the other models (e.g., models that did not include *P*), there remain some lingering doubts as to whether or not this model really does provide the best explanation. One point to remember about path analysis is that the best-fitting model is only one of many possible models that can provide a satisfactory fit. For example, Kendler, Prescott, Myers, and Neale (2003) found that the Internalizing and Externalizing factors are not inherited as a single genetically based syndrome. In this study, 5,600 twins were interviewed on the rate of lifetime DSM-III-R diagnoses for major depression, generalized anxiety disorder, adult antisocial behavior and conduct disorder, any phobia, DSM-IV alcohol dependence, and drug abuse/dependence. They showed that multiple genetic and environmental factors directly influenced each disorder.

So, which is correct? Are syndromes inherited as a unitary entity, or are they convenient names for frequently comorbid disorders that share a common genetic basis? These two studies highlight important strengths and weaknesses of the genetic models used to study comorbidity. On the one hand, the models explain why comorbidity exists and provides, in principle, the means to study the organization of variables. Conversely, they illustrate the phenomenon that two divergent models can provide an equally satisfactory explanation to the same data. A recent multivariate genetic analysis of behavioral disinhibition by Young, Stallings, Corley, Krauter, and Hewitt (2000) nicely illustrates this phenomenon. Levels of substance experimentation, novelty seeking, and DSM-IV symptom counts for conduct disorder and attention-deficit/hyperactivity disorder (ADHD) were assessed on a sample of nearly 400 adolescent twin pairs. Multivariate genetic model-fitting analyses found that either a one-factor common pathways model or a one-factor genetic independent pathway provided an equally good explanation of the covariance between these disorders. In the end, they selected the common pathways model because "this is a more parsimonious model than the independent pathway model and shows no significant decrement in fit by X^2 difference test" (Young et al., 2000, pp. 690–691). One area of behavioral genetics that probably requires more attention is the development of criteria to guide selection between equally well-fitting models. Presently, when statistical guidance is lacking, the choice of model becomes (1) arbitrary, (2) based on one's own theoretical preferences, or (3) based on the principle of parsimony—in which the model with the fewest parameters is the simplest.

THE SCAR MODEL

Last but not least is the scar model. In this model, personality changes are the result of the development of psychopathology and do not contribute to onset. One of the most important elements for a test of the scar model is the element of *time*, specifically, that significant personality changes do not predate the onset of the disorder. Support for the scar model has come from clinical research on Alzheimer's disease, where significant personality change tends to follow the onset of the disorder (Copeland et al., 2003). However, as behavioral genetic research suggests, this may not be sufficient. Referring back to Equation 1, the phenotype represents the *sum* of genetic and environmental action, and it should be clear that genetic factors underlying personality can substantially increase the risk for the development of another disorder, although not reflected in the phenotype. As such, a significant genetic correlation can exist between two variables, but because environmental factors can work in the opposite direction (i.e., r_E is negative), the sum of these effects reflected in phenotypic correlation is zero (Carey, 1999), suggesting that the two variables are unrelated when in fact they are related.

What is important is to examine genetic and environmental influences in the context of time. Longitudinal behavioral genetic research has shown that different etiological factors can operate at different times during development. For example, using data from the well-known Nonshared Environment in Adolescent Development (NEAD) project, Neiderhiser, Reiss, & Hetherington (1996) examined the genetic and environmental factors underlying the development of adolescent adjustment 3 years apart on a sample of 395 families. The first measurement assessed the families during early and the second during middle adolescence. Composite measures of parent reports, adolescent self-reports, and observer ratings of adolescent adjustment (specifically antisocial behavior, autonomy, and social responsibility) were examined. Each one of the three domains was found to have a different pattern of genetic and environmental contributions to stability and change, suggesting that each domain of adolescent adjustment takes different developmental pathways. For example, genetic influences were important for both change and stability in antisocial behavior. Stability in social responsibility, however, was primarily influenced by genetic factors, while nonshared environmental factors were predominantly responsible for change. Finally, genetic and shared environmental influences contributed nearly equally to stability and change in autonomous functioning. Implications from longitudinal studies such as these emphasize the utility of behavior-genetic approaches in explicating the genetic and environmental contributions to developmental pathways that predispose to psychopathology.

CONCLUSIONS

It seems certain that some link exists between personality and psychopathology. It is unclear what role personality plays in different psychopathology, and traditional research methodologies that work solely at the level of the phenotype can produce conflicting results. This chapter suggests that behavior-genetic methods can be used as a means to investigate the role of personality. The concepts of behavior genetics, particularly the concepts of genetic correlation, gene–environment correlation and interaction, and multivariate models such as common and independent pathways models provide a promising approach in answering questions regarding the mechanisms underlying the classic risk, spectrum, and scar models. However, it is important to emphasize that the ideas presented in this chapter are just that—ideas raised to start integrating these domains. There is no doubt that several variations on these ideas exist or can be conceptualized. The major aim of this chapter is to generate discussion on how to understand the ubiquitous relationship between personality and psychopathology.

REFERENCES

American Psychiatric Association. (1994). *Diagnostic and statistical manual of mental disorders* (4th ed.). Washington, DC: Author.

Carey, W. B. (1999). Problems in diagnosing attention and activity. *Pediatrics, 103,* 664–667.

Caspi, A., McClay, J., & Moffitt, T. (2002). Role of genotype in the cycle of violence in maltreated children. *Science, 297*(5582), 851–854.

Copeland, M. P., Daly, E., & Hines, V., Mastromauro, C., Zaitchik, D., Gunther, J., et al. (2003). Psychiatric symptomatology and prodromal Alzheimer's disease. *Alzheimer Disease and Associated Disorders, 17*(1), 1–8.

Costa, P. T., & McCrae, R. R. (1992). *Revised NEO Personality Inventory and NEO Five-Factor Inventory.* Odessa, FL: Psychological Assessment Resources.

Dick, D. M., Rose, R. J., Viken, R. J., Kaprio, J., & Koskenvuo, M. (2001). Exploring gene–environment interactions: Socioregional moderation of alcohol use. *Journal of Abnormal Psychology, 110*(4), 625–632.

Eysenck, H. J., & Eysenck, S. B. G. (1992). *Manual for the Eysenck Personality Questionnaire—Revised.* San Diego, CA: Educational and Industrial Testing Service.

Fauerbach, J. A., Lawrence, J. W., Schmidt, C. W., Jr., Munster, A. M., & Costa, P. T., Jr. (2000). Personality predictors of injury-related posttraumatic stress disorder. *Journal of Nervous and Mental Disease, 188,* 510–517.

Heath, A. C., Bucholz, K. K., Madden, P. A. F., Dinwiddie, S. H., Slutske, W. S., Bierut, L. J., et al. (1997). Genetic and environmental contributions to alcohol dependence risk in a national twin sample: Consistency of findings in women and men. *Psychological Medicine, 27,* 1381–1396.

Heath, A. C., Eaves, L. J., & Martin, N. G. (1989). The genetic structure of personality: III. Multivariate genetic item analysis of the EPQ scales. *Personality and Individual Differences, 10,* 877–888.

Hetherington, E. M., Reiss, D., & Plomin, R. (Eds.). (1994). *Separate social worlds of siblings: The impact of nonshared environment on development.* Hillsdale, NJ: Erlbaum.

Jang, K. L. (2005). *Behavioral genetics of psychopathology: A clinical guide*. Mahwah, NJ: Erlbaum.

Jang, K. L., Stein, M. B., Taylor, S., Asmundson, G., & Livesley, W. J. (2003). Exposure to traumatic events and experience: Aetiological relationships with personality function. *Psychiatry Research, 120*, 61–69.

Jang, K. L., Vernon, P. A., & Livesley, W. J. (2000). Personality disorder traits, family environment, and alcohol misuse: A multivariate behavioural genetic analysis. *Addiction, 95*(6), 873–888.

Jang, K. L., Vernon, P. A., Livesley, W. J., Stein, M. B., & Wolf, H. (2001). Intra- and extra-familial influences on alcohol and drug misuse: A twin study of genetic–environmental correlations. *Addiction, 96*, 1307–1318.

Kendler, K. S. (1996). Major depression and generalized anxiety disorder: Same genes, (partly) different environments—Revisited. *British Journal of Psychiatry, 168*(Suppl. 30), 68–75.

Kendler, K. S., Heath, A. C., Neale, M. C., & Kessler, R. C. (1993). Alcoholism and major depression in women: A twin study of the causes of comorbidity. *Archives of General Psychiatry, 50*, 690–698.

Kendler, K. S., Prescott, C. A., Myers, J., & Neale, M. C. (2003). The structure of genetic and environmental risk factors for common psychiatric and substance use disorders in men and women. *Archives of General Psychiatry, 60*(9), 929–937.

Kilpatrick, D. G., Resnick, H. S., Saunders, B. E., & Best, C. L. (1998). Rape, other violence against women, and posttraumatic stress disorder. In B. P. Dohrenwend (Ed.), *Adversity, stress, and psychopathology* (pp. 161–176). London: Oxford University Press.

Koenen, K. C., Harley, R., Lyons, M. J., Wolfe, J., Simpson, J. C., Goldberg, J., et al. (2002). A twin registry study of familial and individual risk factors for trauma exposure and posttraumatic stress disorder. *Journal of Nervous and Mental Disease, 190*, 209–218.

Koopmans, J. R., Slutske, W. S., Van Baal, C. M., & Boomsma, D. I. (1999). The influence of religion on alcohol use initiation: Evidence for a genotype X environment interaction. *Behavior Genetics, 29*, 445–453.

Krueger, R. F. (1999). The structure of mental disorders. *Archives of General Psychiatry, 56*, 921–926.

Krueger, R. F., Hicks, B. M., Patrick, C. J., Carlson, S. R., Iacono, W. G., & McGue, M. (2002). Etiologic connections among substance dependence, antisocial behavior, and personality: Modeling the externalizing spectrum. *Journal of Abnormal Psychology, 111*, 411–424.

Krueger, R. F., & Tackett, J. L. (2003). Personality and psychopathology: Working toward the bigger picture. *Journal of Personality Disorders, 17*(2), 109–128.

Lewinsohn, P. M., Steinmetz, J. L., Larson, D. W., & Franklin, J. (1981). Depression related cognitions: Antecedents and consequence. *Journal of Abnormal Psychology, 3*, 213–219.

Lysaker, P. H., Bell, M. D., Kaplan, E., Greig, T. C., & Bryson, G. J. (1999). Personality and psychopathology in schizophrenia: The association between personality traits and symptoms. *Psychiatry: Interpersonal and Biological Processes, 62*, 36–48.

Meehl, P. E. (1989). Schizotaxia revisited. *Archives of General Psychiatry, 46*, 935–944.

Moos, R. H., & Moos, B. S. (1974). *Manual for the Family Environment Scale.* Palo Alto, CA: Consulting Psychologist Press.

Neale, M. C., & Cardon, L. R. (1992). *Methodology for genetic studies of twins and families.* London: Kluwer.

Neiderheiser, J. M., Reiss, D., & Hetherington, E. M. (1996). Genetically informative designs for distinguishing developmental pathways during adolescence: Responsible and antisocial behavior. *Development and Psychopathology, 8*(4), 779–791.

Plomin, R., & Daniels, D. (1987). Children in the same family are very different, but why? *Behavioral and Brain Sciences, 10,* 44–59.

Plomin, R., DeFries, J. C., & Loehlin, J. C. (1977). Genotype–environment interaction and correlation in the analysis of human behavior. *Psychological Bulletin, 84*(2), 309–322.

Plomin, R., DeFries, J. C., & McClearn, G. E. (1990). *Behavioral genetics: A primer* (2nd ed.). New York: Freeman.

Plomin, R., DeFries, J. C., McClearn, G. E., & Rutter, M. (1997). *Behavioral genetics* (3rd ed.). New York: Freeman.

Rothbart, M. K. (2004). Commentary: Differential measures of temperament and multiple pathways to childhood disorders. *Journal of Clinical Child and Adolescent Psychology, 33,* 82–87.

Saudino, K. J., Pedersen, N. L., Lichtenstein, P., & McClearn, G. E. (1997). Can personality explain genetic influences on life events? *Journal of Personality and Social Psychology, 72,* 196–206.

Slutske, W. S., Heath, A. C., Madden, P. A. F., Bucholz, K. K., Statham, D. J., & Martin, N. G. (2002). Personality and the genetic risk for alcohol dependence. *Journal of Abnormal Psychology, 111,* 124–133.

Stein, M. B., Jang, K. L., Taylor, S., Vernon, P. A., & Livesley, W. J. (2002). Genetic and environmental influences on trauma exposure and posttraumatic stress disorder symptoms: A twin study. *American Journal of Psychiatry, 159,* 1675–1681.

True, W. R., Rice, J., Eisen, S. A., Heath, A. C., Goldberg, J., Lyons, M. J., et al. (1993). A twin study of genetic and environmental contributions to liability for posttraumatic stress symptoms. *Archives of General Psychiatry, 50*(4), 257–264.

Trull, T. J., Waudby, C. J., & Sher, K. J. (2004). Alcohol, tobacco, and drug use disorders and personality disorder symptoms. *Experimental and Clinical Psychopharmacology, 12*(1), 65–75.

Vernon, P. A., Jang, K. L., Harris, J. A., & McCarthy, J. M. (1997). Environmental predictors of personality differences: A twin and sibling study. *Journal of Personality and Social Psychology, 72,* 177–183.

Vollebergh, W. A. M., Iedema, J., Bijl, R. V., de Graaf, R., Smitt, F., & Ormel, J. (2001). The structure and stability of common mental disorders: The NEMESIS Study. *Archives of General Psychiatry, 58,* 597–603.

Young, S. E., Stallings, M. C., Corley, R. P., Krauter, M. P., & Hewitt, J. K. (2000). Genetic and environmental influences on behavioral disinhibition. *American Journal of Medical Genetics, 96,* 684–695.

Zimmerman, M., Chelminski, J., & McDermut, W. (2002). Major depressive disorder and axis I diagnostic comorbidity. *Journal of Clinical Psychiatry, 68,* 178–193.

Chapter 7

The Construct of Emotion as a Bridge between Personality and Psychopathology

CHRISTOPHER J. PATRICK
EDWARD M. BERNAT

Traditionally, mental disorders have been conceptualized as categorical en
tities into which individuals can be discretely classified. This is the conceptualization on which our current diagnostic nomenclature, the text revision
of the fourth edition of the *Diagnostic and Statistical Manual of Mental
Disorders* (DSM-IV-TR; American Psychiatric Association, 2000), is based.
However, this conceptualization is challenged by the systematic comorbidity
that is known to exist among various psychopathological syndromes within
the DSM (see Clark, Watson, & Reynolds, 1995; Wittchen, 1996). In fact,
recent quantitative structural analyses of the most prevalent mental disorders have revealed two broad spectra of disorders within the DSM: an internalizing spectrum encompassing mood and anxiety disorders and an
externalizing spectrum encompassing child and adult antisocial deviance
and substance abuse/dependence (Kendler, Prescott, Myers, & Neale, 2003;
Krueger, 1999a; Krueger, Caspi, Moffit, & Silva, 1998).[1] Within each of
these spectra, there is a large common factor that disorders share—that is,
reflecting the systematic covariance among them.

An important implication of this finding is that disorders within each of these spectra may arise in part from some common core psychopathological process (see Krueger et al., 1998) that confers a general vulnerability to such disorders. In addition, there may be specific etiological influences that contribute to the unique symptom picture associated with each disorder (e.g., the preoccupation with interpersonal evaluation that is characteristic of social phobia versus the unpredictable episodes of intense physiological hyperarousal associated with panic disorder). This conceptualization has been formalized in recently proposed hierarchical models of the internalizing (Mineka, Watson, & Clark, 1998; Watson, 2005) and externalizing spectra (Krueger et al., 2002). These models propose that there is a broad trait-dispositional factor that disorders within a spectrum share, along with specific etiological influences that determine the unique symptomatic expression of each disorder.

What is the nature of the core underlying processes that account for the shared variance among disorders within internalizing and externalizing spectra? One perspective is that basic personality traits underlie this covariance. For example, the common factor that anxiety disorders and depression share has been interpreted as reflecting the broad personality factor of negative affectivity (Clark & Watson, 1991) or negative emotionality (Tellegen, 1985). In the case of externalizing disorders, there is evidence that a separate trait dimension of impulsivity/disinhibition (Sher & Trull, 1994) or low constraint (Krueger, 1999b) is crucial. However, it is not clear that personality traits can be regarded as more basic etiologically than psychopathological symptoms (Widiger, Verheul, & van den Brink, 1999). Instead, it may be that personality traits like negative affectivity and impulsivity/low constraint are simply alternative phenotypic indicators of the core processes that underlie broad factors of psychopathology (see Krueger et al., 2002).

The position advanced here is that the common and unique elements of disorders within the DSM can be best be understood in terms of underlying brain systems that govern cognitive-affective processing and behavioral control. Our perspective is that individual differences in the functioning of these systems are crucial to an understanding of normal personality dispositions and psychopathological syndromes and to an understanding of links between personality and psychopathology. The primary focus of our review is on brain systems related to emotional reactivity and affective–behavioral control. We believe these functions are of particular relevance to internalizing and externalizing disorders insofar as these disorders involve dysfunction in emotional processing and in the ability to regulate emotional reactivity and to control behavior. We consider how brain motivational systems and individual differences in the functioning of these systems might contribute to these forms of psychopathology and the personality traits with which they are associated. Our formulation emphasizes the functional, action mobilization component of emotion—the component that is most directly assessable, via efferent–physiological response (Lang, Bradley, & Cuthbert, 1990). We argue that a perspective that emphasizes basic brain functions of emotional reactivity and emotional control can lead to new and valuable ways of thinking about the structure of personality and its relationship to psychopathology.

PRIMARY MOTIVATIONAL SYSTEMS

During the 1950s and 1960s, the dominant perspective among psychological theorists interested in emotion and its measurement was the unitary activation perspective. One of the leading figures in this area was Donald Lindsley. Influenced by Morruzi and Magoun's (1949) discovery of the general arousal function of the brainstem reticular formation, Lindsley (1951) advanced an activation theory of emotion in which general level of cortical arousal was considered to be the major determinant of motivational drive. In this model, sympathetic activation and the intensity of expressed emotion were presumed to increase as the level of cortical arousal increased—with the implication that autonomic (electrodermal, cardiovascular) and EEG activity could be used to directly index the main component of emotion, overall drive state. Influenced by this work, Eysenck (1967) incorporated individual differences in arousal (RAS) system functioning into his early neurobiological theory of personality (i.e., as the underlying basis for his extraversion [E] dimension)—which served as inspiration for subsequent biologically based models of personality by Gray (1987), Zuckerman (1979), and others (see the later section titled "Individual Differences in Affective Reactivity and Regulation: Bridging Personality and Psychopathology").

In contrast with this, the prevailing perspective among contemporary emotion theorists is that affective states are differentiated at a basic functional level—that is, distinctive brain activation systems underlie positive-appetitive and negative-defensive emotions. These brain motivational systems are viewed as having evolved through the process of natural selection to promote approach toward life-sustaining opportunities (e.g., nourishment, shelter, reproduction) or withdrawal from life-threatening situations, respectively (Izard, 1993; Lang, 1995; Plutchik, 1984). A number of lines of evidence have contributed to this perspective. Early ethological work by T. C. Schneirla (1959) revealed two general themes in the motivational behavior of animals of a variety of species, corresponding to approach and withdrawal tendencies. Related to this, Konorski (1967) undertook a detailed analysis of exteroceptive reflexes in mammals and concluded that these could be grouped into two fundamental classes, appetitive and defensive, mediated by distinct but interacting brain systems. Subsequently, on the basis of surgical and pharmacological studies with animals, Gray (1987) postulated the existence of distinctive brain systems mediating reward ("behavioral activation system") and punishment learning ("behavioral inhibition system"). Foreshadowing affect-oriented theories of personality (see Watson, Kotov, & Gamez, Chapter 2, this volume), Gray postulated that these same motivational systems anchor major dimensions of personality in humans and contribute to the presence or absence of psychopathology.

The idea of distinctive substrates for positive and negative emotion has also emerged from studies of the structure of self-reported affect in humans. Specifically, factor analyses of verbal descriptors of mood or emotion have consistently revealed two broad dimensions, corresponding to either pleasantness/arousal (Russell & Mehrabian, 1977) or positive affect/ negative affect (PA/NA; Watson & Tellegen, 1985)—with the latter structural model representing a 45-degree rotation of the former. The two models fit mood report data about equally well (Larsen & Diener, 1992) but differ in their conceptual implications. The pleasantness/arousal model implies that appetitive and defensive states oppose each other (see Konorski, 1967) and that general activation varies independently of the pleasantness or unpleasantness of emotional states. The PA/NA model, on the other hand, implies the existence of two separate arousal systems, a positive activation system and a negative activation system (see Tellegen, 1985; Tellegen, Watson, & Clark, 1999).

Interestingly, self-report ratings of discrete (phasic) emotional stimuli yield a dimensional structure that is generally more consistent with the PA/ NA model. For example, Lang and colleagues (e.g., Lang, 1995; Greenwald, Cook, & Lang, 1989; Bradley & Lang, 1994; Lang, Greenwald, Bradley, & Hamm, 1993) have reported results for stimuli from the International Affective Picture System (IAPS; Center for the Study of Emotion & Attention [CSEA], 1999) depicting a wide variety of affective objects and situations, including spiders, snakes, weapons, food, faces, nudes, injury, sports, and the like. When participants rate their affective reactions to these picture stimuli along dimensions of pleasantness (valence) and arousal, the locations of pictures within the two-dimensional affective rating space follow a PA/NA alignment—that is, rated arousal increases systematically as a function of either increasing pleasantness or increasing unpleasantness of pictures. A similar structure has been reported for affective sounds (Bradley, Cuthbert, & Lang, 2000).

However, close inspection of the configuration of discrete emotional stimuli in valence/arousal ratings space (e.g., Lang, 1995, Fig. 1) reveals an important divergence from the PA/NA model. Whereas the two major affective dimensions intersect at their respective midpoints in the formal PA/

NA model, the two dimensions along which the pictures align in valence-arousal space do not cross but rather emanate from a common origin of low arousal and intermediate valence. This basic configuration was replicated in a study that employed actual PA and NA descriptors to rate IAPS pictures (Patrick & Lavoro, 1997). It is notable that this observed pattern coincides with the position, advanced by Cacioppo and Berntson (1994), that increasing arousal or activation arises from mobilization of either the defensive or the appetitive system; from this perspective, low arousal reflects an absence of mobilization in either system. This perspective differs from the conceptualization of positive and negative activation embodied in the classic PA/NA model (Tellegen, 1985; Watson & Tellegen, 1985; Watson, Clark, & Tellegen, 1988), in which states of low activation are represented as inherently pleasant (e.g., contentment) or unpleasant (e.g., sadness). Aside from corresponding more closely to what is known about brain systems underlying basic motivational states (see Cacioppo & Berntson, 1994), the revised perspective on PA/NA that emerges from the IAPS work is potentially more consistent with clinical observation (e.g., dysphoria or depression, which the classic PA/NA model views as fundamentally reflecting a lack of positive activation, typically entails heightened negative activation as well).

Brain Substrates of the Defensive and Appetitive Motivational Systems

A comprehensive review of what is currently known about the neurobiological substrates for negative-defensive and positive-appetitive reactivity is obviously beyond the scope of this chapter. Nevertheless, it is possible to highlight some recent findings of particular relevance to an understanding of affective individual differences and psychopathology. In this section, we focus on the basic subcortical systems that prime defensive and appetitive behavior; in the next section, we consider other brain structures that interact with and regulate these primary motivational systems. Two bodies of work are emphasized in this section. One is the extensive evidence for the amygdala as the heart of the defensive motivational system. Related to this, we discuss findings implicating the central nucleus of the amygdala in fear (i.e., time-limited reactivity to explicit cues signaling punishment), and the extended amygdala—in particular, the bed nucleus of the stria terminalis—in anxiety (i.e., persistent defensive activation not tied to specific environmental cues). The other body of work we consider is evidence for the midbrain dopamine system—comprising dopaminergic neurons in the ventral tegmental area and their projections to structures including the nucleus accumbens, prefrontal cortex, and other regions of the forebrain (for a graphic depiction of this circuitry see, e.g., Heimer et al., 1997, Fig. 14)—in appetitive reactivity and reward learning.

The Defensive Motivational System: Amygdala and Extended Amygdala

A number of contemporary researchers (e.g., Davis, 1992; Fanselow, 1994; LeDoux, 1995, 2000) have characterized the amygdala as the core of the brain's defensive (fear) system. The amygdala is a bilateral subcortical structure located deep within the temporal lobes of the brain that comprises a number of distinct subcomponents ("nuclei"). The motor output system of the amygdala is the central nucleus, which projects to various brain structures that directly mediate fear expression and fear behavior (see Davis, 1992, Fig. 13)—including the central gray (freezing behavior; see below), lateral hypothalamus (sympathetic activation), nucleus reticularis pontis caudalis (reflex facilitation; see below), parabrachial nucleus (enhancement of respiration), and facial motor neurons (facial display of fear). As a function of these outputs, defensive activation occurs when the central nucleus of the amygdala is activated.

Defensive behaviors can be grouped into two broad functional classes: (1) defensive inhibition, which entails immobility ("freezing") and hypervigilance in the presence of cues for punishment, and (2) active defense, characterized by attack or avoidance behavior ("fight or flight") in response to noxious stimulation or immediate danger. It has been suggested that the amygdala participates more directly in the former class of behaviors than the latter. For example, the amygdala projects preferentially to the *ventral* subregion of the midbrain central (periaqueductal) gray, which mediates "freezing" behavior (Fanselow, 1994); indeed, freezing has been commonly used as a measure of fear in studies of amygdala function (see LeDoux, 1995, 2000). In contrast, there is evidence that activation of the dorsal region of the central gray—the region that mediates fight/flight behavior—produces *deactivation* of the amygdala through descending inhibitory connections (Fanselow, DeCola, De Oca, & Landeira-Fernandez, 1995). The implication is that the amygdala may be more important to an understanding of the detection of aversive cues and affiliated preparatory mobilization than to overt defensive behaviors involving active avoidance and aggressive attack.

Sensory input is conveyed to the amygdala primarily through its lateral and basolateral nuclei, which in turn project to the central nucleus. As a function of this, the lateral/basolateral complex has been characterized as the input component of the amygdaloid fear system. For example, LeDoux (1995) noted that the lateral nucleus of the amygdala receives inputs from the sensory thalamus and primary sensory regions of the neocortex. These pathways provide a means by which simple stimuli in the environment can activate the amygdala and evoke defensive (fear) reactivity without a need for higher elaborative processing. However, the lateral and basolateral nuclei of the amygdala also receive inputs from higher brain regions, including the hippocampus, sensory association cortex, and prefrontal cortex, providing a mechanism whereby more complex representations such as declarative memories or images can activate or moderate activity in the amygdala (see below).

Apart from the fact that it receives inputs from simpler and more complex processing regions and that it outputs to various defensive response systems, there are other features of the amygdala that have captured the interest of researchers. The amydgala exhibits a high degree of plasticity, and it has been strongly implicated in fear learning. For example, there is evidence that cells in the lateral nucleus of the amygdala are responsive to both conditioned (CS) and unconditioned stimulus (US) input, and cells of the lateral nucleus show differential patterns of reactivity to a CS after pairing with an aversive US (LeDoux, 2000). In particular, the glutamate receptor N-methyl-D-aspartate (NMDA) appears to play a critical role in long-term potentiation processes within the amygdala that underlie the formation of CS–US associations. For example, it is well established that fear conditioning is blocked by infusion of NMDA receptor antagonists into the amygdala (Davis, Walker, & Myers, 2003; LeDoux, 2000). Thus, the amygdala is not simply an input–output system for fear—it is also a crucial center for learning. Furthermore, recent research indicates that NMDA receptors in the amygdala also play a crucial role in the *extinction* of fear responses acquired through conditioning (Davis et al., 2003).

Another notable feature of the amygdala is the crucial role it plays in attentional processing. Amygdala activation prompts vigilance to the environment, and attention is automatically drawn to stimuli or events that activate the amygdala (Davis & Whalen, 2001). One mechanism for this may be back-projections from the amygdala to primary and secondary sensory cortex (Lang et al., 1998). For example, in primates, there are extensive projections from the amygdala to V1 and V2 regions of visual cortex, such that initial activation of the amygdala by environmental stimuli promotes continued visual processing of those stimuli. There is also evidence for a similar role of the amygdala in attentional processing in humans. For example, depth electrode studies with epileptic patients have shown that early event-related potential responses (200–300 ms) to visual or acoustic stimuli recorded from the amygdala were substantially larger for attended than for ignored stimuli. Elsewhere, Whalen et al. (1998) have demonstrated reactivity of the amygdala to fearful face stimuli in human participants under masking conditions that prevented the faces from being recognized explicitly. These data indicate that in humans the amygdala plays a basic role in the detection of motivationally relevant events and the prioritization of attention to stimuli (see Lang et al., 1997; Sabatinelli, Bradley, Fitzsimmons, & Lang, 2004).

Another closely related structure that has been of interest to investigators studying the brain substrates of defensive reactivity is the bed nucleus of the stria terminalis (BNST). The amygdala and BNST are closely inter-connected with each other, and specific subdivisions of these have been as-sociated together under the rubric of the "extended amygdala" (Alheid, de Olmos, & Beltramino, 1995). In particular, the lateral and medial portions of the BNST can be viewed as the rostral and medial extensions of the cen-tral nucleus of the amygdala, respectively. In addition, the BNST projects to many of the same efferent (motor output) systems as the amygdala, de-scribed above.

However, animal research by Davis and colleagues using the "potenti-ated startle" paradigm (Davis, Walker, & Lee, 1997; Lee & Davis, 1997; Walker & Davis, 1997) has revealed a crucial difference between the roles of the amygdala and BNST in defensive reactivity. "Potentiated startle" re-fers to the increase in the reflexive startle response to an abrupt, intense probe stimulus (e.g., loud noise) that occurs when an individual is exposed to a threatening stimulus or placed in an aversive situation. In animals, the startle reflex is typically measured as the whole body "jump" reaction to a sudden noise probe (see Davis, 1989); in humans, startle is typically mea-sured as the eyeblink (orbicularis EMG) response that occurs to the probe stimulus (see Lang et al., 1990). From their research on the amygdala and BNST, Davis and colleagues concluded that exposure to simple, "explicit" aversive cues in the environment (e.g., a phasic light stimulus previously paired with shock) potentiates the startle reflex because such cues activate the central nucleus of the amygdala, which projects to the nucleus reticularis pontis caudalis (nRPC), a component of the primary brainstem startle circuit.

Other manipulations of negative affect not involving explicit stimulus cues, such as exposure to a threatening or uncertain context for an ex-tended period of time (e.g., a brightly illuminated cage, in the case of a noc-turnal animal like the rat) or intraventricular administration of the anxiogenic peptide corticotropin-releasing hormone (CRH), also produce potentiation of the startle reflex—but in this case the mechanism appears to be a path-way from the BNST to the startle circuit. Thus, infusion of the NMDA re-ceptor antagonist 2,3-dihydroxy-6-nitro-7-sulfamoyl-benzo(f)quinoxaline (NBQX) into the central nucleus of the amygdala blocks startle reflex potentiation associated with exposure to an explicit fear cue (light paired with shock), but not potentiation associated with exposure to an extended aversive context (brightly lit cage), whereas infusion of NBQX into the BNST blocks potentiation associated with exposure to a prolonged aversive context but not potentiation tied to an immediate fear cue (for a summary of this research, see Davis, 1998).

The implication of this work is that the amygdala and BNST, although they are interconnected anatomically and they project to many of the same output systems, play different roles in the activation of defensive states. Specifically, Davis and colleagues conceptualized the central nucleus of the amygdala as a phasic "fear" system that is activated by immediate, specific signals of danger in the environment; the central amygdala mobilizes defensive behavior in the presence of aversive cues, but this mobilization subsides rapidly once the cue is removed. In contrast, the BNST was characterized by these investigators as a tonic "anxiety" system that plays a role in more prolonged negative affective states. Activation of the BNST leads to a more enduring state of defensive mobilization and hypervigiliance that is not tied to explicit cues in the environment. Davis and colleagues theorized that the two systems each have distinctive survival value: when a situation is uncertain or threatening in an ambiguous way, it is adaptive to remain aroused and vigilant until the uncertainty is resolved or the possibility of danger is dispelled; at the same time, because it is important to be able to respond quickly and vigorously to immediate threat, a distinct phasic fear activation system is also adaptive.

Drawing in part on the work of Davis and colleagues, Rosen and Schulkin (1998) formulated a model of the process by which normal adaptive fear reactivity evolves into the maladaptive anxiety that is characteristic of internalizing syndromes such as panic disorder, posttraumatic stress disorder (PTSD), and agitated depression. The crux of the model is that pathological anxiety arises from the sensitization of brain systems (the amygdala and extended amygdala) that underlie normal states of fear and anxious apprehension. Sensitization arises through a process of "kindling" in which repeated elicitation of defensive reactions, or the occurrence of inordinately intense reactions such as those evoked by trauma, induces durable changes in the functioning of the amygdala and BNST, leading to "hyperexcitability" (lowered activation threshold) within these systems. The psychological manifestations of this hyperexcitability are chronic and intense negative affect, associated with a sense of uncontrollability and hypervigilance to the possibility of harmful or otherwise aversive events. Rosen and Schulkin further theorized that sensitization of the brain's fear and anxiety systems is especially likely to occur with experiences that promote kindling in persons who are by nature high in the reactivity of these systems (i.e., individuals who are constitutionally high in trait fearfulness). Thus, the model includes a role for both genes and environment in the pathogenesis of maladaptive anxiety.

The Appetitive Motivational System: Midbrain Dopamine System

Over the past 15 years or so, a revolution has taken place in researchers' thinking about the functioning of the appetitive motivational system. It has long been known that the mesolimbic and mesocortical dopamine systems—encompassing dopaminergic neurons in the ventral tegmental area and their projections to structures including the nucleus accumbens, prefrontal cortex, and other regions of the forebrain—play a crucial role in reward processing and reward behavior. This section focuses primarily on the mesolimbic (midbrain) component of this system. The traditional perspective was that this system mediates the hedonic value (pleasurableness) of reward stimuli. This view emerged from (1) classic brain stimulation studies in which rats implanted with electrodes in these and affiliated neuroanatomic regions would work vigorously to gain electrical pulses to these areas (Olds, 1956; Olds & Milner, 1954; Phillips, 1984; Shizgal, 1999); (2) research demonstrating that structures in the midbrain dopamine system are activated by a wide range of natural and drug rewards; and (3) evidence that deactivation of this system attenuates the behavioral effectiveness of most reinforcers (see Wise, 1985).

The view that the midbrain dopamine system is the seat of "pleasure centers in the brain" (Olds, 1956) was challenged by single-unit recording studies demonstrating that dopaminergic neurons of the ventral tegmental area and substantia nigra in monkeys respond primarily to events that *predict reward* rather than to rewards themselves (Schultz, Apicella, & Ljungberg, 1993; Schultz, 1998). Specifically, within a simple appetitive conditioning task in which a light cue was followed by a food (juice) reward, dopamine cells in these brain regions showed increased firing upon presentation of the reward itself—but only on initial learning trials when the reward was unexpected (i.e., not predicted). As the animal learned the contingency between the light CS and the food reward, dopaminergic neuronal firing at the time of reward delivery subsided, and gave way to firing at the time of light cue presentation. Moreover, once learning was established: (1) if the anticipated reward failed to occur following presentation of the light CS, dopamine neurons showed a *decrease* below their basal rate of firing at the time reward delivery should have occurred; and (2) if the reward was delivered at a time other than when it was expected (i.e., outside the normal delivery point following the light CS), dopamine cells again fired in response to the reward.

The conclusion advanced on the basis of these findings was that neurons in the midbrain dopamine system code for "prediction error"—that is, the degree to which a reward stimulus, or a cue for reward, is unexpected (Montague, Dayan, & Sejnowski, 1996; Schultz, 1998). For example, in the appetitive-conditioning task, dopamine cell firing shifts from the reward to the light CS because the timing of the reward becomes predictable, whereas the occurrence of the CS continues to be unpredictable. The broader implication of this perspective is that the midbrain dopamine system is involved not so much in the hedonic (pleasurable affective) component of reward but in the process of learning to connect rewards to cues in the environment—and thus in the detection of opportunities for reward and in the sequencing of goal-directed actions.

A somewhat different perspective on the role of the midbrain dopamine system in reward processing was advanced by Kent Berridge and colleagues (e.g., Berridge, Venier, & Robinson, 1989; Berridge & Robinson, 1998). These investigators proposed that neurons in the midbrain dopamine system mediate the *incentive salience* of rewards, as opposed to their hedonic value (pleasurableness). A key idea in this theoretic model is the distinct between "wanting" something, and "liking" it. "Wanting" entails attentional saliency accompanied by an active inclination to pursue, whereas "liking" refers to the pleasure that is derived directly from a reward; both processes are posited to include a core implicit element, such that "wanting" or "liking" can be instigated in the absence of conscious awareness. Berridge and colleagues proposed that dopaminergic neurons in the mesolimbic system are critical for the "wanting" component of reward (i.e., the attribution of incentive salience to rewards and reward cues, such that they become objects of desire to be actively pursued) but not for the "liking" component (registering the hedonic impact of reward stimuli). This conceptualization emerged from studies demonstrating that massive destruction of dopamine neurons (via administration of the neurotoxin, 6-hydroxydopamine [6-OHDA]) in key regions of the midbrain dopamine system (nucleus accumbens, neostriatum) eliminated food-seeking behavior in rats without affecting affective reactions to the food itself, as indexed by hedonic facial displays (see Berridge & Robinson, 1998). In other words, according to these investigators, damage to the midbrain dopamine system diminishes "wanting" of rewards (i.e., so they are no longer desired, attended to, and actively pursued) without affecting "liking" (i.e., rewards, when administered, are still "enjoyed"). Other work by these investigators suggests that the core hedonic ("liking") component of reward is mediated by distinct interconnected structures within the basal forebrain and hindbrain—including the opioid-receptor-rich shell of the nucleus accumbens, the ventral pallidum, and the brainstem parabrachial nucleus (see Berridge, 2003).

A key point of divergence between the incentive salience model and the "prediction error" model of Schultz and colleagues, according to Berridge and Robinson (1998), is that the latter model implies an essential role for dopamine in reward learning. Berridge and Robinson presented evidence that rats with extensive 6-OHDA-induced dopamine depletion still showed attenuation and enhancement of hedonic reactivity to a rewarding stimulus, respectively, after the stimulus was paired, on the one hand, with a nausea-inducing agent (lithium chloride) or, on the other, with a palatability-enhancing agent (diazepam). From this, Berridge and Robinson concluded that midbrain dopaminergic neurons are not essential for reward learning, defined as changes in the hedonic value of rewards arising through associative pairings with other pleasurable or aversive stimuli. However, McClure, Daw, and Montague (2003) recently proposed an alternative reward-learning model (the "actor–critic" model) that reconciles the prediction error position with the incentive salience model. In the actor–critic model, the reward-prediction error coded by dopamine neuronal activity serves the dual purpose of imbuing relevant stimuli with incentive value and biasing action selection so as to maximize reward outcomes.

The incentive salience model of Berridge and colleagues, in which "wanting" (mediated by neurons of the midbrain dopamine system) is dissociated from "liking" (mediated by other subcortical structures), was used by these authors as the foundation for an intriguing model of processes underlying drug addiction (Berridge & Robinson, 1995; Robinson & Berridge, 2003). The core idea of the model is that repeated ingestion of drugs causes the midbrain dopamine system to become sensitized; once established, this sensitization is extremely persistent. The evidence for enduring changes in this system as a function of drug taking includes animal studies showing increased effects of stimulant drugs on psychomotor activation with repeated use, and morphologic changes in dopaminergic neurons (e.g., dendritic changes in neurons within the nucleus accumbens), and human neuroimaging studies showing that the midbrain dopamine system is strongly activated when addicts are exposed to drug-associated stimuli as well as when they actually receive the drug (see Robinson & Berridge, 2000). According to these authors, the idea that the "wanting" system is sensitized by repeated drug taking (and potentially by other forms of addictive behavior) helps to explain the inordinate salience that drug cues have for addicts and the compulsive efforts that addicts make to obtain their drug of choice (i.e., craving = "wanting"). The model also accounts for why addicts persist in seeking and ingesting drugs even after the pleasure achieved by taking the drug has waned and aversive consequences have begun to accrue. A further point of the model is that individual differences are presumed to exist in the susceptibility of the "wanting" system to sensitization—as a function of variables such as genes, sex-related hormones, and experience (Robinson & Berridge, 2000).

In summary, contemporary neuroscience research on the midbrain dopamine system points to a novel role for this system in the processing of reward stimuli: this system functions to harness attention in the direction of cues for reward and simultaneously to energize goal-seeking behavior. It provides a mechanism whereby neutral cues in the environment can achieve "incentive salience" through primary and secondary association with rewarding events, and thereby instigate action sequences that promote attainment of reward. Destruction of this system does not appear to eliminate the capacity to "enjoy" rewarding stimuli; however, it does seem to eliminate interest in reward-related cues and in the active pursuit of reward. On the other hand, sensitization of this brain system through repeated, intense stimulation (e.g., repeated ingestion of drugs) can lead to intense feelings of "wanting" (i.e., craving) in relation to drug-related stimuli and compulsive drug-seeking behavior. Although the majority of research on the "reward prediction error" and "incentive salience" models of the midbrain dopamine system has been conducted using food and psychoactive drugs as reward stimuli, there is evidence that this system plays a similar role with respect to other basic appetitive drives (e.g., thirst, sex; Horvitz, Richardson, & Ettenberg, 1993; Fiorino, Coury, & Phillips, 1997). Thus, on the basis of available evidence, there is reason to believe that the midbrain dopamine system comprises the main neural substrate for appetitive motivation, defined as mobilization for approach behavior.

It bears repeating that distinct (albeit interconnected) neural structures appear to mediate the "liking" (hedonic) component of reward—these structures include the shell of the nucleus accumbens and the ventral pallidum and brainstem parabrachial nucleus to which it projects. Berridge (2003) suggested that these structures, which are innervated by the mesolimbic dopamine system, may comprise a core circuit of "liking" that participates in hedonic reactivity to a variety of reward stimuli. It should also be noted that other distinct brain structures contribute to mediation of overt consummatory behaviors tied to specific drive states. For example, fiber tracts running through the lateral and medial divisions of the hypothalamus play a specific crucial role in eating behavior (hunger and satiety, respectively), whereas the medial preoptic area of the hypothalamus appears to be especially crucial for sexual behavior.

AFFECTIVE REGULATION AND CONTROL

At the most basic level, priming of defensive or appetitive motivational behavior can arise through exposure to simple conditioned stimuli in the environment that automatically activate the amygdala or midbrain dopaminergic system. For example, LeDoux (1995, 2000) described a "quick and dirty" processing pathway from the sensory thalamus to the lateral nucleus of the amygdala along which simple acoustic information can be transmitted; because of the existence of this pathway, fear activation can occur to a conditioned tone CS even following massive destruction of the neocortex. A similar fast processing pathway appears to exist for the visual system, involving the basolateral nucleus of the amygdala (Davis & Lee, 1998); this putative pathway has been the focus of human research on "unconscious" processing of visual fear cues including faces (Whalen et al., 1998) and phobic objects (Öhman, 1993). Berridge and Robinson (1998) likewise characterized the midbrain dopamine system as having a low-level implicit processing capacity whereby simple cues in the environment can instigate appetitive mobilization ("wanting") in the absence of "conscious" awareness.

Nevertheless, both the amygdala and midbrain dopamine systems exhibit extensive neural connectivity with various regions of the neocortex. These connections afford a mechanism whereby higher brain processes (e.g., memories, images, plans) can influence processing and reactivity to emotional events, and emotional reactions can in turn influence these higher brain processes. Especially important in the present context are connections between these subcortical affect systems and the prefrontal cortex (PFC). The existence of these connections leads to the question: What specific functional role does the PFC play in emotional processing?

In general, the PFC is thought to be crucial for "top-down" processing, that is, the guidance of behavior by internal representations of goals or states. The PFC is the region of neocortex that is most highly evolved in primates, and it is believed to account for the diversity and flexibility of behavioral strategies exhibited by humans. A number of investigators have proposed that the PFC is especially important for coping with novel or dynamic situations in which selection of appropriate behavioral responses needs to be made on the basis of internal representations of goals and strategies rather than immediate stimulus cues alone (e.g., Cohen & Servan-Schreiber, 1992; Miller, 1999; Wise, Murray, & Gerfen, 1996). Recently, Miller and Cohen (2001) proposed an elegant integrative model of PFC function. According to this model, the control functions of the PFC arise from its specialized capacity for online maintenance of goal representations: by maintaining patterns of activation corresponding to goals and the means needed to achieve them, the PFC provides biasing signals to other regions of the brain with which it connects. These signals serve to prime sensory-attentional, associative, and motor processes that support the performance of a designated task by directing activity along relevant brain pathways. An appealing feature of this model is that it provides a mechanistic account of PFC function that avoids the circularity of mentalistic (i.e., PFC as "executive") accounts.

The major focus of Miller and Cohen's (2001) model is on *cognitive* control functions (i.e., guidance of behavior on the basis of internal representations) associated with the dorsolateral PFC. The dorsolateral PFC has been shown to play a critical role in working memory processes, involving the maintenance of a discrete stimulus representation across a temporal delay (Goldman-Rakic, 1996). For example, in humans, performance of a working memory task that involves matching current stimuli to earlier stimuli in a ongoing stream (the "n-back" task; Cohen et al., 1994) preferentially activates the dorsolateral PFC, with the degree of activation increasing as a function of memory load (Cohen et al., 1997). In addition to its capacity for active maintenance, the dorsolateral PFC is also distinguished by its close connections with sensory association cortices (including occipital, temporal, and parietal); its prominent projections to premotor areas in the medial and lateral frontal lobes, as well other motor structures including the basal ganglia, the cerebellum, and the frontal eye fields; and its ability to encode relations between stimulus events and thus represent rules (mappings) required to perform complex tasks. As a function of these capacities, this region of the PFC also plays a role in more active processes associated with inhibition and regulation of behavioral responses (see Petrides, 2000). For example, the control function of the dorsolateral PFC is important for performance on the Stroop color-naming task (MacDonald, Cohen, Stenger, & Carter, 2000), and for performance of the visual antisaccade task, which entails active inhibition and redirection of reflexive eye movements (Broerse, Crawford, & den Boer, 2001; Muri et al., 1998).

A further intriguing element in the Miller and Cohen (2001) cognitive control model of PFC function is the role they ascribe to dopaminergic neuron activity. Recognizing that patterns of PFC activity that contribute to attainment of a goal (i.e., by biasing other brain systems to respond in goal-relevant ways) must be reinforced in order to recur under appropriate circumstances in the future, these authors suggest that this reinforcing function may be served by dopaminergic projections to the PFC from the midbrain dopamine system, as well as dopamine neurons within the PFC itself. According to the model, the reward prediction error (or "incentive salience") function of dopamine serves in this case to strengthen connections between neurons that signal the *expectation* of reward and representations in the PFC that guide the actions required to *achieve* the reward. In other words, the mesocorticolimbic dopamine activity supplies the incentive for appropriate PFC representations to recur in a task context in which those representations have previously facilitated goal attainment. With regard to pathologic function, Montague, Hyman, and Cohen (2004) proposed—in line with Robinson and Berridge (2000; cited earlier)—that the normal role of the dopamine system as a facilitator of complex PFC-mediated behavior (such as that required to function in a complex work environment, or obtain a college degree) can be "hijacked" by drugs of abuse that sensitize the system and direct its activity toward ritualized maladaptive action patterns. From this perspective, it is reasonable to think that deficits in PFC function arising from genetic and/or experiential factors could render an individual especially vulnerable to this sort of hijacking— i.e., because of a lack of incentive to engage in activities that do not lead to immediate tangible rewards.

Lesser attention is devoted in Miller and Cohen's (2001) model to the ventromedial and orbitofrontal regions of the PFC, which have collectively been termed the orbitomedial PFC (e.g., Blumer & Benson, 1975). These regions connect more directly and extensively than the dorsolateral PFC with medial temporal limbic structures, including the amygdala, hippocampus and associated neocortex, and hypothalamus. As a function of these limbic connections, the orbitomedial PFC appears to play a more dominant role in the anticipation of affective consequences of behavior (Bechara, Damasio, Tranel, & Damasio, 1997; Wagar & Thagard, 2004) and in the unlearning of stimulus-reward associations (i.e., reversal learning; Dias, Robbins, & Roberts, 1996; Rolls, 2000). It should be noted that the dorsolateral and orbitomedial divisions of the PFC are themselves richly interconnected, and thus their functions need to be viewed as interdependent. Nevertheless, as an illustration of the anatomic specificity of different neuro-cognitive measures of PFC function, Bechara, Damasio, Tranel, and Anderson (1998) reported that patients with dorsolateral PFC lesions showed impairments on a working-memory task but not on a "gambling" task involving affect-guided decision making, whereas the reverse was true of patients with ventromedial PFC lesions.

Particular research attention has been devoted in recent years to another key function of the orbitomedial PFC—namely, its role in regulating emotional reactivity and expression. It has long been known that lesions of this brain region are associated with dramatic increases in impulsive, irresponsible, and aggressive behavior. The best-known example of this is the railway worker Phineas Gage, who in 1848 suffered an accident in which an iron tamping rod was driven through his skull from the base to the top, causing extensive damage to the PFC—in particular, the orbitomedial region (Damasio, Grabowski, Frank, Galaburda, & Damasio, 1994). Prior to the accident Gage was described as capable, dependable, and courteous, whereas after he was characterized as impulsive, stubborn, antagonistic, and reckless. This constellation of features arising from damage to the orbitomedial PFC has been labeled "acquired sociopathy" (Damasio, Tranel, & Damasio, 1990). Other more recent cases of this type have been reported on by Anderson, Bechara, Damasio, Tranel, and Damasio (1999) and Blair and Cipolotti (2000). Impulsive aggressive behavior was identified as a prominent feature in each of these cases.

Davidson, Putnam, and Larson (2000) proposed that the orbitomedial PFC functions to suppress emotional activation elicited automatically by cues for reward or punishment. In particular, these authors suggested that deficits in the ability to regulate negative affect associated with orbitomedial PFC impairment may be an important factor underlying impulsive, angry aggression in some individuals. Miller and Cohen (2001) conceptualized this affect suppression function of the orbitomedial PFC in terms of the general biasing function of the PFC: the orbitomedial PFC, with its direct connections to limbic structures, operates to bias task-relevant processes against competition from "hot" (motivationally charged) processes arising in social or emotional contexts. Consistent with this perspective, human neuro-imaging studies have provided evidence that the orbitomedial PFC is selectively activated during efforts to suppress affect evoked by positive or negative emotional stimuli (Beauregard, Levesque, & Bourgouin, 2001;

Ochsner, Bunge, Gross, & Gabrieli, 2002; Ochsner et al., 2004). Human and animal studies also support a role for the orbitomedial PFC in the extinction of fear (e.g., Phelps, Delgado, Nearing, & LeDoux, 2004; Quirk, Russo, Barron, & Lebron, 2000), which has come to be viewed as an active process of relearning rather than a passive process of forgetting (LeDoux, 1995, 2000).

Two other brain regions that appear to be important for regulating emotional behavior are the hippocampus and the anterior cingulate cortex (ACC). The hippocampus connects with the amygdala and midbrain dopamine system as well as the PFC and appears to be important for linking affective responses and goals to complex configural stimuli (contexts). Thus, lesions of the hippocampus block the acquisition of contextual fear conditioning but not simple cue conditioning (LeDoux, 1995). With regard to the PFC, Cohen and O'Reilly (1996) postulated that its connections with the hippocampus provide a mechanism whereby goal representations can be activated dynamically by contextual cues in the environment to guide complex delayed-action sequences (e.g., stopping by the store at the end of the day to pick up groceries needed for dinner). Impairments in hippocampal function would be expected to contribute to a simpler, explicit-cue-driven style of affective processing. On the other hand, the ACC—which connects with premotor and supplementary motor regions as well as with limbic structures (including amygdala and hippocampus) and the PFC—has been conceptualized as a system that invokes the control functions of the PFC as required to successfully perform a task, either by detecting errors in performance as they occur (Scheffers, Coles, Bernstein, Gehring, & Donchin, 1996), by monitoring conflict arising from activation of competing response tendencies (Carter et al., 1998), or by estimating the likelihood of committing an error at the time a response is called for (Brown & Braver, 2005). Impairments in ACC function would be expected to interfere with the ability to inhibit prepotent behavioral responses and to avoid repetition of errors.

INDIVIDUAL DIFFERENCES IN AFFECTIVE REACTIVITY AND REGULATION: BRIDGING PERSONALITY AND PSYCHOPATHOLOGY

Although much has been learned from animal and human research over the past two decades about neural systems mediating emotional reactivity and regulation, the study of individual differences in the functioning of these systems is really only in its infancy. However, consideration of the role these systems play in priming and regulating action strongly suggests that systematic investigation of affective individual differences, and the genetic and experiential factors that underlie them, will be crucial to an understanding of behavior disorders. Recently proposed hierarchical models of internalizing and externalizing disorders within the DSM provide a useful framework for thinking about the sorts of roles these brain systems might play in the most common forms of psychopathology. In this section, we consider, from a general conceptual standpoint, how individual differences in the functioning of these underlying brain systems might play a role in these broad forms of psychopathology and in the personality traits with which they are associated.

It should be noted that the effort to link biological systems to personality and psychopathology has previously been emphasized in major theories advanced by Eysenck (1967), Gray (1987), Tellegen (1985), and Zuckerman (1979), among others. Whereas Eysenck, Tellegen, and Zuckerman first identified major dimensions of personality through analyses of self-report questionnaire data and then speculated about how these dimensions might relate to underlying biological systems, Gray's approach was different. Gray began by delineating broad motivational systems (and affiliated brain structures) involved in reward and punishment learning, based primarily on an analysis of findings from drug and lesion studies with animals, and then postulated how these motivational systems might link to broad personality dimensions (of anxiety and impulsivity) and to psychopathological syndromes (including anxiety, depression, and psychopathy). Based on the conceptualization of motivational systems that emerged from his analysis of animal learning studies, Gray proposed a revision to Eysenck's structural model of personality that he saw as providing a better fit to the biological data. Specifically, Gray rotated Eysenck's neuroticism and extraversion factors by 45 degrees to yield personality dimensions (i.e., anxiety, impulsivity) that corresponded more readily to his two basic motivational systems (i.e., the behavioral inhibition and behavioral activation systems, respectively).

The approach we take here is similar to Gray's in that we begin by considering what is known about basic motivational systems (see above) and then go on to postulate how personality dimensions and psychopathologic syndromes might relate to these systems. However, our approach differs from Gray's in that (1) our conceptualization of brain motivational systems derives from a different, more recent, literature, and (2) our perspective incorporates contemporary ideas about the hierarchical structure of major domains of psychopathology.

Hypothesized Relations among Affect Systems, Personality, and Internalizing Psychopathology

How might the aforementioned affective reactivity and control systems relate to internalizing forms of psychopathology and affiliated personality traits? Mineka et al. (1998) proposed a hierarchical model of internalizing disorders to account for the comorbidity of these disorders as well as the specific symptoms associated with each (see also Brown & Barlow, 1992; Watson, 2005). According to this model, disorders within this spectrum (i.e., anxiety disorders, unipolar depression) share a common broad factor of negative affect reflecting general distress, susceptibility to negative mood states, and hypervigilance to threat. Its personality trait counterpart is the broad Negative Emotionality (Tellegen, 1985; Krueger, McGue, & Iacono, 2001) or Neuroticism factor (Eysenck, 1967; John & Srivastava, 1999). In addition to this, Mineka et al. (1998) postulated that each individual internalizing disorder (with the possible exception of generalized anxiety disorder [GAD], which the authors suggested may reflect primarily high trait negative affect) has a specific etiological factor that accounts for its uniqueness. For example, although depression (like the various anxiety disorders) is associated with heightened negative affect, it is distinguished by a reduced capacity for pleasurable mood states. The personality counterpart to this is low trait Positive Affect (Watson et al., 1988) or Positive Emotionality (Tellegen, 1985). Among the anxiety disorders, panic disorder is distinguished from the others by the presence of physiological hyperreactivity ("anxious arousal"), manifested in the form of acute panic attacks. Likewise, the remaining anxiety disorders are presumably differentiated from one another by other unique etiological determinants—although Mineka et al. were not able to specify on the basis of existing data what these specific determinants might be for disorders other than panic.

With regard to the general negative affectivity factor that the internalizing disorders appear to share, sensitization of the core elements of the defensive motivational system (amygdala and BNST) suggests a plausible biological substrate for this factor. According to Rosen and Schulkin (1998), constitutional differences in the sensitivity of these underlying systems, together with adverse experiences that activate them repeatedly or for prolonged periods, leads to hyperexcitability of these systems—manifested psychologically as intense and persistent negative mood, hypervigilance, and a sense of uncontrollability (i.e., the defining elements of heightened negative affect). As Rosen and Schulkin noted, fear (i.e., defensive mobilization in the presence of imminent threat) is a normal affective state, but there is evidence that individuals differ in core amygdala reactivity (e.g., Hariri et al., 2002)—potentially from a very early age (Goldsmith & Campos, 1982; Kagan, 1994). From this perspective, the crucial individual difference factor underlying internalizing problems may be constitutionally high reactivity of the amygdaloid fear system (i.e., high trait fearfulness).

This position assumes a common underlying substrate to pathological fear and anxiety (i.e., heightened dispositional amygdala reactivity). Consistent with this, fear and anxiety emerge as distinct albeit correlated constructs in the self-report temperament domain when each is defined in terms of emotional reactivity (Buss & Plomin, 1984).[2] Paralleling this, Krueger (1999a) found evidence for separable but correlated "anxious–misery" and "fear" subfactors—the former encompassing major depression, dysthymia, and generalized anxiety disorder, and the latter specific phobia, social phobia, agoraphobia, and panic disorder—within the domain of internalizing psychopathology (see also Krueger & Markon, in press, for meta-analytic evidence of this distinction). Related to this, Mineka et al. (1998) pointed out that the various internalizing disorders differ in terms of the magnitude of involvement of the general negative affect component in relation to specific symptomatic components. For example, available data indicate that disorders within the "anxious–misery" domain (e.g., depression, GAD) show a much larger component of general negative affect than disorders within the "fear" domain (e.g., specific phobia, social phobia).

What variables might lead some high-amygdala reactive individuals to develop disorders marked by high general distress (i.e., chronic anxiety and dysphoria) whereas others develop only focal phobias? The key determinant may be whether enhanced amygdala reactivity interacts with other underlying dispositions and adverse experiences to produce sensitization of not only the core fear system but also its affiliated "anxiety system" (i.e., the extended amygdala/BNST). For example, dispositional factors that enable an individual to limit the intensity and duration of fear episodes or to harness defensive reactions to specific environmental cues would operate against general sensitization. On the other hand, exposure to highly intense, repeated, unpredictable stress (e.g., such as that experienced by military combat personnel) would operate to enhance sensitization (see Rosen & Schulkin, 1998).

Grillon and Davis (1997) provided an experimental demonstration of how conditions of learning can promote generalized fear as opposed to cue-specific fear. The study involved a simple conditioning procedure administered across two separate days of testing. Startle reflex potentiation was used to index defense system activation. In each testing session, participants received either paired or unpaired CS–US presentations; in the paired condition the US (shock) reliably and immediately followed the occurrence of the CS (a light cue), whereas in the unpaired condition the US occurred at times unrelated to the occurrence of the CS. Grillon and Davis found that participants given paired CS–US presentations in conditioning session 1 showed increased fear (as evidenced by startle reflex potentiation) in session 2 only when the CS was present. In contrast, participants exposed to unpaired CS–US presentations showed generally enhanced startle reactivity throughout session 2—even during a baseline phase that preceded the actual conditioning trials. The authors' interpretation of these results was that defensive activation is limited to the core fear (amygdala) system when aversive events are tied to discrete cues, but defensive activation extends to the broader anxiety (BNST) system when aversive events are not predicted reliably by environmental cues.

Subsequently, Grillon and Morgan (1999) demonstrated an intriguing parallel in the responses of patients with posttraumatic stress disorder (PTSD) compared with controls in a differential conditioning procedure in which a CS+ was reliably paired with shock and a CS− was never paired with shock. In this study, the PTSD patients showed a lack of differential conditioning in an initial training session (i.e., a failure to develop enhanced startle reactivity to the CS+ versus the CS− following repeated pairings of the former with shock) and enhanced baseline reactivity in a second training session prior to conditioning trials. The authors interpreted these results as reflecting sensitization of the general anxiety system in patients with PTSD. The findings of this study in turn dovetail with other research indicating that PTSD falls within the "anxious–misery" domain of internalizing disorders (i.e., those that Watson, 2005, has termed "distress disorders") as opposed to the "fear" domain (Cox, Clara, & Ens, 2002; Watson, 2005). Elsewhere, Cuthbert et al. (2003) reported a pattern of enhanced baseline startle reactivity coupled with diminished physiological differentiation between fear-relevant and non-fear-relevant imagery cues in patients meeting criteria for panic disorder with agoraphobic as well as patients with PTSD, in comparison to patients with specific or social phobia as well as healthy controls. These results are consistent with the idea that sensitization of the anxiety system is more generally characteristic of disorders within the "anxious–misery" (aka "distress") domain.

In addition to the concept of a broad negative affect factor that is present to varying degrees in all of the internalizing disorders, a further key element in Mineka et al.'s (1998) hierarchical model is the idea that other factors contribute to the uniqueness of each individual disorder. Particular emphasis was given in their review to low positive affect as a specific factor in depression and dysthymia (see also Clark & Watson, 1991). Furthermore, with regard to the comorbidity between anxiety and depression, Mineka et al. (1998) noted that the onset of prominent anxiety symptoms typically precedes the onset of depressive episodes in anxious individuals who develop depression. How might the relationship between anxiety and depression be understood from the standpoint of underlying appetitive and defensive systems?

The notion that depression is characterized by a lack of pleasurable emotion suggests an abnormality in the functioning of the dopamine ("incentive salience") system. Indeed, a cardinal feature of depression is that cues that instigate reward-seeking behavior in healthy individuals fail to do so in dysphoric individuals. Depression may arise out of chronic anxiety as a function of a shift in the sorts of cues to which incentive salience is assigned in high anxious individuals. When the general anxiety (extended amygdala) system becomes sensitized, priority is naturally assigned to the avoidance of danger and discomfort through active vigilance and anticipation of threat. As a function of this, cues for relief (see Gray, 1987) may achieve a level of incentive salience that supersedes the incentive value of other secondary reward cues (e.g., cues that normally guide one toward fulfillment through work or relationships). As long as such cues continue to effectively predict relief (i.e., avoidance of discomfort), their incentive salience would be maintained. However, under circumstances in which relief cues lose their effectiveness (e.g., when a habitual source of refuge or support is lost), depression would result. This account, although necessarily speculative, is plausible and fits with the typical chronological relationship between anxiety and depression.

Hypothesized Relations among Affect Systems, Personality, and Externalizing Psychopathology

Paralleling the conceptualization of Mineka et al. (1998), Krueger et al. (2002) proposed a hierarchical model of the externalizing spectrum, encompassing DSM syndromes of alcohol dependence, drug dependence, child conduct disorder, and adult antisocial behavior. The database used to formulate the model consisted of symptom scores on these various disorders for a sample of male and female twins recruited from the community ($N = 1,048$). A biometric structural analysis revealed a large common factor ("Externalizing") on which all of these diagnostic variables loaded substantially (.58–.78); more than 80% of the variance in this common factor was attributable to additive genetic influence (see also Young, Stallings, Corley, Krauter, & Hewitt, 2000; Kendler et al., 2003). The remaining variance in each disorder not accounted for by the broad Externalizing factor was attributable primarily to nonshared environmental influence—although for conduct disorder there was also a significant contribution of shared environment.

Based on these findings, Krueger et al. (2002) proposed that a general constitutional factor contributes to the development of various disorders in this spectrum but that the precise expression of this underlying vulnerability (i.e., as antisocial deviance of different sorts, or as alcohol or drug problems) is determined by disorder-specific etiological influences. Although the analysis pointed to unique environmental experience as the main determinant of diagnostic specificity (with some contribution of family environment for conduct disorder), owing to the somewhat modest sample size and large confidence intervals around parameters in the model, reflecting unique etiological contributions to specific syndromes, the authors did not rule out the possibility that specific genetic factors might also contribute to the uniqueness of these disorders. Indeed, Kendler et al. (2003) presented evidence for this in a subsequent study.

What is the underlying basis of the broad Externalizing factor that disorders within this spectrum share? In terms of personality correlates, externalizing psychopathology is associated with traits related to impulsivity, disinhibition, or a lack of constraint (Sher & Trull, 1994; Iacono, Carlson, Taylor, Elkins, & McGue, 1999). In their quantitative model of the externalizing spectrum, Krueger et al. (2002) demonstrated that the higher-order Constraint factor of Tellegen's (in press) Multidimensional Personality Questionnaire, encompassing traits of impulsivity, sensation seeking, and unconventionality (in reverse), loaded significantly and negatively on the broad externalizing factor. Elsewhere, it has been shown that high trait negative affect (or negative emotionality) is characteristic of both internalizing and externalizing psychopathology, whereas low constraint is characteristic of externalizing psychopathology exclusively (Krueger, 1999b; Krueger, Caspi, Moffitt, Silva, & McGee, 1996). However, with regard to negative affectivity, externalizing problems are associated most particularly with elevated aggressiveness, whereas internalizing problems are associated more so with heightened anxiousness (stress reactivity; Krueger et al., 1996). This indicates a differential expression of high negative affect in externalizing syndromes related to a lack of inhibitory control (see Krueger et al., 1998).

With regard to brain systems, the impulsiveness and emotional dysregulation that typify disorders within this spectrum point to prefrontal brain dysfunction as a key mechanism underlying general externalizing vulnerability. As noted earlier, lesions of frontal brain areas are known to result in impulsive externalizing behavior (Blumer & Benson, 1975; Damasio, Tranel, & Damasio, 1990), and in addition deficits on neuropsychological tests of frontal lobe function have been reliably demonstrated for a number of the externalizing syndromes. Morgan and Lilienfeld (2000) reported meta-analytic evidence for deficits on frontal lobe tasks in individuals exhibiting conduct disorder and adult antisocial behavior. Individuals at risk for alcoholism by virtue of a positive parental history also show evidence of impairment on neuropsychological tests of frontal lobe function (Peterson & Pihl, 1990; Tarter, Alterman, & Edwards, 1985). Relatedly, Barkley (1997) proposed on the basis of a review of neuropsychological studies that frontal brain dysfunction characterizes the most prevalent form of ADHD, the hyperactive–impulsive type.

The anterior cingulate cortex (ACC), which functions in tandem with the PFC to guide behavior, is another brain region that seems likely to be involved in externalizing vulnerability. As noted earlier, the ACC functions to monitor ongoing action sequences and to anticipate and detect errors. For example, the error-related negativity (ERN), a brain potential response that occurs following performance errors in a speeded reaction time task, is believed to arise from the ACC (Miltner, Braun, & Coles, 1997; Holroyd, Dien, & Coles, 1998; Luu, Flaisch, & Tucker, 2000). Dikman and Allen (2000) reported that individuals low on socialization, a construct related to externalizing, showed reduced ERN response in a speeded reaction time paradigm. In contrast, individuals with obsessive–compulsive disorder, who conceptually are at the low pole of the inhibition–disinhibition (EXT) continuum (Gray, 1982), show enhanced ERN (Gehring, Himle, & Nisenson, 2000). There is also some evidence that the hippocampus, another structure that operates in conjunction with the PFC to guide behavior (see Miller & Cohen, 2001), may be dysfunctional in some externalizing individuals (e.g., Raine et al., 2004; Soderstrom, Tullberg, Wikkelsoe, Ekholm, & Forsman, 2000).

The consequence of an underlying weakness in the PFC and these affiliated regions with which it interacts would be a propensity to act on the basis of salient cues in the immediate environment rather than on the basis of internal representations of goals and methods for achieving them. In particular, dysfunction in the PFC/ACC systems would compromise an individual's ability to (1) ascribe incentive salience to representations for more complex, distal, but ultimately more fulfilling behavioral goals; (2) anticipate obstacles and formulate strategies for overcoming them before they become overwhelming (e.g., deal proactively with frustrating or threatening circumstances); (3) detect conflict between competing response tendencies (i.e., recognize, on-line, the probability of making an error); and (4) monitor and regulate affective responses in the service of distal goals.

Recent research by Krueger, Markon, Patrick, Benning, and Kramer (2005) indicates that aggressive and addictive tendencies represent the two major thematic expressions of this broad underlying vulnerability. Building upon the work of Krueger et al. (2002), these investigators undertook a fine-grained analysis of problem behaviors and traits within the domain of externalizing in order to delineate more clearly the scope and structure of this spectrum. They began by identifying various constructs embodied in the DSM definitions of the disorders included in the Krueger et al. (2002) analysis, and then developed questionnaire items to tap these constructs. They also surveyed the literature to identify other behavioral and trait constructs linked conceptually or empirically to externalizing; items were also developed to index these constructs. Over three iterative rounds of data collection and analysis (utilizing item response modeling and factor analytic techniques), the authors refined the overall item set to clarify the nature of constructs associated with the broad externalizing factor—and arrived at a final group of 23 constructs (including alcohol, drug, and marijuana use and problems; aggression of various sorts; impulsiveness; irresponsibility; rebelliousness; excitement seeking; blame externalization), each operationalized by a unique subscale. Structural analyses of these 23 subcales revealed evidence of a broad superordinate factor ("External-izing") on which all subscales loaded (with the strongest indicators being "irresponsibility" and "problematic impulsivity") and two subordinate factors accounting for residual variance in particular subscales—one marked by subscales indexing aggression (all forms), callousness, and excitement seeking, and the other marked by subscales indexing substance-related problems.

The findings of this recent work by Krueger et al. (2005) suggest that a broad disinhibitory trait factor (possibly reflecting dysfunction in anterior brain systems that govern affective and behavioral control) contributes to externalizing problems as a whole. A general impulsive/disinhibitory disposition presumably contributes to a broad range of externalizing problems because it entails an active response style that centers on immediate cues in the environment and short-term gratification. High externalizing individuals lack the capacity to attach incentive salience to complex goals and strategies, and thus they seek reward or relief actively, in the current moment. However, the work of Krueger et al. (2005) further suggests that distinct etiological mechanisms underlie externalizing problems involving substance-related problems versus aggressive antisociality.

From the standpoint of the affective systems described earlier, what distinctive brain processes might underlie these alternative expressions of externalizing vulnerability? One intriguing possibility is that addictions and pathological aggression reflect sensitization of alternative dopaminergic pathways supporting distinctive action patterns—one related to drug acquisition and drug taking and the other to active defense behavior. From this perspective, the manifestation of externalizing vulnerability in the form of addictive behavior would arise from unique dispositional factors (e.g., enhanced physiological sensitivity to the pharmacological effects of alcohol or drugs) and experiential factors (e.g., early access to alcohol or drugs) that cause the midbrain dopamine system to become sensitized to drug-related cues (see Berridge & Robinson, 1995; Robinson & Berridge, 2003). On the other hand, the development of aggressive externalization would depend upon distinctive trait factors (e.g., physical strength or size; high trait aggressiveness) and experiential factors (e.g., modeling by others) that promote the use of overt aggression as a means to achieve gratification or relief from immediate distress (i.e., that sensitize the dopamine system to cues for relief or reward obtainable through aggressive acting out).

The idea that addictive behavior entails sensitization of dopaminergic systems to drug-related cues is well developed in the literature (Berridge & Robinson, 1995; Robinson & Berridge, 2003; Montague et al., 2004). The possibility that aggressive externalization entails a parallel sensitization of dopaminergic pathways is more speculative. However, this idea is foreshadowed by the work of Gray (1987), who postulated that active forms of defensive behavior are mediated by the reward ("behavioral activation") system—in contrast to passive forms of defensive behavior, which are mediated by the punishment ("behavioral inhibition") system. There is also abundant evidence in the literature for a role of the dopamine system (together with the serotonin system) in aggressive behavior (see Lee & Coccaro, 2001).

The position advanced here is that the characteristic response to threat or frustration among high aggressive externalizing individuals entails active defense, as opposed to the anxious withdrawal that characterizes the internalizing syndromes. By responding actively in the face of stressors, the aggressive externalizing individual is able to bypass (and potentially inhibit; cf. Fanselow et al., 1995) the fear and anxiety systems and thereby achieve relief, at least in the immediate term. The achievement of relief is experienced as rewarding, resulting in incentive salience being attached to aggression-related environmental cues and action tendencies—which promotes the continuance of aggression. Habitual reliance on aggressive action is further maintained by rewarding outcomes associated with the application of force to achieve goals in nonthreatening situations. This formulation is consistent with evidence indicating that the aggression component of trait negative affectivity is most salient in externalizing disorders, whereas the stress reactivity component is most prominent in internalizing disorders. It is also consistent with data from the temperament literature indicating that anger and fear represent distinct alternative expressions of negative affect (Buss & Plomin, 1984) and with recent psychophysiological research indicating that anger (in contrast to fear or anxiety) constitutes an approach-related defensive state (Harmon-Jones, 2003; Harmon-Jones & Allen, 1998).

SUMMARY AND CONCLUSIONS

In this chapter, we reviewed contemporary conceptualizations of the appetitive and defensive motivational systems, including how these systems operate to influence attentional processing and behavioral response, and we described anterior brain systems that function to control affect, cognition, and behavior. We then considered how these affective reactivity and regulatory systems might play a role in major forms of psychopathology and the personality traits with which they are associated.

We should note that numerous other investigators have formulated hypotheses concerning the role of motivational systems in psychopathology. For example, P. Lang and colleagues have considered how the defensive motivational system in particular may contribute to anxiety disorders (e.g.,

Lang, Bradley, Cuthbert, & Patrick, 1993; Lang, Davis, & Öhman, 2000). Davidson and colleagues have written extensively about the role of cortical and subcortical systems (in particular, the amygdala and PFC) in emotional reactivity and regulatory deficits associated with depression and anxiety (e.g., Davidson, 2002; Davidson, Pizzigalli, Nitschke, & Putnam, 2002). In addition, our own recent research has focused on basic emotional reactivity deficits associated with the syndrome of psychopathy (e.g., Patrick, 1994; Verona, Patrick, Curtin, Bradley, & Lang, 2004). However, the current formulation is novel in that we have focused on recent hierarchical-structural models of psychopathology and their relations with emotion systems.

Considerable attention has also been devoted in prior writings to the association between personality and psychopathology and how affective-motivational systems might mediate this association. Eysenck, Gray, Tellegen, and Zuckerman were mentioned as examples in this regard. However, for the most part, prior theorizing about linkages among emotion, personality, and psychopathology has tended to be "top-down" rather than "bottom-up"—i.e., how do disorders defined on the basis of clinical observation and expert consensus map on to the functioning of these underlying brain systems, or how do dimensions of personality identified on the basis of structural analyses of self-report trait descriptions map on to the functioning of these systems? Accordingly, the typical research strategy has been to examine differences in physiological reactivity (including brain response) associated with individual differences in self-report personality dimensions or psychopathology symptoms.

However, with increasing knowledge of the functioning of brain motivational systems, and disturbances that may occur in this functioning, we also need to begin asking: What individual differences exist in the functioning of these systems, what relations exist between individual differences in functioning across different systems, and how can patterns of individual variation at this lower (neuro-) level lead us to think differently about personality and psychopathology constructs? In other words, it will be increasingly important in future work to allow knowledge of brain function to inform our conceptualizations of individual difference dimensions. We anticipate that this will lead to significant revisions in contemporary thinking about traits and behavior problems, and their structure.

ACKNOWLEDGMENTS

Preparation of this chapter was supported by Grant Nos. MH48657, MH52384, MH65137, and MH072850 from the National Institute of Mental Health; Grant No. R01 AA12164 from the National Institute on Alcohol Abuse and Alcoholism; and funds from the Hathaway endowment at the University of Minnesota.

NOTES

1. It should be noted that lower base rate disorders, including disorders of thought, memory, and perception, were not included in these analyses.
2. However, it should be noted that fear and anxiety tend not to be correlated when fear is defined in terms of willingness to engage in risky behavior to alleviate boredom (i.e., "sensation seeking") rather than as negative affect in the face of danger or threat (Tellegen, 1985; Tellegen & Waller, in press).

REFERENCES

Alheid, G. F., De Olmos, J., & Beltramino, C. A. (1995). Amygdala and extended amygdala. In G. Paxinos (Ed.), *The rat nervous system* (2nd ed., pp. 495–578). London: Academic Press.

American Psychiatric Association. (2000). *Diagnostic and statistical manual of mental disorders* (4th ed., text rev.). Washington, DC: Author.

Anderson, S.W., Bechara, A., Damasio, H., Tranel, D., & Damasio, A. R. (1999). Impairment of social and moral behavior related to early damage in the human prefrontal cortex. *Nature Neuroscience, 2,* 1032–1037.

Barkley, R. A. (1997). Behavioral inhibition, sustained attention, and executive functions: Constructing a unified theory of ADHD. *Psychological Bulletin, 121,* 65–94.

Bechara, A., Damasio, H., Tranel, D., & Anderson, S. W. (1998). Dissociation of working memory from decision making within the human prefrontal cortex. *Journal of Neuroscience, 18,* 428–437.

Bechara, A., Damasio, H., Tranel, D., & Damasio, A. R. (1997). Deciding advantageously before knowing the advantageous strategy. *Science, 275,* 1293–1295.

Beauregard, M., Levesque, J., & Bourgouin, P. (2001). Neural correlates of conscious self-regulation of emotion. *Journal of Neuroscience, 21,* 161–166.

Berridge, K. C. (2003). Pleasures of the brain. *Brain and Cognition, 52,* 106–128.

Berridge, K. C., & Robinson, T. E. (1995). The mind of an addicted brain: Neural sensitization of wanting versus liking. *Current Directions in Psychological Science, 4,* 71–76.

Berridge, K. C., & Robinson, T. E. (1998). What is the role of dopamine in reward: Hedonic impact, reward learning, or incentive salience? *Brain Research Reviews, 28,* 309–369.

Berridge, K. C., Venier, I. L., & Robinson, T. E. (1989). Taste reactivity analysis of 6-hydroxydopamine-induced aphagia: Implications for arousal and anhedonia hypotheses of dopamine function. *Behavioral Neuroscience, 103,* 36–45.

Blair, R. J., & Cipolotti, L. (2000). Impaired social response reversal. A case of "acquired sociopathy." *Brain, 123,* 1122–1141.

Blumer, D., & Benson, D. F. (1975). Personality changes with frontal and temporal lobe lesions. In D. F. Benson & D. Blumer (Eds.), *Psychiatric aspects of neurological disease* (pp. 151–169). New York: Grune & Stratton.

Bradley, M. M., & Lang, P. J. (1994). Measuring emotion: The self-assessment manikin and the semantic differential. *Journal of Behavior Therapy and Experimental Psychiatry, 25,* 49–59.

Bradley, M. M., Cuthbert, B. N., & Lang, P. J. (2000). Affective reactions to acoustic stimuli. *Psychophysiology, 37,* 204–215.

Brown, T. A., & Barlow, D. H. (1992). Comorbidity among anxiety disorders: Implications for treatment and DSM-IV. *Journal of Consulting and Clinical Psychology, 60,* 835–844.

Brown, J. W., & Braver, T. S. (2005). Learned predictions of error likelihood in the anterior cingulate cortex. *Science, 307,* 1118–1121.

Broerse, A., Crawford, T. J., & den Boer, J. A. (2001). Parsing cognition in schizophrenia using saccadic eye movements: A selective overview. *Neuropsychologia, 39,* 742–756.

Buss, A. H., & Plomin, R. (1984). *Temperament: Early developing personality traits.* Hillsdale, NJ: Erlbaum.

Cacioppo, J. T., & Berntson, G. G. (1994). Relationships between attitudes and evaluative space: A critical review with emphasis on the separability of positive and negative substrates. *Psychological Bulletin, 115,* 401–423.

Carter, C. S., Braver, T. S., Barch, D. M., Botvinick, M. M., Noll, D. N., & Cohen, J. D. (1998). Anterior cingulate cortex, error detection, and the online monitoring of performance. *Science, 280,* 747–749.

Center for the Study of Emotion and Attention (CSEA-NIMH). (1999). *The international affective picture system: Digitized photographs.* Gainesville, FL: Center for Research in Psychophysiology, University of Florida.

Clark, L. A., & Watson, D. (1991). Tripartite model of anxiety and depression: Psychometric evidence and taxonomic implications. *Journal of Abnormal Psychology, 100,* 316–336.

Clark, L. A., Watson, D., & Reynolds, S. (1995). Diagnosis and classification of psychopathology: Challenges to the current system and future directions. *Annual Review of Psychology, 46,* 121–153.

Cohen, J. D., Forman, S. D., Braver, T. S., Casey, B. J., Servan-Schreiber, D., & Noll, D. C. (1994). Activation of prefrontal cortex in a nonspatial working memory task with functional MRI. *Human Brain Mapping, 1,* 293–304.

Cohen, J. D., & O'Reilly, R. C. (1996). A preliminary theory of the interactions between prefrontal cortex and hippocampus that contribute to planning and prospective memory. In M. Brandimonte, G. O. Einstein, & M. McDaniel (Eds.), *Prospective memory: Theory and applications* (pp. 267–296). Mahwah, NJ: Erlbaum.

Cohen, J. D., Perlstein, W. M., Braver, T. S., Nystrom, L. E., Noll, D. C., Jonides, J., et al. (1997). Temporal dynamics of brain activation during a working memory task. *Nature, 386,* 604–608.

Cohen, J. D., & Servan-Schreiber, D. (1992). Context, cortex, and dopamine: A connectionist approach to behavior and biology in schizophrenia. *Psychological Review, 99,* 45–77.

Cox, B. J., Clara, I. P., & Enns, M. W. (2002). Posttraumatic stress disorder and the structure of common mental disorders. *Depression and Anxiety, 15,* 168–171.

Cuthbert, B. N., Lang, P. J., Strauss, C., Drobes, D., Patrick, C. J., & Bradley, M. M.

(2003). The psychophysiology of anxiety disorder: Fear memory imagery. *Psychophysiology, 40*, 407–422.

Damasio, H., Grabowski, T., Frank, R., Galaburda, A. M., & Damasio, A. R. (1994). The return of Phineas Gage: Clues about the brain from the skull of a famous patient. *Science, 264*, 1102–1105.

Damasio, A. R., Tranel, D., & Damasio, H. (1990). Individuals with sociopathic behavior caused by frontal damage fail to respond autonomically to social stimuli. *Behavioral Brain Research, 41*, 81–94.

Davidson, R. J. (2002). Anxiety and affective style: Role of prefrontal cortex and amygdala. *Biological Psychiatry, 51*, 68–80.

Davidson, R. J., Pizzigalli, D., Nitschke, J. B., & Putnam, K. M. (2002). Depression: Perspectives from affective neuroscience. *Annual Review of Psychology, 53*, 545–574.

Davidson, R. J., Putnam, K. M., & Larson, C. L. (2000). Dysfunction in the neural circuitry of emotion regulation—A possible prelude to violence. *Science, 289*, 591–594.

Davis, M. (1989). Neural systems involved in fear-potentiated startle. In M. Davis, B. L. Jacobs, & R. I. Schoenfeld (Eds.), Modulation of defined neural vertebrate circuits. *Annals of the New York Academy of Sciences, 563*, pp. 165–183.

Davis, M. (1992). The role of the amygdala in conditioned fear. In J. Aggleton (Ed.), *The amygdala: Neurobiological aspects of emotion, memory and mental dysfunction* (pp. 255–305). New York: Wiley.

Davis, M. (1998). Are different parts of the extended amygdala involved in fear versus anxiety? *Biological Psychiatry, 44*, 1239–1247.

Davis, M., & Lee, Y. (1998). Fear and anxiety: Possible roles of the amygdala and bed nucleus of the stria terminalis. *Cognition and Emotion, 12*, 277–305.

Davis, M., Walker, D. L., & Lee, Y. (1997). Amygdala and bed nucleus of the stria terminalis: Differential roles in fear and anxiety measured with the acoustic startle reflex. *Philosophical Transactions of the Royal Society of London, Series B: Biological Sciences, 352*, 1675–1687.

Davis, M., Walker, D. L., & Myers, K. M. (2003). Role of the amygdala in fear extinction measured with potentiated startle. *Annals of the New York Academy of Sciences, 985*, 218–235.

Davis, M., & Whalen, P. J. (2001). The amygdala: Vigilance and emotion. *Molecular Psychiatry, 6*, 13–34.

Dias, R., Robbins, T. W., & Roberts, A. C. (1996). Dissociation in prefrontal cortex of affective and attentional shifts. *Nature, 380*, 69–72.

Dikman, Z. V., & Allen, J. J. (2000). Error monitoring during reward and avoidance learning in high- and low-socialized individuals. *Psychophysiology, 37*, 43–54.

Eysenck, H. J. (1967). *The biological basis of personality.* Springfield, IL: Thomas.

Fanselow, M. S. (1994). Neural organization of the defensive behavior system responsible for fear. *Psychonomic Bulletin and Review, 1*, 429–438.

Fanselow, M. S., DeCola, J. P., De Oca, B. M., & Landeira-Fernandez, J. (1995). Ventral and dorsolateral regions of the midbrain periaqueductal grey (PAG) control different stages of defensive behavior: Dorsolateral PAG lesions enhance the defensive freezing produced by massed and immediate shock. *Aggressive Behavior, 21*, 63–77.

Fiorino, D. F., Coury, A. G., & Phillips, A. G. (1997). Dynamic changes in nucleus accumbens dopamine efflux during the Coolidge effect in male rats. *Journal of Neuroscience, 17,* 4849–4855.

Gehring, W. J., Himle, J., & Nisenson, L. G. (2000). Action-monitoring dysfunction in obsessive–compulsive disorder. *Psychological Science, 11,* 1–6.

Goldman-Rakic, P. S. (1996). The prefrontal landscape: Implications of functional architecture for understanding human mentation and the central executive. *Philosophical Transactions of the Royal Society of London, Series B: Biological Sciences, 351,* 1445–1453.

Goldsmith, H. H., & Campos, J. J. (1982). Toward a theory of infant temperament. In R. N. Emde & R. J. Harmon (Eds.), *The development of attachment and affiliative systems* (pp. 161–193). New York: Plenum.

Gray, J. A. (1982). *The neuropsychology of anxiety.* New York: Oxford University Press.

Gray, J. A. (1987). *The psychology of fear and stress* (2nd ed.). Cambridge, UK: University of Cambridge Press.

Greenwald, M. K., Cook, E. W., & Lang, P. J. (1989). Affective judgment and psychophysiological response: Dimensional covariation in the evaluation of pictorial stimuli. *Journal of Psychophysiology, 3,* 51–64.

Grillon, C., & Davis, M. (1997). Fear-potentiated startle conditioning in humans: Explicit and contextual cue conditioning following paired versus unpaired training. *Psychophysiology, 34,* 451–458.

Grillon, C., & Morgan, C. A. (1999). Fear-potentiated startle conditioning to explicit and contextual cues in Gulf War veterans with posttraumatic stress disorder. *Journal of Abnormal Psychology, 108,* 134–142.

Hariri, A. R., Mattay, V. S., Tessitore, A., Kolachana, B., Fera, F., Goldman, D., et al. (2002). Serotonin transporter genetic variation and the response of the human amygdala. *Science, 297,* 400–403.

Harmon-Jones, E. (2003). Clarifying the emotive functions of asymmetrical frontal cortical activity. *Psychophysiology, 40,* 838–848.

Harmon-Jones, E., & Allen, J. J. B. (1998). Anger and prefrontal brain activity: EEG asymmetry consistent with approach motivation despite negative affective valence. *Journal of Personality and Social Psychology, 74,* 1310–1316.

Heimer, L., Alheid, G. F., de Olmos, J. S., Groenewegen, H. J., Haber, S. N., Harlan, R. E., et al. (1997). The accumbens: Beyond the core-shell dichotomy. *Journal of Neuropsychiatry and Clinical Neurosciences, 9,* 354–381.

Holroyd, C. B., Dien, J., & Coles, M. G. H. (1998). Error-related scalp potentials elicited by hand and foot movements: Evidence for an output-independent error-processing system in humans. *Neuroscience Letters, 242,* 65–68.

Horvitz, J. C., Richardson, W. B., & Ettenberg, A. (1993). Dopamine receptor blockade and thirst produce differential effects on drinking behavior. *Pharmacology Biochemistry and Behavior, 45,* 725–728.

Iacono, W. G., Carlson, S. R., Taylor, J., Elkins, I. J., & McGue, M. (1999). Behavioral disinhibition and the development of substance-use disorders: Findings from the Minnesota Twin Family Study. *Development and Psychopathology, 11,* 869–900.

Izard, C. E. (1993). Four systems for emotion activation: Cognitive and noncognitive processes. *Psychological Review, 100,* 68–90.

John, O. P., & Srivastava, S. (1999). The Big Five trait taxonomy: History, measurement, and theoretical perspectives. In L. A. Pervin & O. John (Eds.), *Handbook of personality: Theory and research* (2nd ed., pp. 102–138). New York: Guilford Press.

Kagan, J. (1994). *Galen's prophecy: Temperament in human nature.* New York: Basic Books.

Kendler, K. S., Prescott, C. A., Myers, J., & Neale, M. C. (2003). The structure of genetic and environmental risk factors for common psychiatric and substance use disorders in men and women. *Archives of General Psychiatry, 60,* 929–937.

Konorski, J. (1967). *Integrative activity of the brain: An interdisciplinary approach.* Chicago: University of Chicago Press.

Krueger, R. F. (1999a). The structure of common mental disorders. *Archives of General Psychiatry, 56,* 921–926.

Krueger, R. F. (1999b). Personality traits in late adolescence predict mental disorders in early adulthood: A prospective-epidemiological study. *Journal of Personality, 67,* 39–65.

Krueger, R. F., Caspi, A., Moffitt, T. E., & Silva, P. A. (1998). The structure and stability of common mental disorders (DSM-III-R): A longitudinal–epidemiological study. *Journal of Abnormal Psychology, 107,* 216–227.

Krueger, R. F., Caspi, A., Moffitt, T. E., Silva, P. A., & McGee, R. (1996). Personality traits are differentially linked to mental disorders: A multi-trait, multi-diagnosis study of an adolescent birth cohort. *Journal of Abnormal Psychology, 105,* 299–312.

Krueger, R. F., Hicks, B., Patrick, C. J., Carlson, S., Iacono, W. G., & McGue, M. (2002). Etiologic connections among substance dependence, antisocial behavior, and personality: Modeling the externalizing spectrum. *Journal of Abnormal Psychology, 111,* 411–424.

Krueger, R. F., & Markon, K. E. (in press). Reinterpreting comorbidity: A model-based approach to understanding and classifying psychopathology. *Annual Review of Clinical Psychology.*

Krueger, R. F., Markon, K. E., Patrick, C. J., Benning, S. D., & Kramer, M. (2005). *Linking antisocial behavior, substance use, and personality: An integrative quantitative model of the adult externalizing spectrum.* Manuscript submitted for publication.

Krueger, R. F., McGue, M., & Iacono, W. G. (2001). The higher-order structure of common DSM mental disorders: Internalization, externalization, and their connections to personality. *Personality and Individual Differences, 30,* 1245–1259.

Lang, P. J. (1995). The emotion probe: Studies of motivation and attention. *American Psychologist, 50,* 372–385.

Lang, P. J., Bradley, M. M., & Cuthbert, B. N. (1990). Emotion, attention, and the startle reflex. *Psychological Review, 97,* 377–398.

Lang, P. J., Bradley, M. M., & Cuthbert, B. N. (1997). Motivated attention: Affect, activation, and action. In P. J. Lang, R. F. Simons, & M. T. Balaban (Eds.), *Attention and orienting: Sensory and motivational processes* (pp. 97–135). Hillsdale, NJ: Erlbaum.

Lang, P. J., Bradley, M. M., Cuthbert, B. N., & Patrick, C. J. (1993). Emotion and psychopathology: A startle probe analysis. In L. Chapman & D. Fowles (Eds.),

Progress in experimental personality and psychopathology research (Vol. 16, pp. 163–199). New York: Springer.

Lang, P. J., Bradley, M. M., Fitzsimmons, J. R., Cuthbert, B. N., Scott, J. D., Moulder, B., et al. (1998). Emotional arousal and activation of the visual cortex: An fMRI analysis. *Psychophysiology, 35,* 199–210.

Lang, P. J., Davis, M., & Öhman, A. (2000). Fear and anxiety: Animal models and human cognitive psychophysiology. *Journal of Affective Disorders, 61,* 137–159.

Lang, P. J., Greenwald, M. K., Bradley, M. M., & Hamm, A. O. (1993). Looking at pictures: Affective, facial, visceral, and behavioral reactions. *Psychophysiology, 30,* 261–273.

Larsen, R. J., & Diener, E. (1992). Promises and problems with the circumplex model of emotion. In M. S. Clark (Ed.), *Emotion: Review of personality and social psychology* (pp. 25–59). Newbury Park, CA: Sage.

LeDoux, J. E. (1995). Emotion: Clues from the brain. *Annual Review of Psychology, 46,* 209–235.

LeDoux, J. E. (2000). Emotion circuits in the brain. *Annual Review of Neuroscience, 23,* 155–184.

Lee, R., & Coccaro, E. (2001). The neuropsychopharmacology of criminality and aggression. *Canadian Journal of Psychiatry, 46,* 35–44.

Lee, Y., & Davis, M. (1997). Role of the hippocampus, bed nucleus of the stria terminalis and amygdala in the excitatory effect of corticotropin releasing hormone on the acoustic startle reflex. *Journal of Neuroscience, 17,* 6424–6433.

Lindsley, D. B. (1951). Emotions. In S. S. Stevens (Ed.), *Handbook of experimental psychology* (pp. 473–516). New York: Wiley.

Luu, P., Flaisch, T., & Tucker, D. M. (2000). Medial frontal cortex in action monitoring. *Journal of Neuroscience, 20,* 464–469.

MacDonald, A. W., III, Cohen, J. D., Stenger, V. A., & Carter, C. S. (2000). Dissociating the role of dorsolateral prefrontal and anterior cingulate cortex in cognitive control. *Science, 288,* 1835–1838.

McClure, S. M., Daw, N. D., & Montague, P. R. (2003). A computational substrate for incentive salience. *Trends in Neurosciences, 26,* 423–428.

Miller, E. K. (1999). The prefrontal cortex: Complex neural properties for complex behavior. *Neuron, 22,* 15–17.

Miller, E. K., & Cohen, J. D. (2001). An integrative theory of prefrontal cortex function. *Annual Review of Neuroscience, 24,* 167–202.

Miltner, W. H. R., Braun, C. H., & Coles, M. G. H. (1997). Event-related brain potentials following incorrect feedback in a time-estimation task: Evidence for a "generic" neural system for error detection. *Journal of Cognitive Neuroscience, 9,* 788–798.

Mineka, S., Watson, D., & Clark, L. E. A. (1998). Comorbidity of anxiety and unipolar mood disorders. *Annual Review of Psychology, 49,* 377–412.

Montague, P. R., Dayan, P., & Sejnowski, T. J. (1996). A framework for mesencephalic dopamine systems based on predictive Hebbian learning. *Journal of Neuroscience, 16,* 1936–1947.

Montague, P. R., Hyman, S. E., & Cohen, J. D. (2004). Computational roles for dopamine in behavioural control. *Nature, 431,* 760–767.

Morgan, A. B., & Lilienfeld, S. O. (2000). A meta-analytic review of the relation between antisocial behavior and neuropsychological measures of executive function. *Clinical Psychology Review*, 20, 113–136.

Moruzzi, G., & Magoun, H. W. (1949). Brain stem reticular formation and activation of the EEG. *Electroencephalography and Clinical Neurophysiology*, 1, 455–473.

Muri, R. M., Heid, O., Nirkko, A. C., Ozdoba, C., Felblinger, J., Schroth, G., & Hess, C. W. (1998). Functional organization of saccades and antisaccades in the frontal lobe in humans: A study with echo planar functional magnetic resonance imaging. *Journal of Neurology, Neurosurgery, and Psychiatry*, 65, 374–377.

Ochsner, K. N., Bunge, S. A., Gross, J. J., & Gabrieli, J. D. (2002). Rethinking feelings: An fMRI study of the cognitive regulation of emotion. *Journal of Cognitive Neuroscience*, 14, 1215–1229.

Ochsner, K., Ray, R. D., Cooper, J. C., Robertson, E. R., Chopra, S., Gabrieli, J. D., et al. (2004). For better or for worse: Neural systems supporting the cognitive down- and up-regulation of negative emotion. *Neuroimage*, 23, 483–499.

Öhman, A. (1993). Fear and anxiety as emotional phenomena: Clinical phenomenology, evolutionary perspectives, and information processing mechanisms. In M. Lewis & J. M. Haviland (Eds.), *Handbook of emotions* (pp. 511–536). New York: Guilford Press.

Olds, J. (1956). Pleasure centers in the brain. *Scientific American*, 195, 105–116.

Olds, J., & Milner, P. (1954). Positive reinforcement produced by electrical stimulation of septal area and other regions of rat brain. *Journal of Comparative and Physiological Psychology*, 47, 419–427.

Patrick, C. J. (1994). Emotion and psychopathy: Startling new insights. *Psychophysiology*, 31, 319–330.

Patrick, C. J., & Lavoro, S. A. (1997). Ratings of emotional response to pictorial stimuli: Positive and negative affect dimensions. *Motivation and Emotion*, 21, 297–321.

Peterson, J. B., & Pihl, R. O. (1990). Information processing, neuropsychological function, and the inherited predisposition to alcoholism. *Neuropsychology Review*, 1, 343–369.

Petrides, M. (2000). Dissociable roles of mid-dorsolateral prefrontal and anterior inferotemporal cortex in visual working memory. *Journal of Neuroscience*, 20, 7496–7503.

Phelps, E. A., Delgado, M. R., Nearing, K. I., & LeDoux, J. E. (2004). Extinction learning in humans: Role of the amygdala and vmPFC. *Neuron*, 43, 897–905.

Phillips, A. G. (1984). Brain reward circuitry: A case for separate systems. *Brain Research Bulletin*, 12, 195–201.

Plutchik, R. (1984). Emotions: A general psychoevolutionary theory. In K. Scherer & P. Ekman (Eds.), *Approaches to emotion* (pp. 197–219). Hillsdale, NJ: Erlbaum.

Quirk, G. J., Russo, G. K., Barron, J. L., & Lebron, K. (2000). The role of ventromedial prefrontal cortex in the recovery of extinguished fear. *Journal of Neuroscience*, 20, 6225–6231.

Raine, A., Ishikawa, S. S., Arce, E., Lencz, T., Knuth, K. H., Bihrle, S., et al. (2004). Hippocampal structural asymmetry in unsuccessful psychopaths. *Biological Psychiatry*, 55, 185–191.

Robinson, T. E., & Berridge, K. C. (2000). The psychology and neurobiology of addiction: An incentive-sensitization view. *Addiction, 95*, S91–S117.

Robinson, T. E., & Berridge, K. C. (2003). Addiction. *Annual Review of Psychology, 54*, 25–53.

Rolls, E. T. (2000). The orbitofrontal cortex and reward. *Cerebral Cortex, 10*, 284–294.

Rosen, J. B., & Schulkin, J. B. (1998). From normal fear to pathological anxiety. *Psychological Review, 105*, 325–350.

Russell, J. A., & Mehrabian, A. (1977). Evidence for a three-factor theory of emotions. *Journal of Research in Personality, 11*, 273–294.

Sabatinelli, D., Bradley, M. M., Fitzsimmons, J. R., & Lang, P. J. (2004). Parallel amygdala and inferotemporal activation reflect emotional intensity and fear relevance. *NeuroImage, 24*, 1265–1270.

Scheffers, M., Coles, M. G. H., Bernstein, P., Gehring, W. J., & Donchin, E. (1996). Event-related potentials and error-related processing: An analysis of incorrect responses to go and no-go stimuli. *Psychophysiology, 33*, 42–53.

Schneirla, T. C. (1959). An evolutionary and developmental theory of biphasic processes underlying approach and withdrawal. In M. R. Jones (Ed.), *Nebraska Symposium on Motivation* (Vol. 7, pp. 1–42). Lincoln: University of Nebraska Press.

Schultz, W. (1998). Predictive reward signal of dopamine neurons. *Journal of Neurophysiology, 80*, 1–27.

Schultz, W., Apicella, P., & Ljungberg, T. (1993). Responses of monkey dopamine neurons to reward and conditioned stimuli during successive steps of learning a delayed response task. *Journal of Neuroscience, 13*, 900–913.

Sher, K. J., & Trull, T. J. (1994). Personality and disinhibitory psychopathology: Alcoholism and antisocial personality disorder. *Journal of Abnormal Psychology, 103*, 92–102.

Shizgal, P. (1999). On the neural computation of utility: Implications from studies of brain stimulation reward. In D. Kahneman, E. Diener, & N. Schwarz (Eds.), *Well-being: The foundations of hedonic psychology* (pp. 500–524). New York: Russell Sage Foundation.

Soderstrom, H., Tullberg, M., Wikkelsoe, C., Ekholm, S., & Forsman, A. (2000). Reduced regional cerebral blood flow in non-psychotic violent offenders. *Psychiatry Research: Neuroimaging, 98*, 29–41.

Tarter, R. E., Alterman, A. I., & Edwards, K. L. (1985). Vulnerability to alcoholism in men: A behavior-genetic perspective. *Journal of Studies on Alcohol, 46*, 329–356.

Tellegen, A. (1985). Structures of mood and personality and their relevance to assessing anxiety, with an emphasis on self-report. In A. H. Tuma & J. D. Maser (Eds.), *Anxiety and the anxiety disorders* (pp. 681–706). Hillsdale, NJ: Erlbaum.

Tellegen, A. (in press). *Manual for the Multidimensional Personality Questionnaire.* Minneapolis: University of Minnesota Press.

Tellegen, A., & Waller, N. G. (in press). *Exploring personality through test construction: Development of the Multidimensional Personality Questionnaire.* Minneapolis: University of Minnesota Press.

Tellegen, A., Watson, D., & Clark, L. A. (1999). On the dimensional and hierarchical structure of affect. *Psychological Science, 10*, 297–309.

Verona, E., Patrick, C. J., Curtin, J. J., Bradley, M. M., & Lang, P. J. (2004). Psychopathy and physiological response to emotionally evocative sounds. *Journal of Abnormal Psychology, 113*, 99–108.

Wagar, B. M., & Thagard, P. (2004). Spiking Phineas Gage: A neurocomputational theory of cognitive-affective integration in decision-making. *Psychological Review, 111*, 67–79.

Walker, D. L., & Davis, M. (1997). Double dissociation between the involvement of the bed nucleus of the stria terminalis and the central nucleus of the amygdala in light-enhanced versus fear-potentiated startle. *Journal of Neuroscience, 17*, 9375–9383.

Watson, D. (2005). Rethinking the mood and anxiety disorders: A quantitative hierarchical model for DSM-V. *Journal of Abnormal Psychology, 114*, 522–536.

Watson, D., Clark, L. A., & Tellegen, A. (1988). Development and validation of brief measures of positive and negative affect: The PANAS scales. *Journal of Personality and Social Psychology, 54*, 1063–1070.

Watson, D., & Tellegen, A. (1985). Toward a consensual structure of mood. *Psychological Bulletin, 98*, 219–235.

Whalen, P. J., Rauch, S. L., Etcoff, N. L., McInerney, S. C., Lee, M., & Jenike, M. A. (1998). Masked presentations of emotional facial expressions modulate amygdala activity without explicit knowledge. *Journal of Neuroscience, 18*, 411–418.

Widiger, T. A., Verheul, R., & van den Brink, W. (1999). Personality and psychopathology. In L. A. Pervin & O. John (Eds.), *Handbook of personality: Theory and research* (2nd ed., pp. 347–366). New York: Guilford Press.

Wise, R. A. (1985). The anhedonia hypothesis: Mark III. *Behavioral and Brain Sciences, 8*, 178–186.

Wise, S. P., Murray, E. A., & Gerfen, C. R. (1996). The frontal-basal ganglia system in primates. *Critical Reviews in Neurobiology, 10*, 317–356.

Wittchen, H. U. (1996). Critical issues in the evaluation of comorbidity of psychiatric disorders. *British Journal of Psychiatry, 30*(Suppl.), 9–16.

Young, S. E., Stallings, M. C., Corley, R. P., Krauter, K. S., & Hewitt, J. K. (2000). Genetic and environmental influences on behavioral disinhibition. *American Journal of Medical Genetics (Neuropsychiatric Genetics), 96*, 684–695.

Zuckerman, M. (1979). *Sensation seeking: Beyond the optimal level of arousal.* Hillsdale, NJ: Erlbaum.

Chapter 8

A Multidimensional Neurobehavioral Model of Personality Disturbance

RICHARD A. DEPUE
MARK F. LENZENWEGER

The relationship of personality to psychopathology is an exceedingly complex issue with no apparent unifying principles. Not only does the relationship depend on one's model of personality—particularly on how one conceives of the lines of causal influence underlying the structure of personality (Depue & Collins, 1999)—but also on which forms of psychopathology are considered. A modifying role of personality on psychopathology may be the most frequently posited between the two domains. In such cases, a neurobehavioral system underlying a personality trait may serve to *modify* the phenotype and/or course of the disorder. In the case of modifying the course of the disorder, such modification may affect, for instance, the probability of the environmentally elicited onset of the disorder and hence the age of onset or frequency of episodes over time. Examples of this are when variation in the levels of the traits of anxiety (neuroticism, negative emotionality (Tellegen & Waller, in press]) or constraint affect an individual's sensitivity and biologic perturbability to stressful circumstances.

Alternatively, the phenotypic characteristics of the disorder over time may be modified by personality traits, thereby influencing the type of the course of the disorder. For instance, we have suggested that a dopaminergic-facilitated incentive motivation system underlies extraversion (Depue &

Collins, 1999; Depue, Luciana, Arbisi, Collins, & Leon, 1994; Depue & Morrone-Strupinsky, 2005), and that instability in dopamine functioning may yield fluctuations between manic and depressed behavior in some forms of bipolar affective disorder (Depue & Iacono, 1989). To the extent that this is correct, the level of extraversion will reflect in part an individual's level of dopamine functioning. Thus, at times of dopamine instability in people at risk for some forms of bipolar disorder, the *frequency* over time of either hypomanic or depressive episodes may be influenced by trait levels of extraversion/dopamine (high vs. low, respectively). This may represent one source of the heterogeneity of course observed in both subsyndromal and syndromal bipolar disorders—ranging from predominantly depressive episodes, to a balanced frequency of depressed and hypomanic–manic episodes, to predominantly hypomanic–manic episodes.

It is possible, of course, to consider a more direct relationship of personality to psychopathology, and this may take at least two different forms. In a first case, the underlying neurobehavioral system of a personality trait may provide a *foundation* within which a disordered neurobiological variable resides. At times of disordered functioning of that variable, the nature of the *phenotype* of the disorder will partially reflect the behavioral characteristics of the relevant personality trait. For instance, to employ the example used above concerning extraversion, dopamine instability and bipolar disorder, extreme dopamine vascillations between excessive and minimal functioning may be reflected as extremely high extraverted behavioral features (hypomania–mania) or extremely low extraverted features (psychomotor retarded depression), respectively.

A second case of a direct relationship of personality to psychopathology is when so-called *disorder* emerges from natural variation in the neurobehavioral systems underlying personality traits, where disorders represent extreme phenotypes that arise at the tails of naturally occurring behavioral dimensions. Of course, viewing disorder as lying at the extreme of normal personality dimensions is based solely on a phenotypic correlational level of analysis, but no assumption is made herein that phenotypic dimensions are biologically continuous. The phenotypic continuity could well represent several underlying distinct genotypic distributions, as may be the case even within the normal range of variation of some personality traits (Munafo et al., 2003). In no other set of disorders as in the personality *disorders* is this type of direct relationship between personality and psychopathology so often posited. But the manner in which this relationship can be modeled is complex and hotly debated, and typically lacks clarity due to a poorly conceived neurobehavioral foundation of normal personality. Therefore, below we outline what we believe is the best available evidence for the neurobehavioral foundation of normal personality. We then use this foundation to provide a novel model that treats personality disturbance as continuously, emerging phenotypes created by extreme values in the products of multiple interacting dimensions of personality.

THE PROBLEM OF MODELING PERSONALITY DISORDERS

From a scientific perspective, it is really no longer possible to accept the notion that personality disorders represent distinct categorical diagnostic entities. The behavioral features of personality disorders are not organized into discrete diagnostic entities, and multivariate studies of behavioral criteria fail to identify factors that resemble existing diagnostic constructs (Block, 2001; Ekselius, Lindstrom, von Knorring, Bodlund, & Kullgren, 1994; Livesley, 2001; Livesley, Schroeder, Jackson, & Jang, 1994). Indeed, just the opposite is observed: the behavioral features of personality disorders merge imperceptibly in a continuous fashion across diagnostic categories, resulting in (1) significant overlap of behavioral features across categories and hence diagnostic comorbidity within individuals, and (2) symptom heterogeneity within categories and hence frequent (and most common in some studies) application of the ambiguous diagnosis of personality disorders not otherwise specified (Livesley, 2001; Saulsman & Page, 2004). Moreover, aside from schizotypy/schizotypic disorders (Lenzenweger & Korfine, 1992; Korfine & Lenzenweger, 1995), the existing latent class and taxometric analysis literature on personality disorders generally does *not* provide support for distinct entities for the majority of conditions in the personality disorder realm in any compelling fashion (Haslam, 2003), and our reading of that literature suggests that even some provisional taxonic findings for borderline and antisocial personality disorders are open to doubt. It is, accordingly, not surprising that diagnostic membership is not significantly associated with predictive validity as to prognosis or psychological or pharmacological treatments (Livesley, 2001). Such a state of affairs recently led Livesley (2001) to declare that "evidence on these points has accumulated to the point that it can no longer be ignored" (p. 278).

Such a state of affairs supports proponents of a dimensional approach to personality disorders, who note that (1) the behavioral features of personality disorders not only overlap diagnostic categories, but also merge imperceptibly with normality (Livesley, 2001; Saulsman & Page, 2004); and (2) the factorial structure of behavioral traits associated with personality disorders is similar in clinical and nonclinical samples (Livesley, Jackson, & Schroeder, 1992; Reynolds & Clark, 2001). Furthermore, the higher-order structure of personality disorder traits resembles four of the five major traits identified in the higher-order structure of normal personality (Clark & Livesley, 1994; Clark Livesley, Schroeder, & Irish, 1996;

Reynolds & Clark, 2001). These findings suggest that personality disorders may be better understood as emerging at the extremes of personality dimensions that define the structure of behavior in the normal population (for reviews of this position see Costa & Widiger, 1994; Depue & Lenzenweger, 2001; Lenzenweger & Clarkin, 1996, 2005; Livesley, 2001; Reynolds & Clark, 2001; Saulsman & Page, 2004; Widiger, Trull, Clarkin, Sanderson, & Costa, 1994).

This realization has led to innumerable attempts to illustrate the association of personality traits with personality disorder diagnostic categories. Most of these studies have relied on the so-called five-factor model of personality, which defines a structure characterized by the five higher-order traits of extraversion, neuroticism, agreeableness, conscientiousness, and openness to experience. Although Reynolds and Clark (2001) demonstrated that four of these traits (openness shows no consistent relation to personality disorders; Saulsman & Page, 2004) account for a substantial proportion of the variance in interview-based ratings of DSM-IV personality disorder diagnoses, a recent meta-analysis of similar studies demonstrated the limitation of the approach of correlating four traits with personality disorders (Saulsman & Page, 2004). The meta-analysis showed that most such studies illustrate that (1) the correlation of these four traits with personality disorder categories is moderate to weak; (2) the complex "entity" of a personality disorder category is defined by as little as one trait but never by four traits in a significant way; (3) single traits (e.g., neuroticism) characterize more than one and sometimes several putatively distinct personality disorders. For example, how helpful is it to know that histrionic personality disorder is characterized by moderately high extraversion but by no other trait, or, similarly, that dependent personality disorder is associated with moderately high neuroticism but no other trait? To what line of research or clinical intervention does that knowledge lead? Moreover, the traits relate more highly to personality disorder categories that are studied in nonclinical samples, indicating that the traits may be less valuable in defining clinical entities. What the meta-analysis did reveal is that most personality disorders manifest, in common, higher trait levels of neuroticism and lower trait levels of agreeableness, meaning that most individuals with personality disorders are subject to negative emotionality and impaired affiliative or interpersonal behavior. Thus, again, when personality disorder categories serve as the outcome variable, personality traits provide little in the way of power to discriminate between such categories. Overall, then, it is probably not unfair to conclude that such correlational studies have done little to inform the issue of continuity from personality systems to states of disorder, most of them having merely specified correlates of personality disorders and nothing more, and most of these studies lacked an underlying framework for understanding both personality and personality disorders.

The paradox in all of this is that, despite knowing that the personality disorder diagnostic categories are unreliable and lack compelling construct and predictive validity, researchers cling to the approach of relating major personality traits, typically considered at the conceptual level of analysis one trait at a time, to *nonentities* of personality disorders. How can one learn something substantive by relating four higher-order traits to heterogeneous behavioral phenomena that are clustered conceptually (not statistically or theoretically) into diagnostic entities? As Livesley (2001) aptly notes, since personality disorder diagnoses are so fundamentally flawed, it is not important to know whether each personality disorder diagnosis can be accommodated by a dimensional model. Furthermore, the problem in this approach does not appear to be explained simply by use of a small number of broad traits. When the 30 facet scales of the NEO-PI were correlated with personality disorder categories, only modest gains were achieved relative to the use of the four major traits (mean difference in $R^2 \sim .04$) (Dyce & O'Connor, 1998; Millon, 1997).

Perhaps one of the most crucial issues associated with a dimensional personality approach to personality disorders is that the substantive meaning of the four major traits is not clear and generally has been a neglected topic (Block, 2001). Put differently, there is not a clear understanding as to which underlying neurobehavioral systems these traits reflect, which the behavior-genetic literature implies they must (Tellegen et al., 1988). Accordingly, in this chapter we attempt to promote an alternative empirical and theoretical approach to personality disorders. First, we embrace the fact that personality disorders do not exist as *distinct entities*, and, therefore, we refer to the behavioral manifestations that emerge at the extremes of personality dimensions as *personality disturbance* rather than disorders. We exclude schizotypal and paranoid personality disorders from our model, because there is evidence that they may be genetically related to schizophrenia (e.g., Kendler et al., 1993; Lenzenweger & Loranger, 1989), representing an alternative manifestation of schizophrenia liability (Lenzenweger, 1998), and studies of the latent class structure of schizotypy show evidence that its underlying nature is more likely of a taxonic or qualitative nature (Lenzenweger & Korfine, 1992; Korfine & Lenzenweger, 1995; see also Haslam, 2003). The term "disorder," though less formal and regimented than the term "disease," nevertheless connotes a relatively coherent symptomatic entity that, with only more empirical attention, will be characterized by distinct boundaries and underlying dysfunction. We do not believe that, as personality disorders are currently conceived, such a state of scientific credibility will be achieved, and hence they do not warrant the use of the terms "syndrome," "disorder," or "disease." Second, we attempt to delineate the nature of the neurobehavioral systems that we postulate underlie the four major traits of personality. In so doing, we hope to provide a substantive meaning to the four major personality traits that supersedes the extant variation in trait labels and psychological concepts.

The implications of defining personality traits in terms of neurobehavioral systems leads to a third aspect of the chapter, where we derive a model of personality disturbance based on the *interaction* of these neurobehavioral systems. Though, genetically speaking it may be possible to conceive of the neurobiological variables associated with neurobehavioral systems as subject to independent influences, it is impossible to imagine that neurobehavioral systems are independent at a functional level. Similarly, it is impossible to imagine that personality traits can be associated in an independent manner to personality disorders. Neurobehavioral systems, and the personality traits that reflect their influence, interact to produce complex behavior patterns—personality as a whole—in a multivariate fashion. Therefore, our model of personality disturbance rests on a foundation of multivariate interaction of neurobehavioral systems. Such an interaction may yield a phenotypic clustering of behavioral signs or symptoms that could be taken to suggest a demarcation, perhaps indicative of latent threshold effects in the neurobehavioral systems, but the observed clustering represents the end product of underlying continuous dimensional neurobehavioral systems. Such clusterings may be resolved with appropriate statistical methods such as finite mixture modeling. Furthermore, while it is true that our model is dimensional in nature, where personality disturbance lies at the extreme of normal interacting personality dimensions, it is worth noting that no assumption is made herein that phenotypic dimensions of personality are genetically continuous. The phenotypic continuity could well represent several underlying *distinct* genotypic distributions (Gottesman, 1997), as may be the case even within the normal range of variation of some personality traits (Benjamin et al., 1996; Ebstein et al., 1996).

NEUROBEHAVIORAL SYSTEMS UNDERLYING HIGHER-ORDER PERSONALITY TRAITS

The higher-order structure of personality is converging on three to seven factors that account for the phenotypic variation in behavior (Digman, 1997; Tellegen & Waller, in press). Although there is considerable agreement on the robustness of at least four higher-order traits, there is nevertheless substantial variation in the definition of these traits, because researchers emphasize different characteristics depending on their trait concepts. Our model focuses on four higher-order traits that are robustly identified in the psychometric literature and that we define with reference to coherent neurobehavioral systems. Higher-order traits resembling *extraversion* and *neuroticism* (anxiety) are identified in virtually every taxonomy of personality. Affiliation, termed *agreeableness* (Costa & McCrae, 1992; Goldberg & Rosolack, 1994) or *social closeness* (Tellegen & Waller, in press), has emerged more recently as a robust trait, and is composed of affiliative tendencies, cooperativeness, and feelings of warmth and affection (Depue & Morrone-Strupinksy, 2005). Finally, some form of impulsivity, more recently termed *constraint* (Tellegen & Waller, in press) or *conscientiousness* (due to an emphasis on the unreliability, unorderliness, and disorganization accompanying an impulsive disposition [Costa & McCrae, 1992; Goldberg & Rosolack, 1994]), frequently emerges in factor studies.

Agentic Extraversion and Affiliation

Trait Complexities Related to Interpersonal Behavior

Interpersonal behavior is not a unitary characteristic, but rather has two major components. One component, *affiliation*, reflects enjoying and valuing close interpersonal bonds and being warm and affectionate; the other component, *agency*, reflects social dominance, assertiveness, exhibitionism, and a subjective sense of potency in accomplishing goals. These two components are consistent with the two independent major traits identified in the theory of interpersonal behavior: Warm–Agreeable versus Assured–Dominant (Wiggins, 1991). Recent studies have consistently supported a two-component structure of interpersonal behavior in joint factor analyses of multidimensional personality questionnaires (Church, 1994; Church & Burke, 1994; Digman, 1997; Morrone, Depue, Scherer, & White, 2000; Morrone-Strupinsky & Depue, 2004; Tellegen & Waller, in press), where two general traits were identified in each case as affiliation and agency (Depue & Collins, 1999). Lower-order traits of social dominance, achievement, endurance, persistence, efficacy, activity, and energy all loaded much more strongly on agency than on affiliation, whereas traits of sociability, warmth, and agreeableness showed a reverse pattern. Such findings have led trait psychologists to propose that affiliation and agency represent distinct dispositions (Depue & Collins, 1999; Depue & Morrone-Strupinsky, 2005; Tellegen & Waller, in press): whereas affiliation is clearly interpersonal in nature, agency represents a more general disposition that is manifest in a range of achievement-related, as well as interpersonal, contexts (Costa & McCrae, 1992; Goldberg & Rosolack, 1994; Tellegen & Waller, in press; Watson & Clark, 1997; Wiggins, 1991).

Association of Agentic Extraversion and Affiliation with Two Neurobehavioral Systems

Behavioral systems may be understood as behavior patterns that evolved to adapt to stimuli critical for survival and species preservation (Gray, 1973,

1992; MacLean, 1986; Schneirla, 1959). As opposed to specific behavioral systems that guide interaction with very specific stimulus contexts, *general* behavioral systems are more flexible and have less immediate objectives and more variable topographies (Blackburn, Phillips, Jakubovic, & Fibiger, 1989; MacLean, 1986). General systems are activated by broad *classes* of stimulus (Depue & Collins, 1999; Gray, 1973, 1992), and regulate general emotional-behavioral dispositions, such as desire–approach, fear–inhibition, or affiliative tendencies, that modulate goal-directed activity. It is the general systems that directly influence the structure of mammalian behavior at higher-order levels of organization, because, like higher-order personality traits, their pervasive modulatory effects on behavior derive from frequent activation by broad stimulus classes. *Thus, the higher-order traits of personality, which are general and few most likely reflect the activity of the few, general neurobehavioral systems.*

We have suggested that the two traits of agentic extraversion and affiliation reflect the activity of two neurobehavioral systems involved in guiding behavior to *rewarding* goals (Depue & Collins, 1999; Depue & Strupinsky, 2005). Reward involves several dynamically interacting neurobehavioral processes occurring across two phases of goal acquisition: appetitive and consummatory. Although both phases are elicited by unconditioned incentive (reward-connoting) stimuli, their temporal onset, behavioral manifestations, and putative neural systems differ (Berridge, 1999; Blackburn et al., 1989; Depue & Collins, 1999; DiChiara & North, 1992; Wyvell & Berridge, 2000), and are dissociated in factor analytic studies based on behavioral characteristics of animals (Pfaus, Smith, & Coopersmith, 1999).

An appetitive preparatory phase of goal acquisition represents the first step toward attaining biologically important goals (Blackburn et al., 1989; Hillard, Domjan, Nguyen, & Cusato, 1998). It is based on a mammalian behavioral system that is activated by, and serves to bring an animal into contact with, unconditioned and conditioned rewarding incentive stimuli (Depue & Collins, 1999; Gray, 1973; Schneirla, 1959). This system is consistently described in all animals across phylogeny (Schneirla, 1959), and we define this system as *a behavioral approach based on incentive motivation* (Depue & Collins, 1999).

The nature of this behavioral system, as well as the system associated with a consummatory phase of reward (discussed next), can be most efficiently described by using an affiliative object (e.g., a potential mate) as the rewarding goal object. Thus, an affiliative goal is used throughout this and the next sections. In the appetitive phase of affiliation (see Figure 8.1), specific *distal* affiliative stimuli of potential bonding partners—for example, facial features and smiles, friendly vocalizations and gestures, and bodily features (Porges, 1998)—serve as unconditioned incentive stimuli based on their distinct patterns of sensory properties, such as smell, color, shape, and temperature (DiChiara & North, 1992; Hilliard et al., 1998). For instance, Breiter, Aharon, Kanneman, Dale, and Shizgal (2001) and Aharon et al. (2001) have shown that even passive viewing of attractive female faces unconditionally activates the anatomical areas that integrate reward, incentive motivation, and approach behavior in heterosexual males. These incentives are inherently evaluated as positive in valence, and activate incentive motivation, increased energy through sympathetic nervous system activity, and forward locomotion as a means of bringing individuals into close proximity (DiChiara & North, 1992). Moreover, the incentive state is inherently rewarding but in a highly activated manner, and animals will work intensively to obtain that reward without evidence of satiety (Depue & Collins, 1999).

In humans, the incentive state is associated with subjective feelings of desire, wanting, excitement, elation, enthusiasm, energy, potency, and self-efficacy that are distinct from, but typically co-occur with, feelings of pleasure and liking (Berridge, 1999; Watson & Tellegen, 1985). This subjective experience is concordant with the nature of the lower-order traits of social dominance, achievement, endurance, persistence, efficacy, activity, and energy that all load strongly on the *agency* personality factor (see above), and with the adjectives that define the subjective *state* of positive affect that is so closely associated with agentic extraversion (activated, peppy, strong, enthused, energetic; Watson & Tellegen, 1985). Therefore, we have proposed that agentic extraversion reflects the activity of a behavioral approach system based on *positive incentive motivation*.

When close proximity to a rewarding goal is achieved, the incentive–motivational approach gives way to a consummatory phase of goal acquisition (Herbert, 1993). In this phase, specific *interoceptive* and *proximal exteroceptive* stimuli related to critical primary biological aims elicit behavioral patterns that are relatively specific to those conditions (e.g., sexual, social, or food-related) (Blackburn et al., 1989; Hilliard et al., 1998; MacLean, 1986; Timberlake & Silva, 1995). Performance of these behavioral patterns is inherently rewarding (Berridge, 1999). In the case of potential mate acquisition, examples of affiliative behavioral patterns are courtship, gentle stroking and grooming, mating, and certain maternal patterns such as breastfeeding, all of which may include facial, caressive tactile, gestural, and certain vocal behaviors (Polan & Hofer, 1998). Tactile stimulation may be particularly effective in activating affiliative reward processes in animals and humans (Fleming, Korsmit, & Detter, 1994). Significantly, a light pleasant touch that occurs in caress-like skin-to-skin contact between individuals is transmitted by different afferents than a hard or unpleasant touch (Olausson et al., 2002): a light pleasant touch is transmitted by slow-conducting unmyelinated afferents that project to the insular cortex but not to somatosensory areas S1 and S2, whereas a hard unpleasant touch is

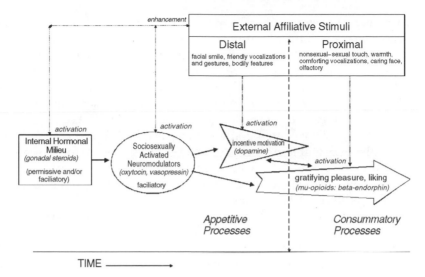

FIGURE 8.1. The development and maintenance of affiliative bonds across two phases of reward. Distal affiliative stimuli elicit an incentive-motivated approach to an affiliative goal, accompanied by strong emotional–motivational feelings of wanting, desire, and positive activation. The approach phase ensures not only sociosexual interaction with an affiliative object but also acquisition of a memory ensemble or network of the context in which approach, reward, and goal acquisition occur. Next, proximal affiliative stimuli emanating from interaction with the affiliative object elicit strong feelings of consummatory reward, liking, and physiological quiescence, all of which become associated with these stimuli as well as the context predictive of reward. As discussed below, dopamine encodes the incentive salience of contextual stimuli predictive of reward during the approach phase and, in collaboration with mu opiate-mediated consummatory reward, encodes the incentive salience of proximal stimuli directly linked to the affiliative object. The end result of this sequence of processes is an incentive-encoded affiliative memory network that continues to motivate approach toward and interaction with the affiliative object. Specialized processes ensure that affiliative stimuli are weighted as significant elements in the contextual ensembles representing affiliative memory networks. These specialized processes include the construction of a contextual ensemble via affiliative stimulus-induced opiate potentiation of dopamine processes, and the influence of permissive and/or facilitatory factors such as gonadal steroids, oxytocin, and vasopressin on (1) sensory, perceptual, and attentional processing of affiliative stimuli and (2) formation of social memories. See Depue and Morrone-Strupinsky (2005) for details.

transmitted by fast-conducting myelinated afferents to S1 and S2 (anterior parietal). The insular cortex is a paralimbic region known to integrate several sensory modalities, including autonomic, gustatory, visual, auditory, and somatosensory, in characterizing the emotional nature of sensory input (Damasio, 2003; Mesulam, 1990).

As opposed to an incentivizing motivational state of activation, desire, and wanting, the expression of *consummatory* behavioral patterns elicits intense feelings of pleasure, gratification, and liking, plus physiological quiescence characterized by rest, sedation, anabolism, and parasympathetic nervous system activity, thereby reinforcing the production and repetition of those behaviors (Berridge, 1999; DiChiara & North, 1992; Porges, 1998, 2001). Thus, whereas appetitive approach processes bring an individual into contact with unconditioned incentive stimuli, consummatory processes bring behavior to a gratifying conclusion (Hilliard et al., 1998). Whether the pleasurable state generated in affiliative interactions shares a common neurobiology with the pleasure generated by other consummatory behaviors (e.g., feeding) is not certain but is assumed by some to be so (DiChiara & North, 1992; Panksepp, 1998).

The core content of affiliation scales seems to reflect the operation of neurobehavioral processes that (1) create a warm, affectionate, gratifying subjective emotional state elicited by others, which in turn (2) motivates close interpersonal behavior. Our hypothesis is that the subjective experience of warmth and affection reflects the *capacity to experience consummatory reward that is elicited by a broad array of affiliative stimuli* (Depue & Morrone-Strupinsky, 2005). This capacity is viewed as providing the key element utilized in additional psychobiological processes that permit the development and maintenance of longer-term affective bonds—defined as long-term selective social attachments observed most intensely between infants and parents and between adult mates, and that are characteristic of social organization in human and other primate societies (Gingrich, Liu, Cascio, Wang, & Insel, 2000; Insel, 1997; Wang et al., 1999). It is important to emphasize that a core capacity for affiliative reward and bonding is not viewed as a sufficient determinant of close social relationships, only as a necessary one, a *sine qua non*. Such affiliative reward is hypothesized to underlie all human social relationships having a positive affective component. Other interpersonal constructs of sociability, attachment, and separation anxiety are accordingly viewed as either broader than affiliation as defined here, and/or as based on different neurobehavioral systems (see Depue & Morrone-Strupinsky, 2005, for a full discussion).

Through Pavlovian associative learning, the experience of reward generated throughout appetitive and consummatory phases is associated with previously affectively neutral stimulus contexts (objects, acts, events, places) in which pleasure occurred, thereby forming conditioned incentive stimuli that are predictive of reward and that have gained the capacity to elicit anticipatory pleasure and incentive motivation (Berridge, 1999; Ostrowski, 1998; Timberlake & Silva, 1995). Because of the predominance of symbolic (conditioned) processes in guiding human behavior in the absence of unconditioned stimuli, conditioned incentives are likely to be particularly important elicitors of *enduring* reward processes (Fowles, 1987). Thus, the acquisition and maintenance of a mate relationship, for example, depends closely on Pavlovian associative learning that links the experience of reward with (1) the salient contextual cues that predict reward during the appetitive phase (e.g., features of a laboratory cage) and (2) a mate's individualistic cues associated directly with consummatory reward (e.g., individual characteristics of a sexually receptive female mate) (Domjan, Cusato, & Villarreal, 2000). Taken together, the above processes support acquisition of affiliative memories, where contextual ensembles are formed and weighted in association with the reward provided by interaction with the potential mate.

Neurobiology of Incentive Motivation and Affiliative Reward

By drawing an association between traits and behavioral systems (i.e., agentic extraversion and incentive motivation, affiliation, and affiliative reward), we are able to utilize the behavioral neurobiology animal literature to discern the neurobiology associated with these behavioral systems and, by analogy, with the personality traits of agentic extraversion and affiliation. As reviewed recently (Depue & Collins, 1999), animal research demonstrates that the positive incentive motivation and experience of reward that underlies a behavioral system of approach is dependent on the functional properties of the midbrain ventral tegmental area (VTA) dopamine (DA) projection system. DA agonists or antagonists in the VTA or nucleus accumbens (NAS), which is a major terminal area of VTA DA projections, in rats and monkeys facilitate or markedly impair, respectively, a broad array of incentive-motivated behaviors. Furthermore, dose-dependent DA receptor activation in the VTA-NAS pathway facilitates the acute rewarding effects of stimulants, and the NAS is a particularly strong site for intracranial self-administration of DA agonists (Le Moal & Simon, 1991; Pich et al., 1997). DA agonists injected in the NAS also modulate behavioral responses to *conditioned* incentive stimuli in a dose-dependent fashion (Cador, Taylor, & Robbins, 1991; Robbins, Cador, Taylor, & Everitt, 1989; Wolterink, Cador, Wolterink, Robbins, & Everitt, 1989). In single-unit recording studies, VTA DA neurons are activated preferentially by appetitive incentive stimuli (Schultz, Dayan, & Montague, 1997). DA cells, most numerously in the VTA, respond vigorously to and in proportion to the magnitude of both conditioned and unconditioned incentive stimuli and in anticipation of reward (Schultz et al., 1997).

Finally, incentive motivation is associated in humans with both positive *emotional* feelings such as elation and euphoria and *motivational* feelings of desire, wanting, craving, potency, and self-efficacy. In humans, DA-activating psychostimulant drugs induce both sets of feelings (Drevets et al., 2001). Also, neuroimaging studies of cocaine addicts found that during acute administration the intensity of a subject's subjective euphoria increased in a dose-dependent manner in proportion to cocaine binding to the DA uptake transporter (and hence to DA levels) in the striatum (Volkow et al., 1997). Moreover, cocaine-induced activity in the NAS was linked equally strongly (if not more strongly) to motivational feelings of desire, wanting, and craving, as to the emotional experience of euphoric rush (Breiter et al., 1997). And the degree of amphetamine-induced DA release in healthy human ventral striatum assessed by positron emission tomography was correlated strongly with feelings of euphoria (Drevets et al., 2001). Hence, taken together, the animal and human evidence demonstrates that the VTA DA–NAS pathway is a primary neural circuit for incentive motivation and its accompanying subjective state of reward.

With respect to consummatory reward and affiliative behavior, a broad range of evidence suggests a role for endogenous opiates. Endogenous opiate release or receptor binding is increased in rats, monkeys, and humans by lactation and nursing, sexual activity, vaginocervical stimulation, maternal social interaction, brief social isolation, and grooming and other nonsexual tactile stimulation (Depue & Morrone-Strupinsky, 2005; Keverne, 1996; Silk, Alberts, & Altmann, 2003). Opiate receptor (OR) antagonists naltrexone or naloxone in small doses apparently reduce the reward derived from social interactions since it increases attempts to obtain such reward, manifested as increases in (1) the amount of maternal contact by young monkeys and (2) solicitations for grooming and frequency of being groomed in mature female monkeys, which has been associated with increased cerebrospinal fluid levels of beta-endorphin (Graves, Wallen, & Maestripieri, 2002; Martel, Nevison, Simpson, & Keverne, 1995). In addition, the endogenous opiate beta-endorphin stimulates play behavior and grooming in juvenile rats, whereas naltrexone leads to reduced grooming of infants and other group members in monkeys and rats and to maternal neglect in monkeys and sheep that is similar to the neglect shown by human mothers who abuse opiates (Keverne, 1996; Martel et al., 1995). Similarly, human females administered the opiate antagonist naltrexone showed an increased amount of time spent alone, a reduced amount of time spent with friends, and a reduced frequency and pleasantness of their social interactions relative to placebo (Jamner & Leigh, 1999). Such findings suggest that opiates provide a critical part of the neural basis on which primate sociality has evolved (Nelson & Panksepp, 1998). Particularly important is the relation between mu opiates and grooming, because the primary function of primate grooming may well be to establish and maintain social bonds (Matheson & Bernstein, 2000).

Perhaps most relevant to affiliative reward is the mu opiate receptor (OR) family, which is the main site of exogenously administered opiate drugs (e.g., morphine) and of endogenous endorphins (particularly, beta-endorphin) (La Buda, Sora, Uhl, & Fuchs, 2000; Schlaepfer et al., 1998; Shippenberg & Elmer, 1998; Stefano et al., 2000; Wiedenmayer & Barr, 2000). Mu ORs also appear to be the main site for the effects of endogenous beta-endorphins and endogenous morphine on the subjective feelings in humans of *increased* interpersonal warmth, euphoria, well-being, and peaceful calmness, as well as of *decreased* elation, energy, and incentive motivation (Schlaepfer et al., 1998; Shippenberg & Elmer, 1998; Stefano et al., 2000; Uhl, Sora, & Wang, 1999).

The facilitatory effects of opiates on affiliative behavior are thought to be exerted by fibers that arise mainly from the hypothalamic arcuate nucleus and terminate in brain regions that typically express mu ORs. Mu ORs may facilitate the rewarding effects associated with many motivated behaviors (Nelson & Panksepp, 1998; Niesink, Vanderschuen, & Van Ree, 1996; Olive, Koenig, Nannini, & Hodge, 2001; Olson, Olson, & Kastin, 1997; Stefano et al., 2000; Strand, 1999). For instance, whereas DA antagonists block appetitive behaviors in pursuit of reward but not the actual consumption of reward (e.g., sucrose; Ikemoto & Panksepp, 1996), mu OR antagonists block rewarding effects of sucrose and sexual behavior, and in neonatal rats persistently impair the response to the inherently rewarding properties of novel stimulation (Herz, 1998). Rewarding properties of mu OR agonists are directly indicated by the fact that animals will work for the prototypical mu agonists morphine and heroin, and that they are dose-dependently self-administered in animals and humans (Di Chiara, 1995; Nelson & Panksepp, 1998; Olson et al., 1997; Shippenberg & Elmer, 1998). There is a significant correlation between an agonist's affinity at the mu OR and the dose that maintains maximal rates of drug self-administration behavior (Shippenberg & Elmer, 1998).

The rewarding effect of opiates may be especially mediated by mu ORs located in the NAS and VTA, both of which support self-administration of mu OR agonists that is attenuated by intracranially administered mu OR antagonists (Davis & Cazala, 2000; Herz, 1998; Schlaepfer et al., 1998; Shippenberg & Elmer, 1998). When opiate and DA-specific antagonists were given prior to cocaine or heroin self-administration the opiate antagonist selectively altered opiate self-administration while DA antagonists selectively altered the response to the DA agonist cocaine (Shippenberg & Elmer, 1998). Destruction of DA terminals in the NAS also showed that opiate self-administration is independent of DA function, at least at the level of the NAS (Dworkin, Guerin, Goeders, & Smith, 1988). Furthermore, NAS DA functioning was specifically related to the incentive salience of reward cues but was unrelated to the hedonic state generated by consuming the rewards (Wyvell & Berridge, 2000). *Thus, DA and opiates appear to functionally interact in the NAS, but they apparently provide independent contributions to rewarding effects.* This appears to be particularly the case for the *acute* rewarding effects of opiates, which are thought to occur through a DA-independent system that is mediated through brainstem reward circuits, including the tegmental pedunculopontine nucleus (Laviolette, Gallegos, Henriksen, & van der Kooy, 2004).

Rewarding effects of opiates are also directly indicated by the fact that a range of mu OR agonists, when injected intracerebroventricularly or directly into the NAS, serve as unconditioned rewarding stimuli in a dose-dependent manner in producing a conditioned place preference, a behavioral measure of reward (Narita, Aoki, & Suzuki, 2000; Nelson & Panksepp, 1998; Shippenberg & Elmer, 1998). VTA-localized mu ORs, particularly in the rostral zone of the VTA (Carlezon et al., 2000), mediate (1) rewarding effects such as self-administration behavior and conditioned place preference (Carlezon, 2000; Shippenberg & Elmer, 1998; Wise, 1998); (2) increased sexual activity and maternal behaviors (Callahan, Baumann, & Rabil, 1996; Leyton & Stewart, 1992; van Furth & van Ree, 1996); and (3) the persistently increased play behavior, social grooming, and social approach of rats subjected to morphine *in utero* (Hol, Niesink, van Ree, & Spruijt, 1996). Indeed, microinjections of morphine or a selective mu OR agonist into the VTA produced marked place preferences, whereas the selective antagonism of mu ORs prevented morphine-induced conditioned place preference (Olmstead & Franklin, 1997). Indeed, transgenic mice lacking the mu OR gene show no morphine-induced place preferences nor physical dependence from morphine consumption, whereas morphine induces both of these behaviors in wild-type mice (Matthes et al., 1996; Simonin et al., 1998). And significantly, opiate but not oxytocin antagonists block the development of partner preference that is induced specifically by *repeated* exposure and *repeated* sexual activity in rodents (Carter, Lederhendler, & Kirkpatrick, 1997).

An *interaction* of DA and mu opiates in the experience of reward throughout appetitive and consummatory phases of *affiliative* engagement appears to involve two processes: During the anticipatory phase of goal acquisition, mu OR activation in the VTA can increase DA release in the NAS and hence the experience of reward (Marinelli & White, 2000). Subsequently, the firing rate of VTA neurons decreases following delivery and consumption of appetitive reinforcers (e.g., food, sex, liquid) (Schultz et al., 1997). At the same time, mu OR activation in the NAS (perhaps by opiate release from higher-threshold NAS terminals that contain both DA and opiates [Le Moal & Simon, 1991]) decreases NAS DA release, creating an opiate-mediated experience of reward associated with consummation that is independent of DA (Churchill, Roques, & Kalivas, 1995). Thus, in contrast to the incentive motivational effects of DA during the anticipation of reward, opiates may subsequently induce calm pleasure and bring consummatory behavior to a gratifying conclusion. This may explain the fact that higher doses of mu OR agonists administered into the NAS can block the self-administration of certain psychostimulant drugs of abuse in animals and reduce appetitive behaviors (Hyztia & Kiianmaa, 2001; Johnson & Ait-Daoud, 2000; Kranzler, 2000).

In sum, as illustrated in Figure 8.1, distal affiliative cues (e.g., friendly smiles and gestures, sexual features) serve as incentive stimuli that activate DA-facilitated incentive–reward motivation, desire, wanting, and approach to affiliative objects. As these objects are reached, more proximal affiliative stimuli (e.g., pleasant touch) strongly activate mu opiate release that promotes an intense state of pleasant reward, warmth, affection, and physiological quiescence and brings approach behavior to a gratifying conclusion. Throughout this entire sequence of goal acquisition, the contextual cues associated with approach to the goal and the cues specifically related to the goal are all associated with the experience of reward. It is beyond the scope of this chapter, but it is worth noting that DA and mu opiates play a critical role in strengthening the association between these contextual cues and reward (Depue & Morrone-Strupinsky, 2005; Gingrich, Cascio, Wang, & Insel, 2000). Thus, these two neuromodulators are critical to establishing our preferences for and memories of particular contexts and affiliative cues predictive of reward.

Individual Differences in DA–Incentive and Mu OR–Reward Processes

Individual differences in agentic extraversion and affiliation are subject to strong genetic influence (Tellegen et al., 1988). If personality disturbance occurs in the region located at the extreme tails of individual difference distributions in the traits of agentic extraversion and affiliation, it is important to show that the neuromodulators associated with incentive motivation and affiliative reward are sources of individual differences in these behavioral systems. Animal research demonstrates that individual differences in DA functioning contribute significantly to variations in incentive-motivated behavior, as does much human work (Depue & Collins, 1999; Depue et al., 1994). Inbred mouse and rat strains with variation in the number of neurons in the VTA DA cell group or in several indicators of enhanced DA transmission show marked differences in behaviors dependent on DA transmission in the VTA–NAS pathway, including levels of spontaneous exploratory activity and DA agonist-induced locomotor activity, and increased acquisition of self-administration of psychostimulants (Depue & Collins, 1999).

Similar findings for mu opiates exist (Depue & Morrone-Strupinsky, 2005). Individual differences in humans and rodents have been demonstrated in levels of mu OR expression and binding that are associated with a preference for mu OR agonists such as morphine (Uhl et al., 1999;

Zubieta et al., 2001). In humans, individual differences in central nervous system mu OR densities show a range of up to 75% between lower and upper thirds of the distribution (Uhl et al., 1999), differences that appear to be related to variations in the rewarding effects of alcohol in humans and rodents (Berrettini, Hoehe, Ferraro, DeMaria, & Gottheil, 1997; McCall, Wand, Eisenberg, Rhode, & Cheskin, 2000a; McCall, Wand, Rhode, & Lee, 2000b; Olson et al., 1997).

Differences of this magnitude in the *expressive* properties of the mu OR gene could contribute substantially to individual variation in mu OR-induced *behavioral* expression via an effect on beta endorphin functional potency. For instance, one source of this individual variation is different single nucleotide polymorphisms (SNPs) in the mu OR gene, OPRM1 (Berrettini et al., 1997; Bond et al., 1998; Gelernter, Kranzler, & Cubells, 1999). The most prevalent of these is A118G, which is characterized by a substitution of the amino acid Asn by Asp at codon 40, with an allelic frequency of 10% in a mixed sample of former heroin abusers and normal controls (Bond et al., 1998). Although this SNP did not bind all opiate peptides more strongly than other SNPs or the normal nucleotide sequence, it did bind beta endorphin three times more tightly than the most common allelic form of the receptor (Bond et al., 1998). Furthermore, beta-endorphin is three times more effective in agonist-induced activation of G-protein-coupled potassium channels at the A118G variant receptor as compared to the most common allelic form (Bond et al., 1998).

Genetic variation in mu OR properties is related to response to rewarding drugs, such as morphine, alcohol, and cocaine, and to opiate self-administration behavior in animals (Berrettini et al., 1997). For instance, when transgenic insertion was used to increase mu OR density specifically in mesolimbic areas thought to mediate substance abuse via VTA DA neurons, transgenic mice showed increased self-administration of morphine compared to wild-type mice, even when the amount of behavior required to maintain drug intake increased 10-fold (Elmer, Pieper, Goldberg, & George, 1995). Thus, the efficacy of morphine as a reinforcer was substantially enhanced in transgenic mice. Conversely, mu OR knockout mice do not develop conditioned place preference and physical dependence on morphine, whereas morphine induces both of these behaviors in wild-type mice (Matthes et al., 1996).

Taken together, these studies suggest that genetic variation in DA and mu OR properties in humans and rodents is (1) substantial, (2) an essential element in the variation in the rewarding value of DA and opiate agonists, and (3) critical in accounting for variation in the Pavlovian learning that underlies the association between contextual cues and reward, as occurs in partner and place preferences (Elmer et al., 1995; Matthes et al., 1996).

Anxiety or Neuroticism

Anxiety and Fear as Two Distinct Behavioral Systems

Adaptation to aversive environmental conditions is crucial for species survival, and at least two distinct behavioral systems have evolved to promote such adaptation. One system is fear (often labeled Harm Avoidance in the trait literature, but this is different from Cloninger, Svrakic, and Przybeck's [1993] Harm Avoidance, which actually assesses anxiety), which is a very specific behavioral system that evolved as a means of escaping unconditioned aversive stimuli that are inherently dangerous to survival, such as tactile pain, injury contexts, snakes, spiders, heights, approaching strangers, and sudden sounds. These stimuli are specific, discrete, and explicit, and in turn elicit specific short-latency, high-magnitude phasic responses of autonomic arousal, subjective feelings of panic, and behavioral escape. Specific, discrete neutral stimuli associated with these unconditioned events elicit conditioned fear. Such conditioned stimuli elicit a different behavioral profile than unconditioned stimuli in that freezing and suppression of operant behavior (i.e., behavioral inhibition), as opposed to active escape, characterize the former, though both response systems involve autonomic arousal, pain inhibition, and reflex potentiation.

There are, however, many aversive circumstances that do not involve specific, discrete, explicit stimuli that evolutionarily have been neurobiologically linked to subjective fear and escape. That is, there are many situations in which specific aversive cues do not exist, but rather the stimulus conditions are associated with an elevated *potential* risk of danger or aversive consequences. In such cases, no explicit aversive stimuli are present to inherently activate escape circuitries. Nevertheless, the stimuli can be unconditioned in nature, as in darkness, open spaces, unfamiliarity, and predator odors, or they can be conditioned contextual cues (general textures, colors, relative spatial locations, sounds) that have been associated with previous exposure to specific aversive stimuli (Davis, Walker, & Lee, 1997; Davis & Shi, 1999; Fendt, Ehdres, & Apfelbach, 2003). Conceptually, these stimuli are characterized in common by unpredictability and uncontrollability—or, more simply, uncertainty. In the social realm, social rejection may constitute an unconditioned aversive cue denoting uncertainty of survival outside the supportive context of a social group (Eisenberger, Lieberman, & Williams, 2003).

In order to reduce the risk of danger in such circumstances, a second behavioral system evolved, *anxiety*. Anxiety is characterized by negative emotion or affect (anxiety, depression, hostility, suspiciousness, distress) that serves the purpose of informing the individual that, though no explicit, specific aversive stimuli are present, conditions are potentially threatening (White & Depue, 1999). This affective state, and the physiological arousal that accompanies it, continues or reverberates until the uncertainty is resolved. Associated responses that may functionally help to resolve the uncertainty are heightened attentional scanning of the uncertain environment and cognitive worrying and rumination over possible response–outcome scenarios. An important point is that no specific motor response is linked to anxiety, because no motor response is specified under stimulus conditions of uncertainty. Caution and locomotor modulation are necessary, but behavioral inhibition will not allow the individual to explore the environment to discover whether danger is indeed lurking. An example is a deer entering an open meadow: caution, slow approach, heightened attentional scanning, and enhanced cognitive activity are optimal, not freezing. This is in direct contradiction to Gray's (1973) theory that the best marker for anxiety is behavioral inhibition; rather, conditioned stimulus fear is associated with such inhibition. Thus, Davis et al. (1997) and Barlow (2002) suggest that the stimulus conditions and behavioral characteristics of fear and anxiety are different, although a similar state of intense autonomic arousal is associated with both emotional states, rendering them similar at the subjective level. The prolonged negative subjective state of anxiety, however, distinguishes its subjective state from the rapid, brief state of panic associated with the presence of a specific fear stimulus.

There is another important difference between fear and anxiety at the trait level of analysis. In personality inventories, fear typically is represented as a primary or facet-level scale, not a higher-order factor (Tellegen & Waller, in press). Fear usually also is associated with a higher-order trait of constraint. In contrast, anxiety, which is typically referred to as neuroticism, is one of the most reliably identified higher-order traits and does not load highly on a constraint higher-order factor. This higher-order nature of anxiety but not fear is related to the fact that, just as with agentic extraversion, the eliciting stimuli for anxiety occur frequently in a civilized society, whereas the specific stimuli that elicit fear do not. This means that anxiety represents a general behavioral system that is activated by a broad class of stimuli, whereas fear represents a more specific behavioral system that evolved to respond to specific stimuli critical for survival.

The trait literature supports the *independence* of anxiety and fear, which as personality traits are subject to distinct sources of genetic variation (Tellegen et al., 1988). As the averaged correlations derived from numerous studies show, the relation between neuroticism (anxiety) and harm avoidance (fear) is essentially zero (Depue & Lenzenweger, 2005; White & Depue, 1999). Moreover, the magnitude of emotional distress and autonomic arousal elicited by discrete stimuli associated with physical harm are significantly related to harm avoidance but not neuroticism, whereas conditions of uncertainty associated with external evaluations of the self are significantly related to neuroticism but not harm avoidance (Depue &

Lenzenweger, 2005; White & Depue, 1999). Furthermore, in contrast to Gray's (1973, 1992) and Cloninger's (Cloninger et al., 1993) theoretical position that anxiety is associated with behavioral inhibition, it is harm avoidance rather than neuroticism that correlates significantly with indices of behavioral inhibition in the context of physical danger. Indeed, one of the most reliable indices of conditioned fear in animals is behavioral inhibition (Davis et al., 1997; Le Doux, 1998; Panksepp, 1998), which is not the case for stimulus-induced anxiety (Davis et al., 1997). Thus, these various findings suggest that anxiety and fear are distinctly different traits, and the analysis of clinical anxiety disorders has reached equivalent conclusions (Barlow, 2002).

NEUROBIOLOGY OF ANXIETY

The psychometric independence of fear and anxiety is mirrored in their dissociable neuroanatomy. Species-specific unconditioned stimuli having an evolutionary history of danger elicit fear and defensive motor escape, facial and vocal signs, autonomic activation, and antinociception specifically from the lateral longitudinal cell column in the midbrain periaquiductal gray (Bandler & Keay, 1996). In turn, periaquiductal gray (PAG) efferents converge on the ventromedial and rostral ventrolateral regions of the medulla, where somatic-motor and autonomic information, respectively, is integrated and transmitted to the spinal cord (Guyenet et al., 1996; Holstege, 1996). Although these processes can occur without a cortex (Panksepp, 1998), association of discrete, explicit neutral stimuli (fear conditioned stimulus) with an unconditioned stimulus and primary negative reinforcement occurs via cortical uni- and polymodal sensory efferents that converge on the basolateral complex of the amygdala (although crude representations of external stimuli can rapidly reach the basolateral amygdala subcortically from the thalamus) (Aggleton, 1992; Davis et al., 1997; LeDoux, 1998). Fear conditioned stimuli elicit a host of behavioral, neuropeptide, and autonomic responses via output from the basolateral amygdala to the central amygdala, which in turn sends functionally *separable* efferents to many hypothalamic and brainstem targets (Aggleton, 1992; LeDoux, Cicchetti, Xagoraris, & Romanski, 1990). In the case of fear conditioned stimuli, as noted above, the motor response is not escape but rather freezing or *behavioral inhibition*, which involves activation of the caudal ventrolateral cell column of the PAG (LeDoux, 1998).

The neuroanatomic distinction between fear and anxiety has been delineated by use of the fear-potentiated auditory-induced startle paradigm. In this paradigm, an established, explicit light conditioned stimulus activates a cell assembly representing the association between conditioned stimulus, unconditioned stimulus (e.g., shock), and tactile pain located in the basolateral amygdala. Excitation of this assembly by the conditioned stimulus activates efferents to the central amygdala, which in turn mono-synaptically potentiates startle reflex circuitry in the reticular nucleus of the caudal pons that is activated simultaneously by, for example, a loud, sudden noise. This potentiation of the startle reflex by a fear conditioned stimulus is *phasic* in nature, occurring almost immediately after light onset but returning to baseline amplitude shortly after light offset (Davis et al., 1997). Lesions of the central amygdala reliably block explicit fear conditioned stimulus-potentiated startle and behavioral inhibition. In contrast, nondiscrete, contextually related aversive stimulation—for example, prolonged *bright light* in an *unfamiliar* environment, which are aversive unconditioned stimuli for nocturnal rats—elicits robust startle potentiation that endures *tonically* as long as the aversive conditions are present, even when the central amygdala is lesioned. These findings suggest that these types of stimulus conditions, which are typically associated with the elicitation of anxiety, rely on a different neuroanatomical foundation in generating an enduring potentiation of the startle reflex (Davis et al., 1997).

The enduring potentiating effects of nondiscrete, contextually related aversive stimuli on the startle reflex is dependent on a group of structures collectively referred to as the *extended amygdala*, which receives massive projections from basolateral and olfactory amygdala complexes, and which represents a macrostructure that is characterized by two divisions, central and medial (Heimer, 2003; McGinty, 1999). As shown in Figure 8.2, these two divisions originate from the central and medial nuclei of the amygdala and consist of cell groups that are distributed throughout the sublenticular area, bed nucleus of the stria terminalis (BNST), around striatal and pallidal structures, and back to merge specifically with the caudomedial region of the NAS. Contextual stimuli are conveyed to the BNST and other central extended amygdala regions via perirhinal and basolateral amygdala (e.g., bright light) and parahippocampal, entorhinal, and hippocampal (contextual stimuli) glutamatergic efferents (Annett, McGregor, & Robins, 1989; Bechara et al., 1995; Everitt & Robbins, 1992; Gaffan, 1992; Heimer, 2003; LeDoux, 1998; Selden, Everitt, Jarrard, & Robbins, 1991; Sutherland & McDonald, 1990). Viewing the sublenticular area and lateral BNST as a foundation for anxiety processes is supported in part by the fact that, in contrast to the central amygdala, (1) neurons in the sublenticular area show maximal prolonged responsiveness specifically to unfamiliar stimuli (Rolls, 1998), and (2) electrical stimulation or lesions of the BNST did not initiate nor block, respectively, the behavioral inhibition elicited by an explicit fear conditioned stimulus (LeDoux et al., 1990), which mirrors the lack of association of behavioral inhibition with trait anxiety, discussed above.

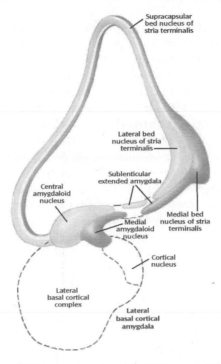

FIGURE 8.2. The central (light gray) and medial (dark gray) divisions of the extended amygdala, shown in isolation from the rest of the brain. From Heimer (2003). Copyright 2003 by the American Psychiatric Association. Reprinted by permission.

Similar to the outputs from the central nucleus of the amygdala, most structures of the central division of the extended amygdala can transmit this motivationally relevant information to some or all hypothalamic and brainstem structures related to emotional expression (Heimer, 2003; Holstege, 1996). Whereas the basolateral complex of the amygdala is involved in pairing positive and negative reinforcement with stimuli that are discrete and explicit and that have been analyzed for their specific characteristics, at least the central division of the extended amygdala appears to associate *general contextual features and nonexplicit, nondiscrete* conditioned and unconditioned stimuli with reinforcement (e.g., light conditions, physical features, spatial relations) (Davis et al., 1997; Davis & Shi, 1999; McDonald, Shammah-Iagnado, Shi, & Davis, 1999). Thus, two emotional learning systems may have evolved: the basolateral amygdala to associate reinforcement with explicit, specific characteristics of objects (i.e., for fear), and the BNST to associate reinforcement with nonexplicit spatial and contextual stimulus aspects (i.e., for anxiety).

A major finding of importance in understanding the association between anxiety and the central extended amygdala is that injection of corticotropin-releasing hormone (CRH) into the BNST potentiates startle in a dose-dependent manner for up to 2 hours' duration (Davis et al., 1997). It is not surprising then that lesions of the BNST, or injection of a CRH antagonist in the BNST, significantly attenuate both bright light- or CRH-enhanced startle without having any effect on discrete fear conditioned stimulus potentiated startle (Davis et al., 1997). In contrast, lesions of the central amygdala eliminate the discrete fear conditioned stimulus-potentiated startle, but have no effect on CRH-enhanced startle. Prolonged bright light-induced startle potentiation is also blocked by (1) lesions of the fornix, which carries hippocampal efferents conveying salient context to the BNST (Amaral & Witter, 1995); (2) glutamatergic antagonists injected into the BNST that block hippocampal efferent input; and (3) buspirone, a potent anxiolytic (Davis et al., 1997). Conversely, lesions of, or glutamate antagonists injected in, the central amygdala blocked fear conditioned stimulus-potentiated startle but had no effect on startle elicited by bright light conditions or on anxiolytic effects in the elevated plus maze, where benzodiazepines have a robust anxiolytic effect (Davis et al., 1997; Treit, Pesold, & Rotzinger, 1993). The basolateral amygdala is involved in both bright light- and conditioned stimulus-potentiated startle due to processing of visual information, but not in CRH-enhanced startle.

Thus, with respect to potentiation of the startle reflex, there is a multivariate double dissociation of the central amygdala and the BNST. As summarized in Figure 8.3 (Davis et al., 1997), the nature of the different stimulus conditions that activate these two structures suggests that the amygdala connects explicit phasic stimuli that predict aversive unconditioned stimuli with rapidly activated evasive responses and subjective fear. In contrast, prolonged contextual and/or unfamiliar stimuli that connote uncertainty about expected outcomes are associated with a neurobehavioral response system that coordinates activation of (1) the negative affective state of anxiety to inform the individual that the current context is uncertain and potentially dangerous; (2) autonomic arousal to mobilize energy for potential action; (3) selective attention in order to maximize sensory input at specified locations in the visual field; and (4) cognition in order to derive a response strategy. Nevertheless, as shown in Figure 8.3, efferents from the BNST and sublenticular area innervate many of the same hypothalamic and brainstem regions as the central amygdala (Heimer, 2003), suggesting that fear and anxiety derive their somewhat similar subjective nature from common neuroendocrine and autonomic response systems (Davis et al., 1997; LeDoux, 1998; Rolls, 1999).

The significance of the prolonged startle-potentiation effects of CRH in the BNST is that CRH and the BNST appear to be integrators of behavioral, neuroendocrine, and autonomic responses to stressful circumstances

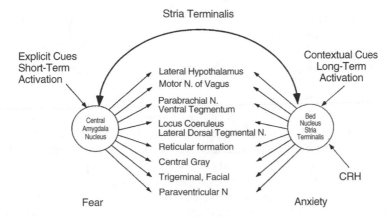

FIGURE 8.3. Hypothetical schematic suggesting that the central nucleus of the amygdala and the bed nucleus of the stria terminalis may be differentially involved in fear versus anxiety, respectively. Both brain areas have highly similar hypothalamic and brainstem targets known to be involved in specific signs and symptoms of fear and anxiety. However, the stress peptide corticotropin releasing hormone (CRH) appears to act on receptors in the bed nucleus of the stria terminalis rather than the amygdala, at least in terms of an increase in the startle reflex. Furthermore, the bed nucleus of the stria terminalis seems to be involved in the anxiogenic effects of a very bright light presented for a long time but not when that very same light was previously paired with a shock. Just the opposite is the case for the central nucleus of the amygdala, which is critical for fear conditioning using explicit cues such as a light or tone paired with aversive stimulation (i.e., conditioned fear). From Davis, Waller, and Lee (1997). Copyright 1997 by the New York Academy of Sciences. Reprinted by permission.

(Leri, Flores, Rodaros, & Stewart, 2002; Pacak, McCarty, Palkovits, Kopin, & Goldstein, 1995; Shaham, Erb, & Stewart, 2000). This integration is accomplished by the activity of both the peripheral and central CRH systems. The peripheral system involves CRH neurons located in the paraventricular nucleus of the hypothalamus, which when activated initiate the series of events that ends in the release of cortisol from the adrenal cortex (Strand, 1999). Cortisol then circulates in the bloodstream and increases energy reserves (gluconeogenesis) and, if not excessive in quantity, enhances neurotransmitters involved in modulating emotion and memory (Kim & Diamond, 2002).

In contrast, the central CRH system is composed of CRH neurons located in many different subcortical brain regions that modulate emotion, memory, and central nervous system arousal (Strand, 1999). Whereas the majority of CRH neurons in the central nervous system do not mediate the effects of stress, some of the CRH-containing regions that are important in mediating stress effects are illustrated in Figure 8.4. For instance, the basolateral amygdala detects discrete aversive stimuli associated with the stressful circumstances and activates the extensive array of CRH neurons located in the central amygdala. These CRH neurons project to many brain regions that modulate emotion, memory, and arousal, including the peripheral CRH neurons in the paraventricular nucleus in the hypothalamus (Strand, 1999). Stress variables associated with context and uncertainty activate CRH neurons in the BNST, which have similar projection targets as the central amygdala (Erb, Salmaso, Rodaros, & Stewart, 2001; Macey, Smith, Nader, & Porrino, 2003; Shaham et al., 2000). Both the central amygdala and the BNST can activate CRH neurons in the lateral hypothalamus, a region that integrates central nervous system arousal. In turn, the lateral hypothalamic CRH projections modulate autonomic nervous system activity. Importantly, as illustrated in Figure 8.4, all three sources of CRH projections—the central amygdala, BNST, and lateral hypothalamus—innervate CRH neurons in the paragiganticocellularis (PGi) (Aston-Jones, Rajkowski, Kubiak, Valentino, & Shiptley, 1996), which is located in the rostral ventrolateral area of the medulla in the brainstem. The PGi is a massive nucleus that provides major integration of central and autonomic

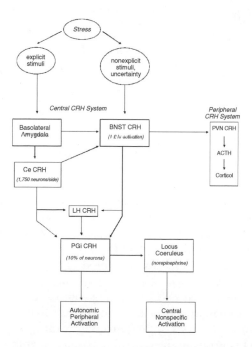

FIGURE 8.4. Components of the central and peripheral corticotropin-releasing hormone (CRH) systems. Ce, central amygdala nucleus; BNST, bed nucleus of the stria terminalis; LH, lateral hypothalamus; PGi, paragiganticocellularis; PVN, paraventricular nucleus of the hypothalamus; ACTH, corticotropic hormone from the anterior pituitary.

arousal and, in turn, coordinates and triggers arousal responses to urgent stimuli via two main pathways eminating from its own population of CRH neurons, which make up 10% of PGi neurons (Aston-Jones et al., 1996). One CRH pathway modulates the autonomic nervous system and hence peripheral arousal effects via projections to the intermediolateral cell column of the spinal cord, activating sympathetic preganglionic autonomic neurons.

The other CRH pathway modulates central arousal effects via activation of the locus coeruleus (LC), where PGi CRH innervation of the LC in humans and monkeys is dense (Aston-Jones et al., 1996). The LC, which is composed of ~20,000 neurons that provide the major source of norepinephrine (NE) in the brain, innervates the entire brain (Oades, 1985). LC neurons that release NE onto beta-adrenergic receptors are responsible for producing a nonspecific emotional activation via broadly collateralizing axons to the central nervous system (Aston-Jones et al., 1996), and this NE release to chronic stress is increased in inbred rat strains with high anxiety (Blizard, 1988) and in posttraumatic stress disorder patients (Charney et al., 1998). This nonspecific emotional activation pattern comprises a global urgent response system that responds to unpredicted events and hence facilitates behavioral readiness alerting (enhanced sensory processing) and attention (enhanced selection of stimuli) (Aston-Jones et al., 1996), which are characteristic of states of anxiety in highly stress-reactive rodents and monkeys (Blizard, 1988; Redmond, 1987). And this central arousal can be enduring: PGi CRH activation of LC neurons endures and peaks 40 minutes after stimulation of the PGi (Aston-Jones et al., 1996). This persistent activation of spontaneous activity in the LC renders the effects of short-lived, nonsalient stimuli of little effect on the LC, such that salient stimuli have an inordinate effect on LC activity and hence, in turn, on central activation. Thus, taken together, the central CRH neuron system is capable of activating a vast array of behaviorally relevant processes during stressful conditions, including activation of the peripheral CRH system.

CRH administration in rodents, as well as in transgenic mice that have an overproduction of CRH centrally (but not peripherally), generates specifically via CRH2 receptors anxiogenic effects, including reduced exploration of unfamiliarity and of the elevated T-maze, reduced sleep, reduced food intake and sexual activity, and increased sympathetic and behavioral signs of anxiety (Nie et al., 2004; Strand, 1999).

These findings taken together suggest that anxiety is essentially a stress response system that relies on a network of CRH neuron populations to modulate behaviorally relevant responses to the stressor. The most potent factors in determining the magnitude of a stressor are the very psychological factors that are eliciting stimuli of the anxiety system: uncontrollability, unpredictability, unfamiliarity, unavoidability, and uncertainty. For example, an animal that can control shock shows little evidence of stress, while the animal that is yoked to the first animal and receives shock without control shows severe behavioral and physiological effects of stress. Thus, it is not the physical nature of the shock that is stressful, but rather the psychological factor of uncontrollability and unpredictability. Furthermore, from the standpoint of trait anxiety or neuroticism, the strongest primary or facet scale in the higher-order factor of anxiety in Tellegen's personality questionnaire is termed "Stress Reactivity" due to the stress-related content of items loading on the scale (Tellegen & Waller, in press).

Nonaffective Constraint or Impulsivity

Delimiting the Heterogeneity of Impulsivity/Constraint

Impulsivity comprises a heterogeneous cluster of lower-order traits that includes sensation seeking, risk taking, novelty seeking, boldness, adventuresomeness, boredom susceptibility, unreliability, and unorderliness. This lack of specificity is reflected in the fact that the content of the measures of impulsivity is heterogeneous, and that not all of these measures are highly interrelated. We (Depue & Collins, 1999) demonstrated elsewhere that at least three different neurobehavioral systems may underlie this trait complex:

1. *Positive incentive motivation*, associated with exploratoration of novel stimulus conditions.
2. *Low fear*, as indicated in risk taking, attraction to physically dangerous activities, and lack of fear of physical harm.
3. *Low levels of a nonaffective form of impulsivity*, which results in disinhibition of the above neurobehavioral systems, as suggested by several researchers (Depue, 1995, 1996; Depue & Spoont, 1986; Panksepp, 1998; Spoont, 1992; Zuckerman, 1994).

As a means of disentangling and clarifying this complexity (see Figure 8.5), we plotted the trait loadings derived in 11 studies (see Depue & Collins, 1999) in which two or more multidimensional personality questionnaires were jointly factor analyzed in order to derive general higher-order traits of personality. All studies identified a higher-order trait of impulsivity that *lacks affective content*, which in Figure 8.5 was labeled as *constraint* following Tellegen (Tellegen & Waller, in press), who introduced the term to emphasize its independence from emotional traits such as extraversion and neuroticism. All studies also found constraint to be orthogonal to a general, higher-order extraversion trait. Figure 8.5 shows a continuous distribution of traits within the two intersecting orthogonal dimensions of extraversion and constraint. Nevertheless, three relatively homogeneous clusterings of traits can be delineated on the basis of the position and content of traits, relative to extraversion and constraint. First, lower-order traits associated with agentic extraversion (sociability, dominance, achievement, positive emotions, activity, energy) cluster at the high end of the extraversion dimension without substantial association with constraint. A tight clustering of most of these traits to extraversion is evident. Second, various traits of impulsivity that *do not incorporate strong positive affect*

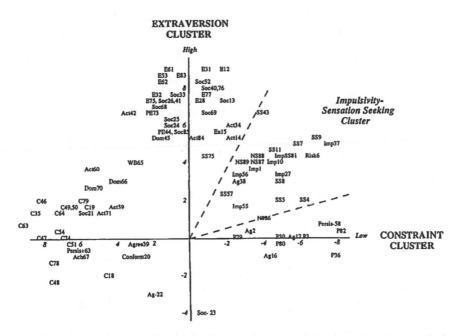

FIGURE 8.5. A plotting of loadings of personality traits derived in 11 studies in which more than one multidimensional personality questionnaire was jointly factor analyzed as a means of deriving general traits of personality. All of these studies defined a general nonaffective impulsivity trait, referred to as constraint (horizontal dimension in the figure), that was separate from the general extraversion trait (vertical dimension in the figure). The figure illustrates three clusterings of traits: an extraversion cluster at the high end of the extraversion dimension; conscientiousness and psychoticism–aggression clusters at the high and low end of the constraint dimension, respectively; and an impulsivity–sensation seeking cluster within the dashed lines. The figure illustrates that extraversion and *non*affective constraint dimensions are generally identified and found to be orthogonal, and that impulsivity–sensation seeking traits *associated with strong positive affect* arise as a joint function of the interaction of extraversion and constraint. See Appendix A in Depue and Collins (1999) for the identity of the trait measure abbreviations with numbers, the questionnaires to which the abbreviations correspond, and the studies providing the trait loadings.

(e.g., Conscientiousness) cluster tightly around the high end of the constraint dimension without substantial association with extraversion; Eysenck's Psychoticism trait and various aggression measures are located at the low end of constraint and show little association with extraversion. Third, all but one trait measure of impulsivity *that incorporate positive affect* (sensation seeking, novelty seeking, risk taking) are located within the dashed lines in Figure 8.5, and are moderately associated with both extraversion and constraint. Thus, currently most trait models of personality separate a nonaffective form of impulsivity and extraversion into distinct traits, although the terms used for the former vary from Conscientiousness (Costa & McCrae, 1992; Goldberg & Rosolack, 1994) to Constraint (Tellegen & Waller in press) and Impulsivity–Unsocialized Sensation Seeking (Zuckerman, 1994).

Conceptually, the complexity of impulsivity can be clarified by hypothesizing that *nonaffective* constraint lacks ties to a specific motivational–emotional system (Depue & Collins, 1999). As discussed below, a vast body of animal and human literature demonstrates that constraint so conceived functions as a central nervous system variable that modulates the threshold of stimulus elicitation of motor behavior, both positive and negative emotions, and cognition (Coccaro & Siever, 1991; Depue, 1995, 1996; Depue & Spoont, 1986; Luciana, Collins, & Depue, 1998; Luciana, Depue, Arbisi, & Leon, 1992; Panksepp, 1998; Spoont, 1992; Zald & Depue, 2001; Zuckerman, 1994). This formulation is consistent with findings that low constraint is associated in both animals and humans with a generalized motor–cognitive–affective impulsivity but is not preferentially associated with any specific motivational system (Depue & Spoont, 1986; Spoont, 1992; Zald & Depue, 2001). Alternatively, *affective* impulsivity emerges from the interaction of nonaffective constraint with other distinct affective–motivational systems, such as positive incentive motivation–agentic extraversion (as in Figure 8.5 above) or anxiety-neuroticism.

Elicitation of behavior can be modeled neurobiologically by use of a minimum threshold construct, which represents a central nervous system weighting of the external and internal factors that contribute to the probability of response expression (Depue & Collins, 1999; Depue & Morrone-Strupinsky, 2005). External factors are characteristics of environmental stimulation, including magnitude, duration, and psychological salience. Internal factors consist of both state (e.g., stress-induced endocrine levels) and trait biological variation.

A response threshold is weighted most strongly by the joint function of two main variables: (1) magnitude of eliciting stimulation and (2) level of postsynaptic receptor activation of the neurobiological variable thought to contribute most variance to the behavioral process in question, such as DA to incentive motivation, mu opiates to affiliative reward, and CRH to anxiety. The relation between these two variables is represented in Figure 8.6 as a trade-off function (White, 1986), where pairs of values (of stimulus magnitude and receptor activation) specify a diagonal representing the minimum threshold value for elicitation of a behavioral process. Findings reviewed above show that agonist-induced *state* changes in DA, mu OR, and CRH activation influence the threshold of incentive-motivated behavior, affiliative reward, and anxiety, respectively. Because the two input variables (stimulus magnitude and receptor activation) are interactive, independent variation in either one not only modifies the probability of eliciting the behavioral process but also simultaneously modifies the value of the other variable that is required to reach a minimum threshold of elicitation.

As illustrated in Figure 8.6, we propose that nonaffective constraint is the personality trait that reflects the greatest central nervous system weight on the construct of a minimum response threshold. As such, constraint exerts a general influence over the elicitation of any emotional behavior, and hence constraint is not preferentially associated with any specific neurobehavioral-motivational system. That is, nonaffective constraint would serve as a source of modulation of the threshold of elicitation of *all* behavioral processes. In this model, other higher-order personality traits would thus reflect the influence of neurobiological variables that strongly contribute to

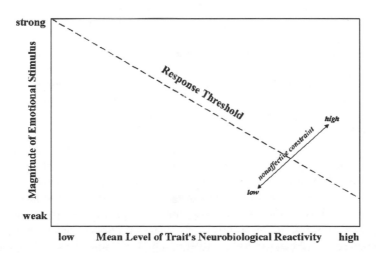

FIGURE 8.6. A minimum threshold for elicitation of a behavioral process (e.g., incentive motivation–positive affect, affiliative reward–affection, anxiety–negative affect) is illustrated as a trade-off function between eliciting stimulus magnitude (left vertical axis) and the mean level of a personality trait's neurobiological reactivity in a biological variable that strongly influences the expression of the trait (e.g., dopamine, mu opiate, CRH) (horizontal axis). Threshold effects due to modulation by nonaffective constraint are illustrated as well.

the threshold for responding, such as DA in the facilitation of incentive motivated behavior, mu opiates in the experience of affiliative reward, and CRH in the potentiation of anxiety.

Neurobiology of Nonaffective Constraint

The important question is what type of central nervous system variables could provide a major weighting of behavioral elicitation thresholds. Functional levels of neurotransmitters that provide a strong, relatively generalized *tonic inhibitory* influence on behavioral responding would be good candidates as significant modulators of a response elicitation threshold, and hence would likely account for a large proportion of the variance in the trait of nonaffective constraint. We and others previously (Coccaro & Siever, 1991; Depue, 1995, 1996; Depue & Spoont, 1986; Panksepp, 1998; Spoont, 1992; Zald & Depue, 2001; Zuckerman, 1994) and Lesch most recently (1998) suggested that serotonin (5-HT), acting at multiple receptor sites in most brain regions, is such a modulator (Azmitia & Whitaker-Azmitia, 1997; Tork, 1990). As reviewed many times in animal and human literatures (Coccaro et al., 1989; Coccaro & Siever, 1991; Depue, 1995, 1996; Depue & Spoont, 1986; Lesch, 1998; Spoont, 1992; Zald & Depue, 2001; Zuckerman, 1994), 5-HT modulates a diverse set of functions—including emotion, motivation, motor, affiliation, cognition, food intake, sleep, sexual activity, and sensory reactivity—such as nociception, sensitization to auditory and tactile startle stimuli, and escape latencies following PAG stimulation—and is associated with many clinical conditions, including violent suicide across several types of disorder, obsessive compulsive disorder, disorders of impulse control, aggression, depression, anxiety, arson, and substance abuse (Coccaro & Siever, 1991; Depue & Spoont, 1986; Lesch, 1998; Spoont, 1992). Furthermore, *reduced* 5-HT functioning in animals (Depue & Spoont, 1986; Spoont, 1992) and humans (Coccaro et al., 1989) is also accompanied by *irritability* and *hypersensitivity* to stimulation in most sensory modalities (Spoont, 1992), which may be due to the important role played by 5-HT in the inhibitory modulation of sensory input at several levels of the brain (Azmitia & Whitaker-Azmitia, 1997; Tork, 1990), as well as to significant 5-HT modulation of the lateral hypothalamic region that activates autonomic reactivity under stressful conditions (Azmitia & Whitaker-Azmitia, 1997). Thus, 5-HT plays a substantial modulatory role in general neurobiological functioning that affects many forms of motivated behavior. In this sense, nonaffective constraint might be viewed as reflecting the influence of the central nervous system variable of 5-HT, which we refer to later as *neural constraint*.

An important but difficult area of research is to determine which personality traits best assess the general modulatory role of 5-HT. As a begin-

ning, we found that 5-HT agonist-induced increases in serum prolactin se-
cretion were correlated significantly and specifically only with the Control/
Impulsivity scale (–.44, $p < .01$) from Tellegen's personality questionnaire
of 11 primary scales (Depue, 1995, 1996).

CONCEPTUALIZING INDIVIDUAL DIFFERENCES UNDERLYING PERSONALITY TRAITS

A more detailed extension of the above threshold model allows behavioral
predictions that help to conceptualize the effects of individual differences in
neurobiological functioning on personality traits. This is because individual
variation in variables that significantly modulate the threshold, especially
biological variables associated with a specific trait as well as 5-HT-related
neural constraint (or nonaffective constraint), will serve as major sources of
modulation of the elicitation of personality traits.

A *trait* dimension of postsynaptic receptor activation of *variable X*
(e.g., DA, mu opiate, or CRH) is represented on the horizontal axis of Figure 8.7, where two individuals with divergent trait levels are demarcated: *A*
(low trait level) and *B* (high trait level). These two divergent individuals
may be used to illustrate the effects of trait differences in variable X receptor
activation on elicitation of behavioral processes (e.g., incentive-motivated
behavior, affiliative reward, or anxiety).

As Figure 8.7 indicates, for any given eliciting stimulus, the degree of
variable X reactivity will, on average, be larger in individual *B* versus *A*.
Hence, the subjective emotional and motivational experiences that are facilitated by variable X (e.g., incentive, affection, anxiety) will also be more
enhanced in B versus A (Depue & Collins, 1999; Depue & Morrone-
Strupinsky, 2005). In addition, the difference between individuals A and B
in magnitude of subjective experience may contribute to variation in the
contemporaneous encoding of a stimulus's intensity or salience (a form of
state-dependent learning) and, hence, in the stimulus's encoded salience in
subsequent memory consolidation. Accordingly, individuals A and B may
develop differences in the capacity of mental representations of (incentive,
affiliative, anxiety) contexts to activate the relevant motivational (incentive,
affiliative, anxiety) processes, which is significant due to the predominant
motivation of behavior in humans by symbolic representations of goals.

If individual differences in encoding apply across the full range of stimulus magnitudes, trait differences in the reactivity of variable X may have
marked effects on the *range* of effective (i.e., eliciting) stimuli. This is illustrated in Figure 8.7, where the right vertical axis represents the range of effective (eliciting) stimuli. Increasing trait levels of variable X (horizontal
axis) are associated with an increasing efficacy of weaker stimuli (left verti-

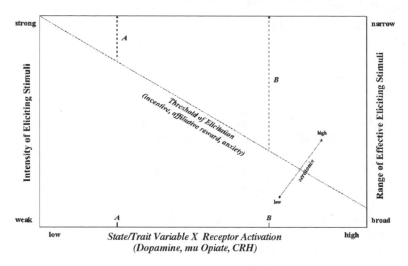

FIGURE 8.7. A minimum threshold for elicitation of a behavioral process (e.g., incentive motivation–positive affect, affiliative reward–affection, anxiety–negative affect) is illustrated as a trade-off function between eliciting stimulus magnitude (left vertical axis) and *variable X* (e.g., dopamine, mu opiate, CRH) postsynaptic receptor activation (horizontal axis). Range of effective (eliciting) stimuli is illustrated on the right vertical axis as a function of level of receptor activation. Two hypothetical individuals with low and high *trait* postsynaptic receptor activation (demarcated on the horizontal axis as *A* and *B*, respectively) are shown to have narrow (*A*) and broad (*B*) ranges of effective stimuli, respectively. Threshold effects due to serotonin modulation are illustrated as well.

cal axis) and, thus, with an increasing range of effective stimuli (right vertical axis). In Figure 8.7 individuals *A* and *B* are shown to have a narrow versus broad range, respectively. Significantly, the broader range for individual *B* suggests that, on average, *B* will experience more frequent elicitation of subjective emotional experiences associated with variable X activity (incentive, affection, anxiety). This means that the probability at any point in time of being in a variable X-facilitated state for individual *B* is higher than for *A*. Therefore, when subsequent relevant stimuli are encountered, their subjectively evaluated magnitude will show a stronger positive bias for *B* than *A*. Thus, trait differences in variable X may *proactively* influence the evaluation and encoding of relevant stimuli, and may not be restricted to *reactive* emotional processes. This raises the possibility of variation in the *dynamics* of behavioral engagement with the environment. A positive relation between *state* variable X activation and stimulus efficacy in the threshold model suggests that, as an initial stimulus enhances variable X activation, the efficacy of subsequently encountered stimuli may be increased proportional to the degree of the initial variable X activation. Under conditions of strong variable X activation, perhaps even previously subthreshold stimuli may come to elicit behavioral processes (incentive, affiliative reward, anxiety).

THE INTERACTIVE NATURE
OF EMOTIONAL TRAITS AND CONSTRAINT

Three of the higher-order personality traits discussed above (agentic extraversion, affiliation, anxiety) provide the qualitative emotional content of comtemporaneous behavior, depending on which neurobehavioral–motivational system is being elicited at any point in time. The fourth trait, nonaffective constraint, modulates the probability of elicitation of all of those systems. As the very construct of personality connotes, however, the affective or emotional *style* of an individual is determined by the interaction of all four higher-order traits. This means that differential strength between these personality traits, or differential reactivity of their underlying neurobehavioral systems, will determine the relative predominance of particular affective or emotional behavior in individuals.

For example, differential relative strength of the traits of agentic extraversion and anxiety has a substantial influence on the predominant affective or emotional style of an individual. Agentic extraversion is associated with a highly positive affective state, whereas anxiety is associated with a negative affective state. Moreover, both traits are associated with *general* neurobehavioral systems, meaning that they both are subject to frequent elicitation by a broad class of stimulus (incentives and uncertainty, respectively). As illustrated in Figure 8.8, the interaction of these two traits leads to various types of affective style depending on the values of the two traits. The upper-right (positive) and lower-left (negative) quadrants manifest the greatest contrast and consistency in affective styles, whereas the affective style of individuals in the upper-left quandrant is mixed, depending on the relative salience of the most recent incentive versus uncertainty context. The lower-right quadrant is characterized by both low positive and negative affective activation, and therefore manifests as impoverished affective-emotional behavior reminiscent of clinical descriptions of schizoid behavior.

A more general effect of the interaction of traits concerns the interaction of nonaffective constraint with other major traits, such as agentic extraversion, anxiety, aggression, and affiliation. A vast body of animal and human evidence consistently associates reduced functioning of 5-HT neurotransmission with *behavioral instability*. This instability is manifested as lability, i.e., a heightened probability of competing behavioral responses due to a reduced threshold of response elicitation (Spoont, 1992). Therefore, instability or lability will increase as a function of increasing stimulus

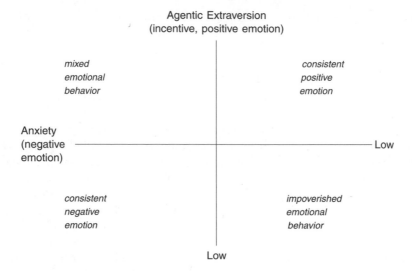

FIGURE 8.8. Combination of the higher-order personality traits of agentic extraversion and anxiety. See text for details.

influences on response elicitation of other behavioral systems (Depue & Spoont, 1986). This means that the effects of constraint depend on interactions with other personality traits that reflect activity in those behavioral systems. That is, the *qualitative content* of unstable behavior will depend on which neurobehavioral–motivational system, or *affective* personality trait, is being elicited at any point in time (Depue & Collins, 1999; Zald & Depue, 2001), although differential strength of various personality traits will obviously produce relative predominance of particular affective behaviors *within individuals*.

An example of the interaction of neurobiological variables associated with constraint (5-HT) and agentic extraversion (DA) helps to illustrate the behavioral instability resulting from low constraint. 5-HT is an inhibitory modulator of a host of DA-facilitated behaviors, including the reinforcing properties of psychostimulants, novelty-induced locomotor activity, the acquisition of self-administration of cocaine, and DA utilization in the NAS (Ashby, 1996; Depue & Spoont, 1986; Spoont, 1992). This modulatory influence arises in large part from the dense dorsal raphe efferents to the VTA and NAS, connections that are known to modulate DA activity (Ashby, 1966; Azmitia & Whitaker-Azmitia, 1997; Spoont, 1992). A 5-HT-related reduction in the threshold of DA facilitation of behavior results in an exaggerated response to incentive stimuli that is most apparent in reward–punishment conflict situations. In such situations, exaggerated responding to incentives results in (1) a greater weighting of immediate versus delayed future rewards; (2) increased reactivity to the reward of safety or relief associated with active avoidance (e.g., suicidal behavior); (3) impulsive behavior, that is, a propensity to respond to reward when withholding or delaying a response may produce a more favorable long-term outcome; and (4) various attempts to experience the increased magnitude and frequency of incentive reward, for example, self-administration of DA-active substances (Babor, Hofmann, & Delboca, 1992; Coccaro & Siever, 1991; Depue & Iacono, 1989; Lesch, 1998). All of these effects impair the ability to sustain long-term goal-directed behavior programs (such as obtaining a college degree) by mental representations of expected rewards that can be repeatedly accessed, held on-line in the prefrontal cortex, and thereby symbolically motivate behavior (Depue & Collins, 1999; Goldman-Rakic, 1987).

A 5-HT–DA interaction is modeled in Figure 8.9 within a personality framework, where the affectively unipolar dimension of agentic extraversion (DA facilitation) is seen in interaction with nonaffective constraint (5-HT inhibition) (Depue, 1996). The interaction of these two traits creates a diagonal dimension of *behavioral stability* that applies equally to affective, cognitive, interpersonal, motor, and incentive processes (Depue & Spoont, 1986; Luciana et al., 1998; Spoont, 1992; Zald & Depue, 2001). The diagonal represents the line of greatest variance in stability, ranging from lability in the upper-left quadrant of the two-space (low 5-HT, high DA) to rigidity in the lower-right (high 5-HT, low DA).

It is important to note that the extent of lability is affected not only by a 5-HT influence, but also by DA's more general facilitative effects on the flow of neural information, where increased DA activity promotes *switching* between response alternatives (i.e., behavioral flexibility) (Depue & Iacono, 1989; Oades, 1985; Spoont, 1992). Indeed, when DA transmission is very low, a problem in exceeding the response facilitation threshold occurs, whereas at very high DA transmission levels, a high rate of switching between response alternatives is seen, which can evolve into a low *variety* of responses when abnormally high (e.g., stereotypy) (Oades, 1985).

This conceptualization of the interaction of 5-HT and DA may be relevant to interpersonal behavior and affiliation. Brothers and Ring (1992) and others (Adolphs, 2003) have argued that humans have an innate cognitive *alphabet* of ethologically significant behavioral signs that signal the emotional intention of others. This alphabet is integrated into its highest representation in human social cognition as a *person* with propensities and dispositions that have valence for the observer, a social construct akin to personality. Personality research has demonstrated that the representation of others exists in two independent, contrasted forms as the *familiar-good other* and the *unfamiliar-evil other*, and the representation of the self is similarly represented in two independent positive and negative forms (Tellegen

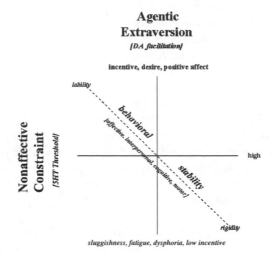

FIGURE 8.9. Combination of the higher-order personality traits of agentic extraversion and nonaffective constraint. See text for details.

& Waller, in press). This is consistent with the fact that most percepts and concepts are represented in the brain as separate unified entities (Squire & Kosslyn, 1998). Interestingly, increased DA activation results in a more rapid switching between contrasting percepts, such as two perceptual orientations of the Necker cube or of an ascending–descending staircase (Oades, 1985). Speculatively, we suggest that the frequent, sometimes rapid, fluctuation between extreme mental representations of others and/or the self as *good* or *bad* that characterize several forms of personality disorders is related primarily to reduced 5-HT functioning (e.g., borderline-like interpersonal disturbance). Furthermore, this condition would be exaggerated when in interaction with increasing DA functioning (e.g., histrionic-like interpersonal disturbance). Such unstable evaluations of others greatly impairs interpersonal relations and may be aggravated in individuals with elevated trait anxiety levels (e.g., borderline-like interpersonal impairment).

A MODEL OF PERSONALITY DISTURBANCE

Illustration of the interactions of two traits taken at a time, as above, is informative, but of course underestimates the complexity of reality. The neurobehavioral systems underlying all of the higher-order traits interact. Therefore, we conceive of personality disturbance as *emergent* phenotypes arising from the interaction of the above neurobehavioral systems underlying major personality traits.

Our multidimensional model is illustrated in Figure 8.10. In the model, the axes are defined by neurobehavioral systems rather than by traits, because traits are only approximate, fallible estimates of these systems, and trait measures vary in content and underlying constructs. In Figure 8.10, behavioral approach based on positive *incentive motivation* (underlying agentic extraversion) and anxiety (underlying neuroticism or trait anxiety) are modeled as a ratio of their relative strength, because the opposing nature of their eliciting stimuli affects behavior in a reciprocal manner, such that the *elicitation* or *expression* of one system is influenced by the strength of the other (Gray, 1973). As discussed above, the interaction of these two systems strongly influences the style of an individual's emotional behavior. The affiliative reward dimension (underlying trait affiliation) in the model largely influences the interpersonal domain, whereas the neural constraint (underlying the trait of nonaffective constraint) dimension modulates the expressive features of the other systems. Due to the limitation of graphing more than three dimensions, it should be noted that the model includes two other systems/traits that we suggest influence the manifestation of personality disturbance. As suggested in the section on trait interactions above, we believe a dimension of affective aggression:fear is necessary to account for the full range of antisocial (high aggression:low fear) behavior and that a dimension of separation anxiety/rejection sensitivity strongly contributes to dependent-, avoidant-, and borderline-like disturbance (all high on this dimension). Taken together, then, the model proposes that the interaction of at least six neurobehavioral systems underlying dimensional personality

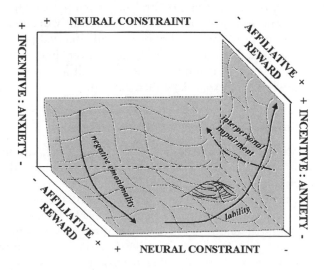

FIGURE 8.10. A multidimensional model of personality disturbance. See text for details.

traits is necessary to account for the emergent phenotypes observed in personality disturbance.

Three significant features of the model that are illustrated in the figure are worth emphasizing. First, the phenotypic expression of personality disturbance, represented by the gray-shaded *reaction* surface in the figure (accounting for ~10% of the population; Lenzenweger, Loranger, Korfine, & Neff, 1997; Livesley, 2001; Torgersen, Kringlen, & Cramer, 2001), is continuous in nature, changing in character gradually but seamlessly across the surface in a manner that reflects the changing product of the multidimensional interactions. It may be that certain areas of the surface are associated with increased probability (risk) of certain features of personality disturbance, and this is represented in the right-back area of the figure as an elevation in the surface that is continuous rather than distinct in contour. Thus, this representation is not meant to imply that a distinct disorder or category exists in that particular area of the surface. Second, the extent and positioning of the reaction surface is weighted most heavily by increasing anxiety, decreasing neural constraint, and decreasing affiliative reward. This weighting is also reflected in the lines with directional arrows overlaying the gray surface in the figure, which illustrate increasing negative emotionality, lability, and interpersonal impairment. These three factors were found to be the most common characteristics of all personality disorders in the meta-analysis of Saulsman and Page (2004), thereby empirically supporting their emphasis in our model. Third, viewing personality disturbance as a *reaction* surface implies that the magnitude of disturbance at any point on the surface is variable, waxing and waning with fluctuations in environmental circumstances, stressors, and interpersonal disruptions, both within and across persons over time. Indeed, we recently demonstrated in a longitudinal assessment of the stability of formally defined personality disorders that phenotypic intensity varied markedly over time, thereby affecting the presence/absence of diagnostic status as well as level of symptomatology (Lenzenweger, Johnson, & Willett, 2004).

Implications of the Model

Several implications of the model can be outlined. First, the model may help to explain sex differences in some forms of personality disturbance. The increased prevalence of males with antisocial behavior may reflect the higher mean of males in the population on the trait of aggression:fear and a lower mean on nonaffective constraint (including 5-HT functioning; Spoont, 1992). Additionally, the increased prevalence of females in clinical populations with borderline- and dependent-like personality disturbance may reflect a combination of (1) their higher mean on both trait anxiety (borderline) and separation distress (dependent); (2) their higher mean on affiliation, thereby increasing the need for social relationships whose loss is feared; (3) their lower mean on agentic extraversion, particularly social dominance, hence enhancing the predominance of high levels of trait anxiety; and (4) their lower mean on aggression:fear, hence decreasing the prevalence of antisocial behavior (Depue & Collins, 1999; Kohnstamm, 1989; Tellegen & Waller, in press).

Second, the model suggests that research on the lines of causal neurobiological influence within the structure of *normal* personality will need to be a primary focus if the neurobiological nature of personality disturbance is to be fully understood. At present, there is a paucity of systematic research in this domain (Depue & Collins, 1999; Depue & Morrone-Strupinsky, 2005). Third, the multidimensional nature of the model indicates that univariate biological research in personality disturbance will inadequately discover the neurobiological nature of personality disturbance. Thus, not only is multivariate assessment suggested, but methods of *combinatorial* representation of those multiple variables—as in profile, finite mixture modeling, latent class, discriminant function, and multivariate taxonomic analyses—will need to be more fully integrated in this area of research. Finally, the trend in development of neurotransmitter-specific drugs may not fully complement the pharmocotherapy requirements of personality disturbance. If personality disturbance represents emergent phenotypes of multiple interacting neurobehavioral systems, then both basic research on the pharmacological modulation of neurobehavioral systems and clinical research on multiregiment pharmacotherapy are greatly needed.

ACKNOWLEDGMENTS

This work was supported by National Institute of Mental Health Research Grant Nos. MH55347 (awarded to Richard A. Depue) and MH-45448 (awarded to Mark F. Lenzenweger).

REFERENCES

Adolphs, R. (2003). Cognitive neuroscience of human social behavior. *Nature Reviews Neuroscience, 4*, 165–178.

Aggleton, J. (1992). *The amygdala: Neurobiological aspects of emotion, memory, and mental dysfunction.* New York: Wiley-Liss.

Agren, G., Olsson, C., Uvnas-Moberg, K., & Lundeberg, T. (1997). Olfactory cues from an oxytocin-injected male rat can reduce energy less in its cagemates. *Neuroreport, 8*, 2551–2555.

Amaral, D., & Witter, M. (1995). Hippocampal formation. In G. Paxinos (Ed.), *The rat nervous system* (pp. 443–494). New York: Academic Press.

Annett, L., McGregor, A., & Robbins, T. (1989). The effects of ibotenic acid lesions of the nucleus accumbens on spatial learning and extinction in the rat. *Behavioral and Brain Research, 31*, 231–242.

Ashby, C. (1996). *The modulation of dopaminergic neurotransmission by other neurotransmitters.* Boca Raton, FL: CRC Press.

Aston-Jones, G., Rajkowski, J., Kubiak, P., Valentino, R., & Shiptley, M. (1996). Role of the locus coeruleus in emotional activation. In G. Holstege, R. Bandler, & C. Saper (Eds.), *The emotional motor system* (pp. 254–279). New York: Elsevier.

Azmitia, E., & Whitaker-Azmitia, P. (1997). Development and adult plasticity of serotonergic neurons and their target cells. In H. Baumgarten & M. Gothert (Eds.), *Serotonergic neurons and 5-HT receptors in the CNS* (Vol. 129, pp. 1–39). New York: Springer.

Babor, T., Hofmann, M., & Delboca, F. (1992). Types of alcoholics: 1. Evidence for an empirically derived typology based on indicators of vulnerability and severity. *Archives of General Psychiatry, 49*, 599–608.

Bandler, R., & Keay, K. (1996). Columnar organization in the midbrain periaqueductal gray and the integration of emotional expression. In G. Holstege, R. Bandler & C. Saper (Eds.), *The emotional motor system.* NY: Elsevier.

Barlow, D. H. (2002). *Anxiety and its disorders: The nature and treatment of anxiety and panic* (2nd ed.). New York: Guilford Press.

Bechara, A., Tranel, D., Damasio, H., Adolphs, R., Rockland, C., & Damasio, A. (1995). Double dissociation of conditioning and declarative knowledge relative to the amygdala and hippocampus in humans. *Science, 269*, 1115–1118.

Benjamin, J., Li, L., Patterson, C., Greenberg, B., Murphy, D., & Hamer, D. (1996). Population and familial association between the D4 dopamine receptor gene and measures of novelty seeking. *Nature Genetics, 12*, 81–84.

Berrettini, W. H., Hoehe, M., Ferraro, T. N., DeMaria, P., & Gottheil, E. (1997). Human mu opioid receptor gene polymorphisms and vulnerability to substance abuse. *Addiction and Biology, 2*, 303–308.

Berridge, K. C. (1999). Pleasure, pain, desire, and dread: Hidden core processes of emotion. In D. Kahneman, E. Diener, & N. Schwarz (Eds.), *Well-being: The foundations of hedonic psychology* (pp. 525–557). New York: Russell Sage Foundation.

Blackburn, J. R., Phillips, A. G., Jakubovic, A., & Fibiger, H. C. (1989). Dopamine and preparatory behavior: II. A neurochemical analysis. *Behavioral Neuroscience, 103*, 15–23.

Blizard, D. A. (1988). The locus ceruleus: A possible neural focus for genetic differences in emotionality. *Experientia, 44*, 491–495.

Block, J. (2001). Millennial contrarianism: The five-factor approach to personality description 5 years later. *Journal of Personality, 69*, 98–107.

Bond, C., LaForge, K. S., Tian, M., Melia, D., Zhang, S., Borg, L., et al. (1998). Single-nucleotide polymorphism in the human mu opioid receptor gene alters ß-endorphin binding and activity: Possible implications for opiate addiction. *Proceedings of the National Academy of Sciences, 95*, 9608–9613.

Breiter, H., Aharon, I., Kahneman, D., Dale, A., & Shizgal, P. (2001). Functional imaging of neural responses to expectancy and experience of monetary gains and losses. *Neuron, 30*, 619–639.

Breiter, H. C., Gollub, R. L., Weisskoff, R. M., Kennedy, D. N., Makris, N., Berke, J. D., et al. (1997). Acute effects of cocaine on human brain activity and emotion. *Neuron, 19*, 591–611.

Brothers, L., & Ring, B. (1992). A neuroethological framework for the representation of minds. *Journal of Cognitive Neuroscience, 4*(2), 107–118.

Cador, M., Taylor, J., & Robbins, T. (1991). Potentiation of the effects of reward-related stimuli by dopaminergic-dependent mechanisms in the nucleus accumbens. *Psychopharmacology, 104*, 377–385.

Callahan, P., Baumann, M., & Rabil, J. (1996). Inhibition of tuberoinfundibular dopaminergic neural activity during suckling: Involvement of mu and kappa opiate receptor subtypes. *Journal of Neuroendocrinology, 8*, 771–776.

Carlezon, W., Haile, C., Coopersmith, R., Hayashi, Y., Malinow, R., Neve, R., et al. (2000). Distinct sites of opiate reward and aversion within the midbrain identified using a herpes simplex virus vector expressing GluR1. *Journal of Neuroscience, 20*, 1–5.

Carter, S., Lederhendler, I., & Kirkpatrick, B. (1997). *The integrative neurobiology of affiliation* (Vol. 807). New York: New York Academy of Sciences.

Charney, D. S., Grillon, C., & Bremner, D. (1998). The neurobiological basis of anxiety and fear: Circuits, mechanisms, and neurochemical interactions (Part I). *Neuroscientist, 4*, 35–44.

Church, A. T. (1994). Relating the Tellegen and five-factor models of personality structure. *Journal of Personality and Social Psychology, 67*, 898–909.

Church, T., & Burke, P. (1994). Exploratory and confirmatory tests of the big five and Tellegen's three- and four-dimensional models. *Journal of Personality and Social Psychology, 66*, 93–114.

Churchill, L., Roques, B. P., & Kalivas, P. W. (1995). Dopamine depletion augments endogenous opioid-induced locomotion in the nucleus accumbens using both μ1 and d opioid receptors. *Psychopharmacology, 120*, 347–355.

Clark, L. A., & Livesley, W. J. (1994). Two approaches to identifying the dimensions of personality disorder. In P. T. Costa, Jr. & T. A. Widiger (Eds.), *Personality disorders and the five factor model of personality*. Washington, DC: American Psychological Association.

Clark, L. A., Livesley, W. J., Schroeder, M. L., & Irish, S. L. (1996). Convergence of two systems for assessing personality disorder. *Psychological Assessment, 8*, 294–303.

Clarkin, J. F., & Lenzenweger, M. F. (Eds.). (1996). *Major theories of personality disorder*. New York: Guilford Press.

Cloninger, C. R., Svrakic, D., & Przybeck, T. (1993). A psychobiological model of temperament and character. *Archives of General Psychiatry, 50*, 975–990.

Coccaro, E., & Siever, L. (1991). *Serotonin and psychiatric disorders*. Washington, DC: American Psychiatric Association Press.

Coccaro, E., Siever, L., Klar, H., Maurer, G., Cochrane, K., Cooper, T., et al. (1989). Serotonergic studies in patients with affective and personality disorders. *Archives of General Psychiatry, 46,* 587–599.

Costa, P., & McCrae, R. (1992). Revised *NEO Personality Inventory (NEO-PI-R) and NEO Five-Factor Inventory (NEO-FFI) professional manual.* Odessa, FL: Psychological Assessment Resources.

Costa, P. T., Jr., & Widiger, T. A. (1994). *Personality disorders and the five factor model of personality.* Washington, DC: American Psychological Association.

Damasio, D. (2003). *Looking for Spinoza.* New York: Harcourt.

David, V., & Cazala, P. (2000). Anatomical and pharmacological specificity of the rewarding effect elicited by microinjections of morphine into the nucleus accumbens of mice. *Psychopharmacology, 150,* 24–34.

Davis, M., & Shi, C. (1999). The extended amydala: Are the central nucleus of the amygdala and the bed nucleus of the stria terminalis differentially involved in fear versus anxiety? In J. F. McGinty (Ed.), Advancing from the ventral striatum to the extended amygdala: Implications for neuropsychiatry and drug use. *Annals of New York Academy of Sciences, 877,* 281–291.

Davis, M., Walker, D., & Lee, Y. (1997). Roles of the amygdala and bed nucleus of the stria terminalis in fear and anxiety measured with the acoustic startle reflex. *Annals of the New York Academy of Sciences, 821,* 305–331.

Depue, R. (1995). Neurobiological factors in personality and depression. *European Journal of Personality, 9,* 413–439.

Depue, R. (1996). Neurobiology and the structure of personality: Implications for the personality disorders. In J. Clarkin & M. Lenzenweger (Eds.), *Major theories of personality disorders* (pp. 165–192). New York: Guilford Press.

Depue, R. A., & Collins, P. F. (1999). Neurobiology of the structure of personality: Dopamine, facilitation of incentive motivation, and extraversion. *Behavioral and Brain Sciences, 22,* 491–569.

Depue, R., & Iacono, W. (1989). Neurobehavioral aspects of affective disorders. *Annual Review of Psychology, 40,* 457–492.

Depue, R. A., & Lenzenweger, M. F. (2001). A neurobehavioral dimensional model of personality disorders. In W. J. Livesley (Ed.), *Handbook of personality disorders* (pp. 136–176). New York: Guilford Press.

Depue, R. A., & Lenzenweger, M. F. (2005). A neurobehavioral dimensional model of personality disturbance. In M. F. Lenzenweger & J. Clarkin (Eds.), *Major theories of personality disorders* (2nd ed.). New York: Guilford Press.

Depue, R., Luciana, M., Arbisi, P., Collins, P., & Leon, A. (1994). Dopamine and the structure of personality: Relation of agonist-induced dopamine activity to positive emotionality. *Journal of Personality and Social Psychology, 67,* 485–498.

Depue, R. A., & Morrone-Strupinsky, J. V. (2005). A neurobehavioral model of affiliative bonding: Implications for conceptualizing a human trait of affiliation. *Behavioral and Brain Sciences, 28,* 313–395.

Depue, R., & Spoont, M. (1986). Conceptualizing a serotonin trait: A behavioral dimension of constraint. *Annals of the New York Academy of Sciences, 487,* 47–62.

Di Chiara, G. (1995). The role of dopamine in drug abuse viewed from the perspective of its role in motivation. *Drug and Alcohol Dependence, 38,* 95–137.

Di Chiara, G., & North, R. A. (1992). Neurobiology of opiate abuse. *Trends in the Physiological Sciences, 13,* 185–193.

Digman, J. M. (1997). Higher-order factors of the big five. *Journal of Personality and Social Psychology, 73,* 1246–1256.

Domjan, M., Cusato, B., & Villarreal, R. (2000). Pavlovian feed-forward mechanisms in the control of social behavior. *Behavioral and Brain Sciences, 23,* 1–29.

Drevets, W. C., Gautier, C., Price, J. C., Kupfer, D. J., Kinahan, P. E., Grace, A. A., et al. (2001). Amphetamine-induced dopamine release in human ventral striatum correlates with euphoria. *Biological Psychiatry, 49,* 81–96.

Dworkin, S., Guerin, G., Goeders, N., & Smith, J. (1988). Kainic acid lesions of the nucleus accumbens selectively attenuate morphine self-administration. *Pharmacology Biochemistry and Behavior, 29,* 175–181.

Dyce, J. A., & Connor, B. P. (1998). Personality disorders and the five-factor model: A test of facet-level predictions. *Journal of Personality Disorders, 12,* 31–45.

Ebstein, R., Novick, O., Umansky, R., Priel, B., Osher, Y., Blaine, D., et al. (1996). Dopamine D4 receptor (DRD4) exon III polymorphism associated with the human personality trait of novelty seeking. *Nature Genetics, 12,* 78–80.

Ekselius, L., Lindstrom, E., von Knorring, L., Bodlund, O., & Kullgren, G. (1994). A principal component analysis of the DSM-III R axis II personality disorders. *Journal of Personality Disorders, 8,* 140–148.

Eisenberger, N., Lieberman, M., & Williams, K. (2003). Does rejection hurt?: An fMRI study of social exclusion. *Science, 302,* 290–292.

Elmer, G. I., Pieper, J. O., Goldberg, S. R., & George, F. R. (1995). Opioid operant self-administration, analgesia, stimulation and respiratory depression in μ-deficient mice. *Psychopharmacology, 117,* 23–31.

Erb, S., Salmaso, N., Rodaros, D., & Stewart, J. (2001). A role for the CF-containing pathway from central nucleus of the amygdala to the bed nucleus of the stria terminalis in the stress-induced reinstatement of cocaine seeking in rats. *Psychopharmacology, 158,* 360–365.

Everitt, B., & Robbins, T. (1992). Amygdala-ventral striatal interactions and reward-related processes. In J. Aggleton (Ed.), *The amygdala: Neurobiological aspects of emotion, memory, and mental dysfunction.* New York: Wiley-Liss.

Fendt, M., Endres, T., & Apfelbach, R. (2003). Temporary inactivation of the bed nucleus of the stria terminalis but not of the amygdala blocks freezing induced by trimethylthiazoline, a component of fox feces. *Journal of Neuroscience, 23,* 23–28.

Fleming, A. S., Korsmit, M., & Deller, M. (1994). Rat pups are potent reinforcers to the maternal animal: Effects of experience, parity, hormones, and dopamine function. *Psychobiology, 22*(1), 44–53.

Fowles, D. C. (1987). Application of a behavioral theory of motivation to the concepts of anxiety and impulsivity. *Journal of Research in Personality, 21,* 417–435.

Gaffan, D. (1992). Amygdala and the memory of reward. In J. Aggleton (Ed.), *The amygdala: Neurobiological aspects of emotion, memory, and mental dysfunction.* New York: Wiley-Liss.

Gelernter, J., Kranzler, H., & Cubells, J. (1999). Genetics of two μ opioid receptor gene (OPRM1) exon I polymorphisms: Population studies, and allele frequencies in alcohol- and drug-dependent subjects. *Molecular Psychiatry, 4*, 476–483.

Gingrich, B., Liu, Y., Cascio, C., Wang, Z., & Insel., T. R. (2000). Dopamine D2 receptors in the nucleus accumbens are important for social attachment in female prairie voles *(Microtus ochrogaster). Behavioral Neuroscience, 114*(1), 173–183.

Goldberg, L., & Rosolack, T. (1994). The big five factor structure as an integrative framework. In C. Halverson, G. Kohnstamm, & R. Marten (Eds.), *The developing structure of temperament and personality from infancy to adulthood.* Hillside, NJ: Erlbaum.

Goldman-Rakic, P. S. (1987). Circuitry of the prefrontal cortex and the regulation of behavior by representational memory. In V. Mountcastle (Ed.), *Handbook of physiology.* American Physiological Society.

Gottesman, I. I. (1997). Twins: En route to QTLs for cognition. *Science, 276,* 1522–1523.

Graves, F. C., Wallen, K., & Maestripieri, D. (2002). Opioids and attachment in rhesus macaque abusive mothers. *Behavioral Neuroscience, 116,* 489–493.

Gray, J. A. (1973). Causal theories of personality and how to test them. In J. R. Royce (Ed.), *Multivariate analysis and psychological theory.* New York: Academic Press.

Gray, J. (1992). Neural systems, emotion and personality. In J. Madden, S. Matthysee, & J. Barchas (Eds.), *Adaptation, learning and affect.* New York: Raven Press.

Guyenet, P., Koshiqa, N., Huangfu, D., Baraban, S., Stornetta, R., & Li, Y.-W. (1996). Role of medulla oblongata in generation of sympathetic and vagal outflows. In G. Holstege, R. Bandler, & C. Saper (Eds.), *The emotional motor system.* New York: Elsevier.

Haslam, N. (2003). The dimensional view of personality disorders: A review of the taxometric evidence. *Clinical Psychology Review, 23,* 75–93.

Heimer, L. (2003). A new anatomical framework for neuropsychiatric disorders and drug abuse. *American Journal of Psychiatry, 160,* 1726–1739.

Herbert, J. (1993). Peptides in the limbic system: Neurochemical codes for coordinated adaptive responses to behavioural and physiological demand. *Progress in Neurobiology, 41,* 723–791.

Herz, A. (1998). Opioid reward mechanisms: A key role in drug abuse? *Canadian Journal of Physiology and Pharmacology, 76,* 252–258.

Hilliard, S., Domjan, M., Nguyen, M., & Cusato, B. (1998). Dissociation of conditioned appetitive and consummatory sexual behavior: Satiation and extinction tests. *Animal Learning and Behavior, 26*(1), 20–33.

Hol, T., Niesink, M., van Ree, J., & Spruijt, B. (1996). Prenatal exposure to morphine affects juvenile play behavior and adult social behavior in rats. *Pharmacology, Biochemistry, and Behavior, 55,* 615–618.

Holstege, G. (1996). The somatic motor system. In G. Holstege, R. Bandler, & C. Saper (Eds.), *The emotional motor system*. New York: Elsevier.

Hyztia, P., & Kiianmaa, K. (2001). Suppression of ethanol responding by centrally administered CTOP and naltrindole in AA and Wistar rats. *Alcohol Clinical and Experimental Research, 25,* 25–33.

Ikemoto, S., & Panksepp, J. (1996). Dissociations between appetitive and consummatory responses by pharmacological manipulations of reward-relevant brain regions. *Behavioral Neuroscience, 110,* 331–345.

Insel, T. R. (1997). A neurobiological basis of social attachment. *American Journal of Psychiatry, 154*(6), 726–733.

Johnson, B., & Ait-Daoud, N. (2000). Neuropharmacological treatments for alcoholism: Scientific basis and clinical findings. *Psychopharmacology, 149,* 327–344.

Kalivas, P., Churchill, L., & Klitenick, M. (1993). The circuitry mediating the translation of motivational stimuli into adaptive motor responses. In P. Kalivas & C. Barnes (Eds.), *Limbic motor circuits and neuropsychiatry*. Boca Raton, FL: CRC Press.

Kendler, K. S., McGuire, M., Gruenberg, A. M., O'Hare, A., Spellman, M., & Walsh, D. (1993). The Roscommon Family Study: III. Schizophrenia-related personality disorders in relatives. *Archives of General Psychiatry, 50,* 781–788.

Keverne, E. B. (1996). Psychopharmacology of maternal behaviour. *Journal of Psychopharmacology, 10*(1), 16–22.

Kim, J., & Diamond, D. (2002). The stressed hippocampus, synaptic plasticity and lost memories. *Nature Reviews Neuroscience, 3,* 453–462.

Kohnstamm, G. (1989). Temperament in childhood: Cross-cultural and sex differences. In G. Kohnstamm, J. Bates, & M. Rothbart (Eds.), *Temperament in childhood*. New York: Wiley.

Korfine, L., & Lenzenweger, M. F. (1995). The taxonicity of schizotypy: A replication. *Journal of Abnormal Psychology, 104,* 26–31.

Kranzler, H. R. (2000). Pharmacotherapy of alcoholism: Gaps in knowledge and opportunities for research. *Alcohol and Alcoholism, 35,* 537–547.

La Buda, C., Sora, I., Uhl, G., & Fuchs, P. N. (2000). Stress-induced analgesia in mu-opioid receptor knockout mice reveals normal function of the delta-opioid receptor system. *Brain Research, 869,* 1–10.

Laviolette, S. R., Gallegos, R. A., Henriksen, S. J., & van der Kooy, D. (2004). Opiate state controls bi-directional reward signaling via GABA-A receptors in the ventral tegmental area. *Nature Neuroscience, 10,* 160–169.

LeDoux, J. (1998). *The emotional brain*. New York: Simon & Schuster.

LeDoux, J., Cicchetti, P., Xagoraris, A., & Romanski, L. (1990). The lateral amygdaloid nucleus: Sensory interface of the amygdala in fear conditioning. *Journal of Neuroscience, 10,* 1062–1069.

Le Moal, M., & Simon, H. (1991). Mesocorticolimbic dopaminergic network: Functional and regulatory roles. *Physiological Reviews, 71,* 155–234.

Lenzenweger, M. F. (1998). Schizotypy and schizotypic psychopathology: Mapping an alternative expression of schizophrenia liability. In M. F. Lenzenweger & R. H. Dworkin (Eds.), *Origins and development of schizophrenia: Advances in ex-*

perimental psychopathology (pp. 93–121). Washington, DC: American Psychological Association.

Lenzenweger, M. F., & Clarkin, J. F. (1996). The personality disorders: History, development, and research issues. In J. F. Clarkin & M. F. Lenzenweger (Eds.), *Major theories of personality disorder* (pp. 1–35). New York: Guilford Press.

Lenzenweger, M. F., & Clarkin, J. F. (2005). The personality disorders: History, development, and research issues. In J. F. Clarkin & M. F. Lenzenweger (Eds.), *Major theories of personality disorder* (2nd ed., pp. 1–42). New York: Guilford Press.

Lenzenweger, M. F., Johnson, M. D., & Willett, J. B. (2004). Individual growth curve analysis illuminates stability and change in personality disorder features: The Longitudinal Study of Personality Disorders. *Archives of General Psychiatry, 61*, 1015–1024.

Lenzenweger, M. F., & Korfine, L. (1992). Confirming the latent structure and base rate of schizotypy: A taxometric analysis. *Journal of Abnormal Psychology, 101*, 567–571.

Lenzenweger, M. F., & Loranger, A. W. (1989). Detection of familial schizophrenia using a psychometric measure of schizotypy. *Archives of General Psychiatry, 46*, 902–907.

Lenzenweger, M. F., Loranger, A. W., Korfine, L., & Neff, C. (1997). Detecting personality disorders in a nonclinical population: Application of a two-stage procedure for case identification. *Archives of General Psychiatry, 54*, 345–351.

Leri, F., Flores, J., Rodaros, D., & Stewart, J. (2002). Blockade of stress-induced but not cocaine-induced reinstatement by infusion of noradrenergic antagonists into the bed nucleus of the stria terminalis or the central nucleus of the amygdala. *Journal of Neuroscience, 22*, 5713–5718.

Lesch, K.-P. (1998). Serotonin transporter and psychiatric disorders. *The Neuroscientist, 4*, 25–34.

Lesch, K., Bengel, D., & Heils, A. (1996). Association of anxiety-related traits with a polymorphism in the serotonin transporter gene regulatory region. *Science, 274*, 1527–1531.

Livesley, W. J. (2001). Commentary on reconceptualizing personality disorder categories using trait dimensions. *Journal of Personality, 69*, 277–286.

Livesley, W. J., Jackson, D. N., & Schroeder, M. L. (1992). Factorial structure of traits delineating personality disorders in clinical and general population samples. *Journal of Abnormal Psychology, 101*, 432–440.

Livesley, W. J., Schroeder, M. L., Jackson, D. N,, & Jang, K. L. (1994). Categorical distinctions in the study of personality disorder: Implication for classification. *Journal of Abnormal Psychology, 103*, 6–17.

Luciana, M., Collins, P., & Depue, R. (1998). Opposing roles for dopamine and serotonin in the modulation of human spatial working memory functions. *Cerebral Cortex, 8*, 218–226.

Luciana, M., Depue, R. A., Arbisi, P., & Leon, A. (1992). Facilitation of working memory in humans by a D2 dopamine receptor agonist. *Journal of Cognitive Neuroscience, 4*, 58–68.

Macey, D., Smith, H., Nader, M., & Porrino, L. (2003). Chronic cocaine self-administration upregulates the norepinephrine transporter and alters functional activity in the bed nucleus of the stria terminalis of the Rhesus monkey. *Journal of Neuroscience, 23,* 12–16.

MacLean, P. (1986). Ictal symptoms relating to the nature of affects and their cerebral substrate. In E. Plutchik & H. Kellerman (Ed.), *Emotion: Theory, research, and experience: Vol. 3. Biological foundations of emotion.* New York: Academic Press.

Marinelli, M., & White, F. (2000). Enhanced vulnerability to cocaine self-administration is associated with elevated impulse activity of midbrain dopamine neurons. *Journal of Neuroscience, 20,* 8876–8885.

Martel, F., Nevison, C., Simpson, M., & Keverne, E. (1995). Effects of opioid receptor blockade on the social behavior of rhesus monkeys living in large family groups. *Developmental Psychobiology, 28,* 71–84.

Matheson, M. D., & Bernstein, I. S. (2000). Grooming, social bonding, and agonistic aiding in rhesus monkeys. *American Journal of Primatology, 51,* 177–186.

Matthes, H. W., Maldonado, R., Simonin, F., Valverde, O., Slowe, S., Kitchen., I., et al. (1996). Loss of morphine-induced analgesia, reward effect and withdrawal symptoms in mice lacking the μ-opioid-receptor gene. *Nature, 383,* 819–823.

McCall, M., Wand, G., Eissenberg, T., Rohde, C., & Cheskin, I. (2000a). Naltrexone alters subjective and psychomotor responses to alcohol in heavy drinking subjects. *Neuropsychopharmacology, 22,* 480–492.

McCall, M., Wand, G., Rohde, C., & Lee, S. (2000b). Serum 6-beta-naltrexol levels are related to alcohol responses in heavy drinkers. *Alcoholism: Clinical and Experimental Research, 24,* 1385–1391.

McDonald, A., Shammah-Iagnado, S., Shi, C., & Davis, M. (1999). Cortical afferents to the extended amygdala. *Annals of New York Academy of Sciences, 877,* 309–338.

McGinty, J. F. (1999). Regulation of neurotransmitter interactions in the ventral striatum. In J. F. McGinty (Ed.), Advancing from the ventral striatum to the extended amygdala: Implications for neuropsychiatry and drug use. *Annals of New York Academy of Sciences, 877,* 129–139.

Mesulam, M. (1990). Large-scale neurocognitive networks and distributed processing for attention, language, and memory. *Annals of Neurology, 28,* 597–613.

Millon, T. (1997). *The Millon inventories: Clinical and personality assessment.* New York: Guilford Press.

Morrone, J., Depue, R., Scherer, J., & White, T. (2000). Film-induced incentive motivation and positive affect in relation to agentic and affiliative components of extraversion. *Personality and Individual Differences, 29,* 199–216.

Morrone-Strupinsky, J. V., & Depue, R. A. (2004). Differential relation of two distinct, film-induced positive emotional states to affiliative and agentic extraversion. *Personality and Individual Differences, 36,* 1109–1126.

Munafo, M. R., Clark, T. G., Moore, L. R., Payne, E., Walton, R., & Flint, J. (2003). Genetic polymorphisms and personality: A systematic review and meta-analysis. *Molecular Psychiatry, 8,* 471–484.

Narita, M., Aoki, T., & Suzuki, T. (2000). Molecular evidence for the involvement of NR2B subunit containing N-methyl-D-aspartate receptors in the development of morphine-induced place preference. *Neuroscience, 101,* 601–606.

Nelson, E. E., & Panksepp, J. (1998). Brain substrates of infant–mother attachment:

Contributions of opioids, oxytocin, and norepinephrine. *Neuroscience and Biobehavioral Reviews, 22*(3), 437–452.

Nie, Z., Schweitzer, P., Roberts, A., Madamba, S., Moore, S., & Siggins, G. (2004). Ethanol augments GABAergic transmission in the central amygdala via CRF1 receptors. *Science, 303,* 1512–1514.

Niesink, R. J. M., Vanderschuen, L. J. M. J., & van Ree, J. M. (1996). Social play in juvenile rats in utero exposure to morphine. *NeuroToxicology, 17*(3–4), 905–912.

Oades, R. (1985). The role of noradrenaline in tuning and dopamine in switching between signals in the CNS. *Neuroscience Biobehavioral Review, 9,* 261–282.

Olausson, H., Lamarre, Y., Backlund, H., Morin, C., Wallin, B. G., Starck, G., et al. (2002). Unmyelinated tactile afferents signal touch and project to insular cortex. *Nature Neuroscience, 5,* 900–904.

Olive, M., Koenig, H., Nannini, M., & Hodge, C. (2001). Stimulation of endorphin neurotransmission in the nucleus accumbens by ethanol, cocaine, and amphetamine. *Journal of Neuroscience, 21*(RC184), 1–5.

Olmstead, M., & Franklin, K. (1997). The development of a conditioned place preference to morphine effects of microinjections into various CNS sites. *Behavioral Neuroscience, 111,* 1324–1334.

Olson, G., Olson, R., & Kastin, A. (1997). Endogenous opiates: 1996. *Peptides, 18,* 1651–1688.

Ostrowski, N. L. (1998). Oxytocin receptor mRNA expression in rat brain: Implications for behavioral integration and reproductive success. *Psychoneuroendocrinology, 23*(8), 989–1004.

Pacak, K., McCarty, R., Palkovits, M., Kopin, I., & Goldstein, D. (1995). Effects of immobilization on in vivo release of norepinephrine in the bed nucleus of the stria terminalis in conscious rats. *Brain Research, 688,* 242–246.

Panksepp, J. (1998). *Affective neuroscience: The foundations of human and animal emotions.* New York: Oxford University Press.

Pfaus, J. G., Smith, W. J., & Coopersmith, C. B. (1999). Appetitive and consummatory sexual behaviors of female rats in bilevel chambers: I. A correlational and factor analysis and the effects of ovarian hormones. *Hormones and Behavior, 35,* 224–240.

Pich, E., Pagliusi, S., Tessari, M., Talabot-Ayer, D., van Huijsduijnen, R., & Chiamulera, C. (1997). Common neural substrates for the addictive properties of nicotine and cocaine. *Science, 275,* 83–86.

Polan, H. J., & Hofer, M. A. (1998). Olfactory preference for mother over home nest shavings by newborn rats. *Developmental Psychobiology, 33,* 5–20.

Porges, S. (1998). Love: An emergent property of the mamalian autonomic nervous system. *Psychoneuroendocrinology, 23,* 837–861.

Porges, S. (2001). The polyvagal theory: Phylogenetic substrates of a social nervous system. *International Journal of Psychophysiology, 42,* 123–146.

Redmond, D. E. (1987). Studies of the nucleus locus coeruleus in monkeys and hypotheses for neuropsychopharmacology. In J. Y. Meltzer (Ed.), *Psychopharmacology: The third generation of progress* (pp. 967–975). New York: Raven Press.

Reynolds, S. K., & Clark, L. A. (2001). Predicting dimensions of personality disorder from domains and facets of the five-factor model. *Journal of Personality, 69,* 199–222.

Robbins, T., Cador, M., Taylor, J., & Everitt, B. (1989). Limbic-striatal interactions in reward-related processes. *Neuroscience and Biobehavioral Reviews, 13,* 155–162.

Rolls, E. T. (1999). *The brain and emotion.* New York: Oxford University Press.

Saulsman, L. M., & Page, A. C. (2004). The five-factor model and personality disorder empirical literature: A meta-analytic review. *Clinical Psychology Review, 23,* 1055–1085.

Schlaepfer, T. E., Strain, E. C., Greenberg, B. D., Preston, K. L., Lancaster, E., Bigelow, G. E., et al. (1998). Site of opioid action in the human brain: Mu and kappa agonists' subjective and cerebral blood flow effects. *American Journal of Psychiatry, 155*(4), 470–473.

Schneirla, T. (1959). An evolutionary and developmental theory of biphasic processes underlying approach and withdrawal. In M. Jones (Ed.), *Nebraska Symposium on Motivation* (pp. 14–35). Lincoln: University of Nebraska Press.

Schultz, W., Dayan, P., & Montague, P. (1997). A neural substrate of prediction and reward. *Science, 275,* 1593–1595.

Selden, N., Everitt, B., Jarrard, L., & Robbins, T. (1991). Complementary roles of the amygdala and hippocampus in aversive conditioning to explicit and contextual cues. *Neuroscience, 42,* 335–350.

Shaham, Y., Erb, S., & Stewart, J. (2000). Stress-induced relapse to heroin and cocaine seeking in rats: A review. *Brain Research Reviews, 33,* 13–33.

Shippenberg, T. S., & Elmer, G. I. (1998). The Neurobiology of Opiate Reinforcement. *Critical Reviews in Neurobiology, 12*(4), 267–303.

Silk, J. B., Alberts, S. C., & Altmann, J. (2003). Social bonds of female baboons enhance infant survival. *Science, 302,* 1231–1234.

Simonin, F., Valverde, O., Smadja, C., Slowe, S., Kitchen, I., Diierich, A., et al. (1998). Disruption of the kappa-opioid receptor gene in mice enhances sensitivity to chemical visceral pain, impairs pharmacological actions of the selective kappa agonist U-50,488H and attenuates morphine withdrawal. *European Journal of Molecular Biology, 17,* 886–897.

Spoont, M. (1992). Modulatory role of serotonin in neural information processing: Implications for human psychopathology. *Psychological Bulletin, 112,* 330–350.

Squire, L., & Kosslyn, S. (1998). *Findings and current opinion in cognitive neuroscience.* Cambridge, MA: MIT Press.

Stefano, G., Goumon, Y., Casares, F., Cadet, P., Fricchione, G., Rialas, C., et al. (2000). Endogenous morphine. *Trends in Neuroscience, 23,* 436–442.

Strand, F. L. (1999). *Neuropeptides: Regulators of physiological processes.* Cambridge, MA: MIT Press.

Sutherland, R., & McDonald, R. (1990). Hippocampus, amygdala and memory deficits in rats. *Behavioral and Brain Research, 37,* 57–79.

Tellegen, A., Lykken, D. T., Bouchard, T. J., Wilcox, K. J., Segal, N. L., & Rich, S. (1988). Personality similarity in twins reared apart and together. *Journal of Personality and Social Psychology, 54,* 1031–1039.

Tellegen, A., & Waller, N. G. (in press). Exploring personality through test construction: Development of the multidimensional personality questionnaire. In S. Briggs & J. Cheek (Eds.), *Personality measures: Development and evaluation* (Vol. 1). New York: JAI Press.

Timberlake, W., & Silva, K. (1995). Appetitive behavior in ethology, psychology, and behavior systems. In N. Thompson (Ed.), *Perspectives in ethology: Vol. 11. Behavioral design* (pp. 211–253). New York: Plenum.

Torgersen, S., Kringlen, E., & Cramer, V. (2001). The prevalence of personality disorders in a community sample. *Archives of General Psychiatry, 58*, 590–596.

Tork, I. (1990). Anatomy of the serotonergic system. *Annals of the New York Academy of Science, 600*, 9–32.

Treit, D., Pesold, C., & Rotzinger, S. (1993). Dissociating the anti-fear effects of septal and amygdaloid lesions using two pharmacologically validated models of rat anxiety. *Behavioral Neuroscience, 107*, 770–785.

Uhl, G. R., Sora, I., & Wang, Z. (1999). The μ opiate receptor as a candidate gene for pain: Polymorphisms, variations in expression, nociception, and opiate responses. *Proceedings of the National Academy of Sciences, 96*, 7752–7755.

van Furth, W., & van Ree, J. (1996). Sexual motivation: Involvement of endogenous opioids in the ventral tegmental area. *Brain Research, 729*, 20–28.

Volkow, N., Wang, G., Fischman, M., Foltin, R., Fowler, J., Abumrad, N., et al. (1997). Relationship between subjective effects of cocaine and dopamine transporter occupancy. *Nature, 386*, 827–829.

Wang, Z., Yu, G., Cascio, C., Liu, Y., Gingrich, B., & Insel, T. R. (1999). Dopamine D2 receptor-mediated regulation of partner preferences in female prairie voles (*Microtus ochrogaster*): A mechanism for pair bonding? *Behavioral Neuroscience, 113*(3), 602–611.

Watson, C., & Clark, L. (1997). Extraversion and its positive emotional core. In S. Briggs, W. Jones, & R. Hogan (Eds.), *Handbook of personality psychology.* New York: Academic Press.

Watson, D., & Tellegen, A. (1985). Towards a consensual structure of mood. *Psychological Bulletin, 98*, 219–235.

White, N. (1986). Control of sensorimotor function by dopaminergic nigrostriatal neurons: Influence on eating and drinking. *Neuroscience and Biobehavioral Reviews, 10*, 15–36.

White, T. L., & Depue, R. A. (1999). Differential association of traits of fear and anxiety with norepinephrine- and dark-induced pupil reactivity. *Journal of Personality and Social Psychology, 77*(4), 863–877.

Widiger, T. A., Trull, T. J., Clarking, J. F., Sanderson, C., & Costa, P. T., Jr. (1994). A description of the DSM-III-R and DSM-IV personality disorders with the Five Factor Model of personality. In P. T. Costa, Jr. & T. A. Widiger (Eds.), *Personality disorders and the five factor model of personality.* Washington, DC: American Psychological Association.

Wiedenmayer, C., & Barr, G. (2000). Opioid receptors in the ventrolateral periaqueductal gray mediate stress-induced analgesia but not immobility in rat pups. *Behavioral Neuroscience, 114*, 125–138.

Wiggins, J. (1991). Agency and communion as conceptual coordinates for the understanding and measurement of interpersonal behavior. In D. Cicchetti & W.

Grove (Eds.), *Thinking clearly about psychology: Essays in honor of Paul Everett Meehl* (pp. 89–113). Minneapolis: University of Minnesota Press.

Wise, R. (1998). Drug-activation of brain reward pathways. *Drug and Alcohol Dependence, 51*, 13–22.

Wolterink, G., Cador, M., Wolterink, I., Robbins, T., & Everitt, B. (1989). Involvement of D1 and D2 receptor mechanisms in the processing of reward-related stimuli in the ventral striatum. *Society of Neuroscience, 15*, 490.

Wyvell, C. L., & Berridge, K. C. (2000). Intra-accumbens amphetamine increases the conditioned inventive salience of sucrose reward: Enhancement of reward "wanting" without enhanced "liking" or response reinforcement. *Journal of Neuroscience, 20*, 8122–8130.

Young, L. J., Wang, Z., & Insel, T. R. (1998). Neuroendocrine bases of monogamy. *Trends in the Neurosciences, 21*, 71–75.

Zald, D., & Depue, R. (2001). Serotonergic modulation of positive and negative affect in psychiatrically healthy males. *Personality and Individual Differences, 30*, 71–86.

Zubieta, J.-K., Smith, Y., Bueller, J., Xu, Y., Kilbourn, M., Jewett, D., et al. (2001). Regional Mu opioid receptor regulation of sensory and affective dimensions of pain. *Science, 293*, 311–315.

Zuckerman, M. (1994). An alternative five-factor model for personality. In C. Halverson, G. Kohnstamm & R. Marten (Eds.), *The developing structure of temperament and personality from infancy to adulthood.* Hillsdale, NJ: Erlbaum.

Chapter 9

Developing Treatments That Bridge Personality and Psychopathology

BJÖRN MEYER
PAUL A. PILKONIS

Developing treatments for patients with chronic personality pathology (Axis II) and accompanying acute conditions (Axis I) is important, primarily because personality disorders rarely occur in "pure form," especially in tertiary care settings. For example, out of more than 18,000 patients at an academic medical center, only 2.8% were diagnosed exclusively with an Axis II diagnosis (Fabrega, Ulrich, Pilkonis, & Mezzich, 1992); most presented with complex patterns of "comorbidity" (although this term has been criticized because it implies the co-occurrence of categorically distinct disease entities rather than integrated personality–psychopathology processes; see also Dolan-Sewell, Krueger, & Shea, 2001; Lilienfeld, Waldman, & Israel, 1994).

In our view, treatments for these complex cases ought to be based on conceptual models that elucidate the relationship between Axis I and II disorders. Instead of attempting to treat Axis I and II conditions "sequentially" (e.g., first the depression, then the dependent personality disorder), such treatments should be informed by an awareness that common risk factors and vulnerability processes influence both enduring and acute forms of psychopathology. Four such processes and their implications for treatment development are described in this chapter: (1) biologically based temperament dispositions that may place individuals at risk simultaneously for Axis

I and II disorders (e.g., neuroticism/threat responsiveness; hyporesponsiveness to rewards); (2) early adverse experiences and resulting attachment disturbances; (3) cognitive and emotional disturbances; and (4) failures to engage with need-fulfilling developmental tasks. After considering these processes and their treatment implications, strategic processes in the treatment of co-occurring Axis I and II conditions are briefly described in the second part of our chapter. As in a previous chapter (Pilkonis, 2001), we emphasize throughout the importance of approaching treatments in developmental terms, that is, organizing treatment around goals beyond symptom relief, with a focus on facilitating engagement with normative developmental tasks, including attachment and interpersonal relationships, autonomy and identity formation, and generativity on behalf of others.

CONCEPTUAL MODELS OF AXIS I AND AXIS II ASSOCIATIONS

The conceptual and empirical overlap between personality disorders and syndrome disorders (i.e., Axis I disorders) is extensive. One review estimated that between 66 and 97% of patients with personality disorders can be diagnosed with concurrent syndrome disorders; conversely, 13–81% of those with Axis I disorders may be diagnosable with a co-occurring personality disorder (Dolan-Sewell et al., 2001). This may differ, of course, by specific Axis II disorder; for example, as many as 8 of 10 individuals with borderline personality disorder may suffer from major depressive disorder at some point in their lives (Zanarini et al., 1998); strong associations are also documented between antisocial personality disorder and alcohol/substance use disorders (e.g., Morgenstern, Langenbucher, Labouvie, & Miller, 1997) and between avoidant personality disorder and generalized social phobia (Alden, Laposa, Taylor, & Ryder, 2002), among others. Regardless of the reasons for Axis I and II co-occurrences, it is clear that many patients frequently experience both chronic personality dysfunction and acute syndromes, which justifies efforts to develop integrated treatments for these patients.

Clinically, the simultaneous occurrence between Axis I and II disorders often indicates poor symptom course, higher functional impairment, and suboptimal treatment response (e.g., Reich & Green, 1991). For example, patients with posttraumatic stress disorder (PTSD) tend to improve less from treatment if they are also diagnosable with borderline personality disorder (Feeny, Zoellner, & Foa, 2002), and depressed patients recover more slowly if they are diagnosable with a Cluster C personality disorder (Viinamäki et al., 2003). The presence of obsessive–compulsive personality traits also predicts suboptimal response to pharmacological treatment of obsessive–compulsive Axis I symptoms (Cavedini, Erzegovesi, Ronchi, & Bellodi, 1997). Similarly, Hardy and colleagues (1995) found that Cluster C personality disorders among depressed patients predicted poor response to psychodynamic–interpersonal but not to cognitive-behavioral psychotherapy. In a sample of 149 psychiatric patients with various Axis I disorders, borderline personality disorder features predicted less optimal psychosocial functioning and recovery from depression over a 6-month period (Meyer, Pilkonis, Proietti, Heape, & Egan, 2001), and in the National Institute of Mental Health Treatment of Depression Collaborative Research Program, patients with personality disorders also showed poorer social functioning following treatment (Shea et al., 1990). In yet another study, borderline features were associated with less optimal response to electroconvulsive therapy (Sareen, Enns, & Guertin, 2000). Conversely, the presence of syndromal depression among patients with borderline personality disorder has been linked with poorer treatment response (Goodman, Hull, Clarkin, & Yeomans, 1998).

In summary, a body of literature is emerging to document that personality disorders are often accompanied by concurrent syndrome disorders and that such co-occurrences have negative prognostic implications. Despite such evidence, the questions of whether, how much, and why personality dysfunction might complicate treatment are by no means settled; some evidence even suggests that personality pathology may not significantly worsen treatment response (Mulder, 2002). One way forward will be to take a more fine-grained look at which specific personality disorder characteristics and behaviors mediate the treatment process. For example, Hilsenroth, Holdwick, Castlebury, and Blais (1998) found that five specific cluster B symptoms "were independent and nonredundant predictors of the number of psychotherapy sessions attended by a patient" (p. 168). Specifically, patients with borderline fears of abandonment and anger management problems and those with a histrionically exaggerated sense of relationship intimacy tended to seek more psychotherapy sessions, whereas those with antisocial interpersonal indifference and narcissistic needs for admiration tended to terminate sooner (Hilsenroth et al., 1998).

UNDERSTANDING AND TREATING PERSONALITY AND PSYCHOPATHOLOGY RISK

Various theoretical models that aim to elucidate the co-occurrence of personality and syndrome disorders have been presented in the literature (e.g., Dolan-Sewell et al., 2001; Lyons, Tyrer, Gunderson, & Tohen, 1997; Millon & Davis, 1996). In a recent article, Krueger and Tackett (2003) described four such models: (1) the predisposition/vulnerability model, according to which maladaptive personality traits enhance the likelihood of developing syndrome disorders; (2) the complication/scar model, according to which syndrome disorders exert enduring negative effects upon the patient's personality; (3) the pathoplasty/exacerbation model, which holds that Axis I versus Axis II disorders have independent etiologies although maladaptive personality traits can influence the expression or course of the syndrome disorder; and (4) the spectrum model, which argues that syndrome and personality disorders are not distinct in quality but, rather, represent different points on a continuum ("spectrum") of severity. Given the complexity and heterogeneity of personality and syndrome disorders, our question in this chapter is not so much which of these models is "more correct" than others for specific Axis I/Axis II combinations. Indeed, these models are probably best viewed not as mutually exclusive but as complementary and compatible, and in some cases indicative of different aspects of complex personality–psychopathology relations over time. For example, a (genetically linked) neuroticism predisposition might enhance the likelihood of developing repeated major depressive episodes, which in turn could further exacerbate enduring emotional vulnerability traits in such a person. From a treatment development perspective, the crucial point is that various factors and processes may simultaneously influence personality dysfunction and syndromal status. Four such processes are described in the following section.

BIOLOGICAL/GENETIC VULNERABILITIES

There is an increasing consensus that a relatively small number of genetically based fundamental personality traits are associated with vulnerability to Axis I and II disorders. For example, Livesley, Jang, and Vernon (1998) showed that four higher-order dimensions—dysregulation, dissocial behavior, inhibitedness, and compulsivity—appear to underlie personality disorder risk; each of these dimensions emerged in both psychiatric and control samples and may have a substantial genetic basis. Similar models have been described by Siever and Davis (1991) and Cloninger, Svrakic, and Przybeck (1993), among others.

Jang and Livesley (1999) also showed in a twin study that some of the "Big Five" personality dimensions share a genetic basis with dimensions of personality disorder pathology; the closest association was found between neuroticism and personality disorder risk. Such findings are consistent with a large number of previous studies; more than 50 studies have reported consistent links between the "Big Five" traits and personality disorders (cf. Costa & Widiger, 2002). Experts are now converging on the specific associations between big five facets and specific personality disorders; for example, antisocial personality disorder can be construed as a "particular combination of high antagonism; low deliberation, dutifulness, and self-discipline; low anxiety and self-consciousness; and high impulsiveness, excitement seeking, and angry hostility" (Lynam & Widiger, 2001, p. 410). To provide a contrasting example, avoidant personality disorder is thought to be generally linked with high levels of introversion and neuroticism (e.g., Alden et al., 2002; Meyer, 2002), and more specifically avoidant personality disorder can be characterized by neuroticism facets such as anxiousness, self-consciousness and vulnerability, and by introversion facets such as low assertiveness and excitement seeking (Lynam & Widiger, 2001). Nevertheless, evidence also suggests that residual personality disorder variance—above that which can be explained by the five factors—sometimes predicts important aspects of patients' history, concurrent functioning, and symptom course (Morey & Zanarini, 2000).

Clark, Watson, and Mineka (1994), among many others, also reiterated that basic personality or temperament traits can be viewed as general risk factors for diverse forms of psychopathology. According to their review, which focused on Axis I rather than II psychopathology, neuroticism, construed as "temperamental sensitivity to negative stimuli" (p. 104), confers vulnerability to anxiety disorders such as phobias, generalized anxiety disorder, and PTSD. Neuroticism is often linked to sensitivity in the behavioral inhibition system (BIS), one of Gray's (e.g., 1987) basic motivational systems that has been studied extensively across many species. Individuals with high levels of BIS sensitivity tend to respond with intense distress to perceived threats (Carver & White, 1994). For example, in a recent study, BIS was strongly linked to distress among women who imagined that their romantic partner might leave them for an attractive rival (high threat condition); among those in a low threat condition, BIS and distress were unrelated (Meyer, Olivier, & Roth, 2005). BIS sensitivity also appears to predict distress following unpleasant events in experimental (Heponiemi, Keltikangas-Jaervinenm, Puttonen, & Ravana, 2003) and naturally occurring situations (Gable, Reis, & Elliot, 2000). The BIS may also be directly relevant to Axis I and II psychopathology. Caseras, Torrubia, and Farré (2001), for instance, reported that a BIS self-report scale distinguished among patients with (1) cluster C, (2) cluster A and B, and (3) no personality disorders. Johnson, Turner, and Iwata (2003) found in an epidemiological study that BIS sensitivity was linked with anxiety and depressive disorder symptoms.

Gray's (1987) second major motivational system, the behavioral activation or approach system (BAS), is thought to govern positive affect and approach behavior in response to appetitive stimuli. Low BAS sensitivity levels are often linked to Axis I conditions such as depression (Beevers & Meyer, 2002; Henriques & Davidson, 2000; Kasch, Rottenberg, Arnow, & Gotlib, 2002; Mineka, Watson, & Clark, 1998). In one study with a clinical sample of depressed outpatients, Kasch and colleagues (2002) showed that BAS sensitivity correlated strongly and inversely with depression severity, was stable over time (i.e., independent of depression state fluctuations), and predicted recovery from depression over an 8-week period, which the authors interpreted as "consistent with formulations positing that an underactive BAS, or lowered responsiveness to reward and decreased motivational drive to pursue rewarding stimuli, may cause and/or maintain depression" (p. 595).

The relationship of the BAS to personality disorders has received little systematic attention. In one study using a college student sample (Meyer, 2002), however, features of both schizoid and avoidant personality disorder correlated inversely with BAS (avoidant, unlike schizoid, personality disorder also correlated positively with BIS). Dependent personality disorder, by contrast, correlated more weakly or not at all with the subscales of a BAS questionnaire. These findings are consistent with the idea that more introverted, withdrawn, depression-prone personality disorder variants (e.g., avoidant and schizoid) share a low BAS-related temperamental vulnerability, whereas the more extraverted, sociable, impulsive personality disorders (such as antisocial, borderline, and histrionic) may be linked to heightened BAS sensitivity.

In some Axis I and II disorders, interactions between the BIS and BAS may also play a role. For example, mania in bipolar disorder has been construed as a high BAS/low BIS phenomenon: "low activity in the behavioral inhibition system accompanied by high activity in the approach system [BAS] might be thought of as underlying mania" (Gray, 1991, p. 300; see also Fowles, 1993, for similar arguments), and empirical evidence at least partially supports such ideas (e.g., Meyer, Johnson, & Winters, 2001). Low BIS/high BAS combinations may also play a role in antisocial personality (e.g., Arnett, Smith, & Newman, 1997; Fowles, 1980), although a third core trait—constraint versus disinhibition (Krueger et al., 1994)—may be even more relevant in this context. The specific links between basic temperamental dispositions and specific Axis I and II disorders continue to be debated and empirically refined, but for the purposes of this chapter the key point is the recognition that common vulnerability traits, which probably have a substantial genetic component and demonstrable biological bases, appear to facilitate risk for both acute and chronic forms of psychopathology. Which conclusions might clinicians draw from this recognition?

WORKING WITH TEMPERAMENTAL VULNERABILITIES

An important treatment implication from these lines of research is that the genetically based personality traits underlying personality and syndrome vulnerability are probably not easily changed through therapeutic intervention. We agree, then, with Harkness and Lilienfeld's (1997) assertion that "The single greatest misconception that patients (and perhaps some therapists) hold about therapy is the expectation that a high-NE (negative emotionality) person can be turned into a low-NE person" (p. 356). A treatment goal more realistic than fundamental personality change would be to improve the fit between a patient's "hard-wired" trait profile and their social environment. That is, a chronic disease model may be appropriate; efforts to change neuroticism, introversion, or other temperamental vulnerabilities—especially in short-term interventions—are probably naive.

Another obvious implication from this research is that pharmacotherapy might be considered in efforts to target the biologically based temperament vulnerabilities underlying Axis I and II risk. For example, depressive symptoms in borderline personality disorder are often treated with selective serotonin reuptake inhibitors (SSRIs), mood swings with antiepileptic medication, and psychotic symptoms with atypical antipsychotics (Markovitz, 2004). The increasingly widespread use of pharmacotherapy to change the temperamental "core" of personality will undoubtedly rekindle debates about the ethical implications of such approaches (see Kramer, 1993).

Several studies suggest that it is indeed possible to alter the basis of personality through pharmacological intervention, even in nondisordered individuals. Knutson and colleagues (1998), for example, found reductions in neuroticism/negative emotionality and increases in extraversion and social-affiliative behavior in a group of healthy volunteers treated with SSRIs. In another study with 20 healthy volunteers, Tse and Bond (2001) also found that administration of citalopram triggered increases in self-directedness, as measured by Cloninger's Temperament and Character Inventory (TCI). Thus, there is mounting evidence that some of the temperamental foundations conferring risk for various forms of Axis I and II pathology can be targeted by pharmacological intervention. The question of whether psychotherapy can directly alter these core dimensions, by contrast, remains largely unaddressed.

Some theorists have also offered suggestions for how therapeutic approaches could be modified to fit patients' predominant temperament. Patients with a highly sensitive BIS tend to overreact to threats and avoid potentially punishing experiences; somewhat ironically, the therapeutic challenge might be to gently but persistently facilitate exposure to the events or situations they fear. That is, exposure-based approaches would seem to be indicated among patients with BIS-related vulnerability. Consistent with this idea, Caseras and colleagues (2001), who found that high BIS levels characterized cluster C disorders, suggested that "treatment of cluster C patients should involve the modification of their evasive behavioural style, so reducing their sensitivity to aversive stimuli, even when this might mean the greater temporary presence of an anxiety state" (p. 357).

The treatment of BAS-related vulnerability, by contrast, remains even more speculative. However, a strong case can be made, in our view, for viewing behavioral activation interventions (e.g., Martell, Addis, & Jacobson, 2001) as promising leads to target low-BAS-related clinical phenomena. In these treatments, clients and therapists work together to identify and schedule engaging activities that increase clients' contact with positive reinforcers and broaden their behavioral repertoires. There is good evidence that such interventions are among the most effective and efficient in reducing depression (e.g., Jacobson et al., 1996), but the implications and applications of behavioral activation treatments in the context of personality disorders have not yet been explored.

EARLY ADVERSITY
AND ATTACHMENT DISTURBANCES

Beyond the biological/temperamental vulnerabilities described in the preceding section, another risk factor for both Axis I and II psychopathology is early psychosocial adversity, such as abuse and neglect. There is a wealth of literature showing that early adversity increases risk for later maladjustment, including Axis I syndromes (e.g., PTSD) as well as personality disorders (e.g., Yen et al., 2002; Zanarini et al., 1997). It is generally recognized that early maltreatment is probably neither necessary nor sufficient for the later development of personality disorder, but such adverse experiences can increase vulnerability, especially when combined with temperamental predispositions (e.g., Meyer & Carver, 2000; Millon & Davis, 1996). Despite the tenuous links between early trauma and later personality pathology, it seems increasingly well established that certain personality disorders are consistently linked with reports of early maltreatment, especially borderline personality disorder (Battle et al., 2004). Perhaps most famously, Linehan (1993) hypothesized that a common developmental antecedent of borderline personality disorder is "an invalidating environment . . . in which communication of private experiences is met by erratic, inappropriate, and extreme responses. . . . [T]he expression of private experiences is not validated; instead, it is often punished and/or trivialized" (p. 49).

The links between early adversity and later personality maladjustment are often conceptualized from an attachment perspective (Bartholomew et al., 2001; Lyddon & Sherry, 2001; Meyer & Pilkonis, 2005). In such views, early experiences of caregiver insensitivity and unresponsiveness (or even abuse and neglect) interfere with the formation of positive, integrated mental representations of the self, others, and relationships in general. Such negatively biased "internal working models" (Bretherton & Munholland, 1999) can give rise to the variants of insecure attachment, such as anxious–preoccupied, fearful–avoidant, or dismissive–avoidant, which in turn appear to confer risk for specific personality disorders. Dependent, borderline, and histrionic personalities, for instance, can be understood as variants of pre-occupied attachment, and avoidant personality as a variant of fearful at-tachment (Meyer & Pilkonis, 2005). In one recent study, borderline and avoidant personality disorder features were linked with a measure of anx-ious adult attachment, which in turn was associated with tendencies to evaluate emotionally neutral faces more negatively (Meyer, Pilkonis, & Beevers, 2004), pointing to the potential utility of attachment theory for understanding personality pathology.

This idea is also supported by studies that show, for example, that chil-dren with anxious-ambivalent attachment are at increased risk for later anxiety-related problems, whereas those with disorganized/disoriented at-tachment are at risk for anger- and aggression-related problems (e.g., Weinfield, Sroufe, Egeland, & Carlson, 1999). Secure attachment, by con-trast, is thought to protect against such pathways into psychopathology, as securely attached children may be relatively better at responding sensitively to emotional cues, being empathic, and forming stable friendships. Early attachment relationships may also influence children's trajectory for acquir-ing effective emotion regulation interpersonal skills, which in turn influ-ences their vulnerability for developing Axis I and II disorders. A continu-ing challenge in this area is to clarify which specific early experiences result in the formation of the cognitive–affective–motivational constellations that characterize the various personality disorders (Meyer & Pilkonis, 2005).

TREATING THE SEQUELAE OF EARLY ADVERSITY

The treatment of psychological sequelae of early (and more recent) adver-sity and trauma is a complex issue (e.g., Foa & Rothbaum, 1998; Resick & Schnicke, 1993), beyond the scope of this chapter. Nevertheless, new treat-ments targeting concurrent Axis I and II psychopathology would be well advised to take into account the lessons learned from established interven-tions. The more established and validated psychological interventions in this domain increasingly converge on the view that two types of interven-tion are necessary to treat the adult consequences of trauma: (1) exposure-based approaches, in which patients are asked to reexperience, relive, or retell aspects of the trauma in vivid detail, so that habituation to the unwanted, feared memories can be achieved, and (2) insight-oriented, sup-portive approaches in which patients consciously process the implications and consequences of the trauma and renegotiate their self-image in the context of their environment. These two approaches are linked with, and grow out of, current theoretical perspectives on the cognitive processing of traumatic memories (e.g., Brewin, Dalgleish, & Joseph, 1996).

According to dual processing theory, for example (Brewin et al., 1996), traumatic memories are encoded in two distinct memory systems: verbally accessible memory (VAM) and situationally accessible memory (SAM). According to the theory, VAM can be altered by deliberate cognitive reprocessing: "On the one hand, the person needs to actively reduce the secondary negative affects generated by the implications of the trauma by consciously reasserting perceived control, reattributing responsibility, and achieving an integration of the new information with preexisting concepts and beliefs. This . . . may involve substantial editing of autobiographical memory (VAMs) in order to bring perceptions of the event into line with prior expectations" (Brewin et al., 1996, p. 678). Changing SAM, by contrast, is more likely to occur through exposure-based treatments, in which patients vividly retell and reexperience details of the trauma, so that the reactivated feared memories can be paired with noncatastrophic information in the safety of the therapist's office: "Following activation and emergence into consciousness, SAMs will be automatically altered or added to whenever some or all of the information they contain happens to be paired with changes in concurrent bodily states or contents of consciousness" (Brewin et al., 1996, p. 678).

In our view, integrated treatments for personality disorders and concurrent symptom disorders would incorporate these two components. Many patients with personality disorders—especially those with borderline personality disorder—report traumatic memories of early abuse and neglect, and it would seem logical to use both exposure and conscious reprocessing-based interventions to target these symptoms, regardless of whether the primary problems are coded on Axis I or II. Such a dual-focused approach would also be consistent with common factor models of the therapeutic process, according to which these two elements—direct experiential exposure to feared memories or events, and conscious reframing/reprocessing—are among the universally processes of effective therapeutic intervention (e.g., Weinberger, 1995).

In the context of discussing the treatment of Axis I and II sequelae of early adversity, it should also be noted that attachment theory has much to say about this process (see Meyer & Pilkonis, 2002). One of the consequences of early adversity, after all, is later attachment insecurity, which in turn influences not only patients' symptom experience but also their ability to engage in and benefit from treatment. For example, patients' attachment patterns appear to influence the quality of the therapeutic alliance (Mallinckrodt, Gantt, & Coble, 1995) and treatment outcome (Fonagy et al., 1996; Meyer et al., 2001). Those with secure forms of attachment may find it easier to engage in the treatment process and thus ultimately benefit more from treatment, although the greatest relative improvements may sometimes be seen among insecurely attached patients, perhaps because of their initially poorer functioning (e.g., Fonagy et al., 1996). Therapists working from an attachment perspective—regardless of whether their patients carry Axis I, II, or both diagnoses—may be well advised to (1) assess patients' attachment patterns, (2) learn how balance patient attachment style with congruent and complementary therapeutic action, (3) aim to directly change insecure patient attachment to secure ones, and (4) develop awareness of their own attachment style and its potential effects on the therapeutic process (see Meyer & Pilkonis, 2002, for an elaborated discussion of these treatment recommendations).

NEGATIVE COGNITION AND EMOTION IN AXIS I AND AXIS II

Temperament-related predispositions and early-life adversity are probably important distal predictors of both Axis I and II psychopathology, but concurrent disturbances in cognitive and emotional functioning can be regarded as the more relevant proximal predictors. In terms of emotional dysregulation as a key vulnerability factor, perhaps the most well-known example is Linehan's (1993) conceptualization of borderline personality disorder: "BPD is primarily a dysfunction of the emotion regulation system; it results from biological irregularities combined with certain dysfunctional environments" (p. 42). In this view, "high sensitivity to emotional stimuli, emotional intensity, and slow return to emotional baseline" (p. 43) constitutes a biologically based vulnerability, which—when coupled with emotionally invalidating environments—is thought to increase subsequent risk for the borderline personality disorder symptoms.

Some aspects of this model have received support by experimental research. For example, it appears that patients with borderline personality disorder may exhibit characteristically low thresholds for amygdala activation, which puts them at greater risk for extreme emotional responses (Herpertz, Dietrich, et al., 2001). At the same time, evidence indicates that patients with borderline personality disorder may actually be physiologically less responsive than others to emotional stimuli. According to Herpertz and colleagues (2000), this emotional unresponsiveness may result in compensatory stimulus-seeking and disinhibition: "Low autonomic reactivity found in BPD and antisocial subjects may be a common risk factor for developing nonadaptive, impulsive modes of behavior" (pp. 348–349). Consistent with such a view, patients with antisocial personality disorder or psychopathy have been found to be abnormally unresponsive to emotional and especially fear/punishment-related stimuli (Herpertz, Werth, et al., 2001). By contrast, those with avoidant personality disorder—and anxious individuals more generally—may exhibit heightened baseline physiological reactivity (Herpertz et al., 2000).

In terms of cognitive disturbances in Axis II disorders, studies are beginning to show that patients with personality disorders often harbor negative beliefs and show distinctive biases in the processing of social information. There is evidence, for instance, that patients with borderline personality disorder may be more likely than others to think in extreme terms, especially in borderline personality disorder-relevant contexts, such as when thinking about relationship crises, interpersonal desertion, rejection, or abuse (Veen & Arntz, 2000). There is also evidence that those with borderline personality disorder evaluate others in negative, simplistic terms (Arntz & Veen, 2001). Furthermore, individuals with borderline personality disorder features may tend to evaluate neutral or ambiguous social cues—such as faces—more negatively than others, which then might motivate or prompt hostility (Meyer et al., 2004; Wagner & Linehan, 1999). Data also suggest that individuals with personality disorders harbor distinctive maladaptive beliefs (e.g., Arntz, Dietzel, & Dreessen, 1999; Arntz, Dreessen, Schouten, & Weertman, in press; Beck et al., 2001; Butler, Brown, Beck, & Grisham, 2002); for example, those with avoidant personality disorder features appear to hold beliefs such as "If others really get to know me, they will reject me." The strength with which such beliefs are held, in turn, predicts how negatively versus positively ambiguous social situations are interpreted (Dreessen, Arntz, Hendriks, Keune, & van den Hout, 1999).

The literature on cognitive and emotional processes in personality disorders is of course dwarfed by the much larger literature on such processes in Axis I syndromes. Cognitive processes have been studied for decades across many Axis I disorders, such as depression (Clark, Beck, & Alford, 1999), social phobia (Clark & Wells, 1995), and posttraumatic stress disorder (Dalgleish, 2004), to name just a few examples. This body of literature is of course extremely extensive and heterogeneous; any brief summary here would be superficial and trivial (i.e., "negative cognition has been implicated in most Axis I disorders"). Nevertheless, the important point is that the cognitive approach to Axis I syndromes has been singular in terms of inspiring research and clinical applications. Although some cognitive approaches to treating personality disorders have been described (e.g., Beck, Freeman, & Associates, 1990), research on cognitive processes in chronic personality pathologies is still lagging behind.

Emotion-related processes, such as emotional responsiveness and emotion regulation have also been studied in several Axis I disorders, although these areas have generally received less attention than cognitive processes in

Axis I. For example, there is evidence that depressed individuals have different attitudes and cognitive responses to their emotions than their nondepressed counterparts (Rude & McCarthy, 2003). Additionally, depressed individuals may differ in the physiological mechanisms that normally regulate negative emotion, for example, during crying (Rottenberg et al., 2003). Other work on emotional/mood functioning and its implications for Axis I syndromes has focused on topics such as diurnal mood variation (Rusting & Larsen, 1998), attention to arousal versus valence aspects of mood (Diener, Colvin, Pavot, & Allman, 1991), and emotional responsiveness to pleasant and unpleasant situations (e.g., Meyer, Johnson, & Winters, 2001). Again, although a detailed review of the research on emotional processes in Axis I disorders is beyond the scope of this chapter, our points are that such research (1) is being actively pursued, (2) should be extended beyond Axis I to chronic forms of personality pathology, and (3) has implications for the development of integrated treatments.

TREATING NEGATIVE COGNITION AND EMOTION IN AXIS I AND AXIS II DISORDERS

There is, of course, a long and distinguished history of targeting negative cognitions in Axis I disorders; the treatments developed by A. T. Beck and colleagues for depression (e.g., Beck, Rush, Shaw, & Emery, 1979) and anxiety disorders (Beck, Emery, & Greenberg, 1985) could perhaps be listed as the classic examples. Over the past 15 years, these cognitive approaches have been systematically extended to Axis II conditions (e.g., Beck et al., 1990; Cottraux & Blackburn, 2001; Young, Klosko, & Weishaar, 2003). These therapies include cognitive strategies such as identifying negative schemas; examining evidence to disconfirm negative beliefs; rating and reevaluating problematic beliefs; reinterpreting early experiences; and using worksheets and flashcards to practice the refuting of dysfunctional beliefs and the use of more adaptive beliefs (for a brief overview, see Cottraux & Blackburn, 2001). Although initial tests are promising (Cottraux & Blackburn, 2001), much remains to be done to test the specific efficacy of these interventions for the various personality disorders (and much less for the many Axis I and II combinations). Because of their recognized clinical utility and established efficacy in treating Axis I conditions, however, it would seem prudent for integrative personality disorder interventions to include specific cognitive intervention strategies. This approach would also be consistent with common factor approaches that regard cognitive reframing as one of the universal—and perhaps a key—process from which therapies derive their general effectiveness (Weinberger, 1995).

A recent trend in cognitive therapies is the development of less "control-oriented" cognitive change strategies. These methods recognize experimental and correlational findings that, for most clients, negative cognitions are very difficult to change voluntarily. In fact, this literature suggests that attempts to control negative cognitions can often backfire; the effects of thought suppression tend to be ironic or paradoxical, especially under conditions of strain, cognitive load, or stress (Beevers & Meyer, 2004; Wegner, Schneider, Carter, & White, 1987; Wenzlaff & Wegner, 2000; Wenzlaff, Wegner, & Roper, 1988). Such findings have inspired the development of acceptance- rather than control-oriented cognitive strategies, in which clients learn to adopt a more open, "mindful," and less combative attitude toward their own problematic cognitions (e.g., Hayes, Strosahl, & Wilson, 1999; Segal, Williams, & Teasdale, 2002). These new interventions tend to use meditative exercises, metaphors, and paradoxical stories rather than the more traditional (and presumably more control-oriented) therapeutic dialogue in order to facilitate this kind of passive observer stance toward problematic cognitions, memories, and emotions. Evidence suggests that these new treatments are very effective across various diagnoses and clinical problems (e.g., Bach & Hayes; 2002; Bond & Bunce, 2000; Ma & Teasdale, 2004), although they have not yet been tested specifically in the context of Axis I and II co-occurring disorders. Nevertheless, the point can be made that integrative personality disorder treatment ought to consider the potential utility of these new developments, and some such treatments have already incorporated acceptance-based and mindfulness-based techniques (e.g., Linehan, 1994).

Beyond the classic cognitive techniques and the more recent acceptance/mindfulness-based approaches, there are of course also many established interventions that aim to correct or optimize cognitive and emotional dysfunction, and our selection here is admittedly somewhat arbitrary. For example, such other approaches include Greenberg's emotion-focused therapy (Greenberg, 2002) and techniques from Gestalt therapy (Wagner-Moore, 2004). Current cognitive therapies for personality disorders also often already include emotion-focused interventions, such as psychodrama and "playing devil's advocate" (Cottraux & Blackburn, 2001).

Broadly speaking, all these strategies have in common that they aim to optimize information processing (i.e., reduce or correct maladaptive attention to or elaboration of negative content); examine and undermine the stranglehold of rigid, counterproductive beliefs; and facilitate flexible, adaptive emotional experience and regulation. These interventions can be said to differ in the degree to which they use emotionally engaging, contemplative–meditative, or rational–deliberative techniques, but the important point is that integrative treatments ought to incorporate such procedures to address the negative cognitive and emotional processes shared by Axis I and II disorders.

FACILITATING ENGAGEMENT
WITH VALUED LIFE TASKS

A final point that deserves attention, in our view, is that Axis II patients often are so entangled in their current symptoms that they "default" on the normative tasks of adulthood (Pilkonis, 2001). It would perhaps be easy for many therapists to focus exclusively on the roles of predisposing temperament, developmental antecedents, and current cognitive and emotional dysfunction. What such an approach would miss, though, is a future orientation: Where should the patient go from here? How can the patient engage with developmental tasks such as the establishment of mutually nurturing relationships and the autonomous pursuit of productive activity?

Such a future focus on life tasks, meanings, and values has been emphasized in various recent treatments, some of which emphasize the importance of identifying "valued life directions" (ACT; Hayes et al., 1999), and some of which focus more on identifying concrete goals the patient is motivated to pursue (Kanfer & Schefft, 1988). A common theme, perhaps, is that the idea that it is important to facilitate patients' engagement with activities that promise to maximize autonomy, mastery, and relatedness—processes that are so commonly valued and beneficial that they can be regarded as universal psychological needs (Deci & Ryan, 2002). Studies have shown that pursuing activities that facilitate the attainment of these needs tends to improve well-being (e.g., Reis, Sheldon, Gable, Roscoe, & Ryan, 2000; Sheldon, Ryan, & Reis, 1996), which provides additional justification for explicitly including such foci in integrative treatments.

In this context, we have also emphasized in a previous chapter the importance of facilitating patients' engagement with the challenges of normal adult development, such as those described in Erikson's classic theoretical model (1968, 1974, 1980). Many of the personality disorders can be characterized by their failures at several development stages, including early ones. According to Erikson's theory, the first developmental stage (infancy; first year of life) concerns the struggle between basic trust versus mistrust. Inconsistent, cold, and unresponsive parenting during this period is thought to result in chronic interpersonal mistrust and pessimism (cf. Carver & Scheier, 2004), consistent with the attachment–theoretical notion that such forms of early adversity can result in insecure attachment and heightened risk for later personality pathology (e.g., Lyddon & Sherry, 2001). Individuals with personality disorders also often struggle with later developmental tasks, such as the quest to attain a coherent identity during adolescence, to achieve the capacity for intimacy and establish mutually nurturing relationships during young adulthood, and to move beyond narrow self-centeredness and attain generativity in adulthood (Erikson, 1968, 1974, 1980).

In one of the few empirical studies on the links between Erikson's stages and psychological adjustment, Vandewater, Ostrove, and Stewart (1997) reported that identity and generativity in adulthood were robustly related to well-being. In that study, more than 100 women were followed over time, and measures of identity and generativity were derived from Q-sort analyses of comprehensive personality questionnaires and raters' judgments of responses to a projective test. These measures were linked to indices of subjective well-being and psychosocial functioning, even though personality disorders were not directly assessed. In our view, the question of how failures to resolve normative developmental struggles facilitate the formation of personality disorders, then, remains one of the least explored and most promising avenues for future research in this area.

In summary, beyond targeting temperamental predispositions, consequences of early adversity, and current cognitive–emotional disturbances, integrative treatments could include future-oriented interventions that help patients identify valued life directions and personally meaningful goals. The pursuit of these goals is likely to be more beneficial and health-enhancing to the degree that they fulfill basic psychological needs, such as autonomy, mastery, and relatedness, and to the degree that they facilitate patients' successful engagement with the normative tasks of adult development.

IMPLEMENTING COMPLEX TREATMENTS FOR COMPLEX PATIENTS

The preceding sections, to summarize once again, suggest that temperament, early adversity, cognitive–emotional dysfunction, and failure to engage in valued and need-fulfilling life tasks should all be taken into account, and each of these processes has some relatively straightforward treatment implications (e.g., to assess temperament, modify interventions to fit temperament, consider pharmacotherapy, adjust expectations). However, how should one translate all these consequences and recommendations into a coherent treatment, especially in the current climate of managed health care?

Our goal here is not to propose yet another specific "type" of therapy for personality disorders—several others have already articulated treatments from cognitive (e.g., Beck et al., 1990, Cottraux & Blackburn, 2001; Young, 1994), cognitive-behavioral/dialectical (e.g., Linehan, 1993); interpersonal (Benjamin, 1996), supportive (Winston, Rosenthal, & Muran, 2001), psychoanalytic (Gabbard, 2001), and several other perspectives. The comparative merit of these various "brand-name" therapies is of course not resolved, and—more importantly in this context—these therapies have typically not been designed specifically to treat patients who experience both syndrome and personality pathology. An integrative treatment model was described by Livesley (2001), who emphasized the importance of general therapeutic strategies such as building a strong alliance, maintaining stability in the treatment process, offering validation, and facilitating motivation. Livesley's suggestions distill many of the findings that have emerged in recent years in the area of psychotherapy integration and common factors research. Traditionally, this research has drawn on treatment studies of syndrome rather than personality disorders; it is clear, however, that the principles that have been harnessed from this work are more broadly applicable. We agree with Livesley's (2001) adamant point that *"evidence-based treatment of personality disorder should seek to maximize the effect of common factors"* (p. 571, emphasis in original).

A common factors model that is perhaps particularly compelling was articulated by Weinberger (1995), who in turn based his views on the classic writings of Frank (1973), among others. What adds to the heuristic appeal of Weinberger's analysis is his focus on just five core factors or processes: (1) forming a strong working alliance, (2) facilitating positive expectations of therapeutic success, (3) helping the patient confront or face the problem, (4) providing opportunities for patient mastery or cognitive control experiences, and (5) ensuring that the patient attributes the success of treatment to his or her own efforts. In the treatment of patients who experience complex chronic as well as acute psychopathologies, the importance of skillfully implementing these processes is likely to be even more important than in straightforward interventions for circumscribed Axis I conditions.

MAXIMIZING THE COMMON FACTORS AND PROCESSES

Before patients even enter treatment, they form a particular set of relatively more positive or negative expectations about the treatment, and these, in turn, are known to influence their motivation for and engagement with the treatment, which later is reflected in the quality of the alliance and overall outcome (e.g., Meyer et al., 2002; Joyce, Ogrodniczuk, Piper, & McCallum, 2003). Diagnosis-related individual differences probably exist in the valence and strength of patients' pretreatment expectations and their motivation to seek and engage in treatment. For example, Tyrer, Mitchard, Methuen, and Ranger (2003) reported that patients with some personality disorders commonly seek treatment whereas others tend to reject it. Patients with paranoid, schizoid, and antisocial personality disorders rarely seek treatment, but those with Cluster C disorders (e.g., avoidant, dependent) may be much more open and motivated (Tyrer et al., 2003).

Negative expectations can be targeted initially by providing an overall physical context that conveys confidence, optimism, and trustworthiness. For example, patients who enter an appealing, culture-appropriate, warm, and welcoming therapist office might immediately form a very different set of expectations than those who come to a foreboding and sterile clinic. Beyond these initial—physical—expectations modifiers, therapists can also use simple therapeutic exercises in the first session to instill a sense of hope and confidence. Such exercises are commonly recommended, in fact, across various therapies, such as cognitive therapy (CT; Beck et al., 1979) and interpersonal therapy for depression (IPT; Weissman, Markowitz, & Klerman, 2000). In CT, for example, therapists aim to demonstrate right away how cognitive techniques can bring about immediate mood relief, which then "helps to increase . . . confidence in the efficacy of therapy" (Beck et al., 1979, p. 95). In IPT, patients are also confidently told that "the outlook for your recovery is excellent" and "you are going to be actively engaged in therapy" (Weissman et al., 2000, p. 40), in the hope that this enhances positive expectancies, motivation, and overall engagement.

Other interventions, such as in motivational interviewing (MI; Miller & Rollnick, 2002), also focus directly on improving motivation for change. In this approach, one of the ways to clarify and potentially enhance motivation is by conducting a thorough intake assessment and then providing and discussing feedback. In the context of treating combined Axis I and II conditions, such routine assessments could serve the useful function of clarifying, beyond diagnostic categories, the roles played in each case by temperament, early adversity and attachment styles, cognitive–emotional disturbances, and engagement in meaningful life tasks. The results of such assessment could be discussed collaboratively with the patient, and MI strategies— such as clarifying goals, supporting self-efficacy, and practicing empathy— could be used to enhance the patient's motivation to engage with the treatment.

One of the key tasks at the next stage is then to ensure that the early alliance develops optimally. There is of course a wealth of literature documenting the importance of the alliance, which is commonly regarded as the strongest predictor of outcome (e.g., Horvath & Bedi, 2002; Orlinsky, Grawe, & Parks, 1994). Supporting this view, Wampold (2001) concluded that "the relationship accounts for dramatically more of the variability in outcomes than the totality of specific ingredients" (p. 158), and he estimated that the alliance alone accounts for as much as 5% of outcome variance. It may be particularly difficult—and important—to develop strong alliances with patients who present with borderline personality disorder and other forms of personality pathology (e.g., Yeomans, Gutfreund, Selzer, & Clarkin, 1994). Therapists who are more interpersonally skillful, empathic, and open appear generally better able to establish optimal alliances (Horvath & Bedi, 2002). One of the key skills in this context is therapists' ability to sensitively respond to and adjust their interventions based on patients' personalities and their subtly fluctuating in-session behaviors (Stiles, Honos-Webb, & Surko, 1998). Many measures have been developed that can be used to monitor the quality of the alliance in routine treatment; most of them appear to measure aspects of the alliance such as energetic collaborative engagement and agreement on the goals and tasks of treatment (Horvath & Bedi, 2002).

As the alliance is developing and individual patient needs and problems are crystallizing, specific, patient-tailored intervention techniques become a more dominant focus. These include the strategies described earlier in this chapter, such as exposure-based interventions, behavioral activation and activity scheduling, restructuring of attachment styles and close relationships, teaching of cognitive refutation techniques, experiential exercises to facilitate acceptance and mindfulness, and clarification of as well as facilitation of engagement with valued life tasks. In Weinberger's (1995) common factor model, some of these processes could be subsumed under the categories of (1) helping the patient confront the problem (e.g., through exposure exercises) and (2) providing opportunities for mastery or cognitive control experiences (e.g., through behavioral activation, acceptance/mindfulness exercises, cognitive restructuring, and clarification of values and goals). Throughout the treatment process—and particularly toward the end—it is important that the patient experiences treatment gains as internally caused (Weinberger, 1995). Attributing therapeutic success to external factors but failure to the self would indicate greater likelihood of relapse and symptom exacerbation (DeRubeis & Hollon, 1995).

PROVIDING OPTIMAL CARE FOR COMPLEX PATIENTS IN THE MANAGED CARE CULTURE

The preceding sections presented a brief overview of some of the principles we regard as important in providing optimal treatment for patients with complex co-occurring Axis I and II pathologies. However, in this era of managed care and accountability, it is clear that not every clinician will be in a position to offer optimal and exhaustive treatment for each patient, and the choices and strategies of which treatments are selected and how they are implemented will likely require increasing levels of empirical justification. One of the central questions that we (as treatment providers) face, then, is whether we have an obligation to reduce variability in the behavior of both patients and providers—that is, should we (or can we) create contingencies in the health care system that move mental health treatment from being less of a freelance art to more of an evidence-based craft? If one accepts the premise that we should move in this direction and that the current constraints in the system are not likely to change dramatically, then we need to reconsider seriously what we can hope to accomplish with any single treatment episode and, more to the present point, how any single treatment episode fits into a longer-term, even lifetime, plan for the care of patients with personality disorders—which, by definition, are chronic and pervasive. The challenge is to find appropriate models that allow clinicians who operate within these constraints to work meaningfully with patients' chronic temperamental vulnerabilities, to help them process the harmful consequences of their adverse learning histories, to reoptimize their cognitive and emotional functioning, and to facilitate their engagement with need-fulfilling life tasks.

As we confront this issue, some unexpected consequences emerge. First, the role of assessment and formulation and the need to negotiate collaboratively with patients about the conceptualization of their problems become even more critical. This may seem paradoxical; given the time constraints for any individual episode of care, but it may be effective to spend more rather than less time in assessment and "diagnosis." We may be unable to "cure" personality problems in 10 or 20 sessions (although we can often provide important symptomatic relief). However, one of the critical things we can give patients even in a brief intervention is a better understanding of themselves and various skills and strategies for establishing, maintaining, and generalizing effective self-management.

On the basis of case formulations that flow from this assessment, treatment providers need to make selective decisions about which goals to try to accomplish in the current treatment episode (e.g., stabilize acute symptoms or focus on more chronic vulnerabilities). Beyond this, providers also need to educate patients about the longitudinal nature of self-management over time. That is, because of the tenacious and recurrent nature of these complex pathologies, patients need to be provided with a blueprint about when and how to seek additional future care, about how to recognize and triage problems, and so on. The general point is that our treatment goals for Axis II disorders need to become more process-oriented, even as we attack the "content" problems posed by different symptoms and diagnoses on Axis I.

To deliver optimal care to patients with these complex disorders, we also need "staged" models of treatment in which different stages or sequences are identified, operationalized, and offered in flexible ways (either consecutively or separated in time) "in the context of patient preferences and readiness." Thus, it may be useful to develop models of sequential changes in treatment that can be measured reliably, that signal positive long-term outcomes, that include "dosage" guidelines, and that include rules for when to stop or to shift focus.

There are at least three "families" of treatment alternatives: (1) continuous treatment, at different intensities; (2) acute treatment, followed by maintenance strategies; and (3) primary care models (i.e., brief acute treatments at the patient's discretion, provided in the context of a stable relationship over time and a willingness to treat many different kinds of problems). There are suggestions in the literature on somatoform disorders (Bass & Benjamin, 1993), however, that being proactive, even without highly intensive outpatient treatments, can be beneficial (e.g., scheduling regular brief appointments in advance rather than relying on requests for care initiated by patients).

For patients with severe personality disorders, such stages are likely to involve (1) the achievement of physical safety and evidence of day-to-day emotional stability, (2) articulation and emotional processing of adverse concurrent and historical circumstances, and (3) efforts at personal growth and improvements in the quality of life. Examples of attempts at such models include dialectical behavior therapy (Linehan, 1993) for patients with borderline personality disorder, where stage I is focused on life-threatening and treatment-interfering behavior, stage II can then involve emotional processing of earlier developmental adversity, and stage III focuses on quality-of-life issues. There are similar suggestions in the literature on the treatment of trauma and early abuse (Herman, 1992) where the first stage is stabilization of the patient, stage 2 is the "working through" of the trauma, and stage 3 is promotion of greater involvement with current life circumstances and relationships.

In this context, it must be recognized that the chronic and recurrent conditions with which these patients present require sustained and collaborative efforts, involving treatment providers (therapists), the patients themselves, and the patients' families. De facto, patients and their families are the primary caregivers for chronic illness. Today this stance is increasingly sanctioned, implicitly and explicitly, by changes in the managed health care system, as illustrated in this quote by Von Korff, Gruman, Schaefer, Lurry, and Wagner (1997):

> Self-care and medical care are sometimes viewed as competing rather than complementary strategies. When self-care implies limited access to health care, it may carry negative connotations for patients and health care providers. At the same time, medical care for chronic illness is rarely effective in the absence of adequate self-care. . . . Collaborative management occurs when patients and care providers have shared goals, a sustained working relationship, mutual understanding of roles and responsibilities, and requisite skills for carrying out their roles. (p. 1097)

To practice effectively, then, we must develop innovative models of care that incorporate state-of-the-art principles of chronic disease management, adapted to mental disorders, including a primary emphasis on collaboration with the patient and members of his or her social network.

TOWARD INTEGRATED TREATMENTS FOR PERSONALITY AND SYNDROMAL PSYCHOPATHOLOGY

In this chapter, we have briefly outlined common processes and principles that influence syndrome as well as personality disorders. We pointed here to the importance of biologically based temperament predispositions, early forms of psychosocial adversity and resulting attachment disturbances, cognitive and emotional dysregulation, as well as failures to engage with developmental challenges and meet basic psychological needs. Each of these processes has straightforward treatment implications, and a set of broad recommendations—which of course need to be tailored to the individual case—was articulated. These interventions should not be administered as disembodied techniques; instead, they must be implemented by skilled and talented therapists who can effectively maximize the effectiveness of the common therapeutic processes, such as enhancing expectations, forming and maintaining strong alliances, facilitating exposure and cognitive control, and ensuring internal attributions of treatment gains. Delivering optimal treatments for patients with complex problems will be increasingly difficult unless flexible treatment models are developed that are appropriate to the chronic nature of these patients' conditions. To this end, staged treatment models, involvement of the family and patient context, and flexible treatment delivery will become increasingly important.

REFERENCES

Alden, L. E., Laposa, J. M., Taylor, C. T., & Ryder, A. G. (2002). Avoidant personality disorder: Current status and future directions. *Journal of Personality Disorders, 16,* 1–29.

Arnett, P. A., Smith, S. S., & Newman, J. P. (1997). Approach and avoidance motivation in psychopathic criminal offenders during passive avoidance. *Journal of Personality and Social Psychology, 72,* 1413–1428.

Arntz, A., Dietzel, R., & Dreessen, L. (1999). Assumptions in borderline personality disorder: Specificity, stability and relationship with etiological factors. *Behaviour Research and Therapy, 37,* 545–557.

Arntz, A., Dreessen, L., Schouten, E., & Weertman, A. (2004). Beliefs in personality disorders: A test with the Personality Disorder Belief Questionnaire. *Behaviour Research and Therapy, 42,* 1215–1225.

Arntz, A., & Veen, G. (2001). Evaluations of others by borderline patients. *Journal of Nervous and Mental Disease, 189,* 513–521.

Bach, P., & Hayes, S. C. (2002). ACT in prevention of re-hospitalization in psychotic inpatients. *Journal of Consulting and Clinical Psychology, 70,* 1129–1139.

Bartholomew, K., Kwong, M. J., & Hart, S. D. (2001). Attachment. In W. J. Livesley (Ed.), *Handbook of personality disorders: Theory, research, and treatment* (pp. 196–230). New York: Guilford Press.

Bass, C., & Benjamin, S. (1993). The management of chronic somatisation. *British Journal of Psychiatry, 162,* 472–480.

Battle, C. L., Shea, M. T., Johnson, D. M., Yen, S., Zlotnick, C., Zanarini, M. C., et al. (2004). Childhood maltreatment associated with adult personality disorders: Findings from the collaborative longitudinal personality disorders study. *Journal of Personality Disorders, 18,* 193–211.

Beck, A. T., Butler, A. C., Brown, G. K., Dahlsgaard, K. K., Newman, C. F., & Beck, J. S. (2001). Dysfunctional beliefs discriminate personality disorders. *Behaviour Research and Therapy, 39,* 1213–1225.

Beck, A. T., Emery, G., & Greenberg, R. L. (1985). *Anxiety disorders and phobias: A cognitive perspective.* New York: Basic Books.

Beck, A. T., Freeman, A. M., & Associates (1990). *Cognitive therapy of personality disorders.* New York: Guilford Press.

Beck, A. T., Rush, J., Shaw, B. F., & Emery, G. (1979). *Cognitive therapy of depression.* New York: Guilford Press.

Beevers, C. G., & Meyer, B. (2002). Lack of positive experiences and positive expectancies mediate the relationship between BAS responsiveness and depression. *Cognition and Emotion, 16,* 549–564.

Beevers, C. G., & Meyer, B. (2004). Thought suppression and depression risk. *Cognition and Emotion, 18,* 859–867.

Benjamin, L. S. (1996). *Interpersonal diagnosis and treatment of personality disorders.* New York: Guilford Press.

Bond, F. W., & Bunce, D. (2000). Mediators of change in emotion-focused and problem-focused worksite stress management interventions. *Journal of Occupational Health Psychology, 5,* 156–163.

Bretherton, I., & Munholland, K. A. (1999). Internal working models in attachment relationships: A construct revisited. In J. Cassidy & P. R. Shaver (Eds.), *Handbook of attachment: Theory, research, and clinical applications* (pp. 89–111). New York: Guilford Press.

Brewin, C. R., Dalgleish, T., & Joseph, S. (1996). A dual representation theory of posttraumatic stress disorder. *Psychological Review, 103,* 670–686.

Butler, A. C., Brown, G. K., Beck, A. T., & Grisham, J. R. (2002). Assessment of dysfunctional beliefs in borderline personality disorder. *Behaviour Research and Therapy, 40,* 1231–1240.

Carver, C. S., & Scheier, M. F. (2004). *Perspectives on personality* (5th ed.). Boston: Allyn & Bacon.

Carver, C. S., & White, T. L. (1994). Behavioral inhibition, behavioral activation, and affective responses to impending reward and punishment: The BIS/BAS scales. *Journal of Personality and Social Psychology 67,* 319–333.

Caseras, X., Torrubia, R., & Farré, J. M. (2001). Is the behavioural inhibition system the core vulnerability for cluster C personality disorders? *Personality and Individual Differences, 31,* 348–359.

Cavedini, P., Erzegovesi, S., Ronchi, P., & Bellodi, L. (1997). Predictive value of obsessive–compulsive personality disorder in antiobsessional pharmacological treatment. *European Neuropsychopharmacology, 7,* 45–49.

Clark, D. A., & Beck, A. T., & Alford, B. A. (1999). *Scientific foundations of cognitive theory and therapy of depression.* New York: Wiley.

Clark, D. M., & Wells, A. (1995). A cognitive model of social phobia. In R. G. Heimberg, M. Liebowitz, D. Hope, & F. Scheier (Eds.), *Social phobia: Diagnosis, assessment, and treatment* (pp. 69–93). New York: Guilford Press.

Clark, L. A., Watson, D., & Mineka, S. (1994). Temperament, personality, and the mood and anxiety disorders. *Journal of Abnormal Psychology, 103,* 103–116.

Cloninger, C. R., Svrakic, D. M., & Przybeck, T. R. (1993). A psychobiological model of temperament and character. *Archives of General Psychiatry, 50,* 975–990.

Costa, P. T., Jr., & Widiger, T. A. (2002). *Personality disorders and the five-factor model of personality* (2nd ed.). Washington, DC: American Psychological Association.

Cottraux, J., & Blackburn, I.-M. (2001). Cognitive therapy. In W. J. Livesley (Ed.), *Handbook of personality disorders: Theory, research, treatment* (pp. 377–399). New York: Guilford Press.

Dalgleish, T. (2004). Cognitive approaches to posttraumatic stress disorder: The evolution of multirepresentational theorizing. *Psychological Bulletin, 130,* 228–260.

Deci, E. L., & Ryan, R. M. (2000). The "what" and "why" of goal pursuits: Human needs and the self-determination of behavior. *Psychological Inquiry, 11,* 227–268.

DeRubeis, R. J., & Hollon, S. D. (1995). Explanatory style in the treatment of depression. In G. M. Buchanan & M. E. P. Seligman (Eds.), *Explanatory style* (pp. 99–111). Hillsdale, NJ: Erlbaum.

Diener, E., Colvin, C. R., Pavot, W. G., & Allman, A. (1991). The psychic costs of intense positive affect. *Journal of Personality and Social Psychology, 61,* 492–503.

Dolan-Sewell, R. T., Krueger, R. F., & Shea, M. T. (2001). Co-occurrence with syndrome disorders. In W. J. Livesley (Ed.), *Handbook of personality disorders: Theory, research, and treatment* (pp. 84–104). New York: Guilford Press.

Dreessen, L., Arntz, A., Hendriks, T., Keune, N., & van den Hout, M. (1999). Avoidant personality disorder and implicit schema-congruent information processing bias: A pilot study with a pragmatic inference task. *Behaviour Research and Therapy, 37,* 619–632.

Erikson, E. H. (1968). *Identity: Youth and crisis.* New York: Norton.

Erikson, E. H. (1974). *Dimensions of a new identity.* New York: Norton.

Erikson, E. H. (1980). *Identity and the life cycle.* New York: Norton.

Fabrega, H., Jr., Ulrich, R., Pilkonis, P. A., & Mezzich, J. E. (1992). Pure personality disorders in an intake psychiatric setting. *Journal of Personality Disorders, 6,* 153–161.

Feeny, N. C., Zoellner, L. A., & Foa, E. B. (2002). Treatment outcome for chronic PTSD among female assault victims with borderline personality characteristics: A preliminary examination. *Journal of Personality Disorders, 16,* 30–40.

Foa, E. B., & Rothbaum, B. O. (1998). *Treating the trauma of rape*. New York: Guilford Press.

Fonagy, P., Leigh, T., Steele, M., Steele, H., Kennedy, R., Mattoon, G., et al. (1996). The relation of attachment status, psychiatric classification, and response to psychotherapy. *Journal of Consulting and Clinical Psychology, 64*, 22–31.

Fowles, D. C. (1980). The three arousal model: Implications of Gray's two-factor learning theory for heart rate, electrodermal activity, and psychopathy. *Psychophysiology, 17*, 87–104.

Fowles, D. C. (1993). Biological variables in psychopathology: A psychobiological perspective. In P. B. Sutker & H. E. Adams (Eds.), *Comprehensive handbook of psychopathology* (2nd ed., pp. 57–82). New York: Plenum Press.

Frank, J. D. (1973). *Persuasion and healing*. Baltimore: Johns Hopkins University Press.

Gabbard, G. O. (2001). Psychoanalysis and psychoanalytic psychotherapy. In W. J. Livesley (Ed.), *Handbook of personality disorders: Theory, research, and treatment* (pp. 359–376). New York: Guilford Press.

Gable S. L., Reis, H. T., & Elliot, A. J. (2000). Behavioral activation and inhibition in everyday life. *Journal of Personality and Social Psychology, 78*, 1135–1149.

Goodman, G., Hull, J. W., Clarkin, J. F., & Yeomans, F. E. (1998). Comorbid mood disorders as modifiers of treatment response among inpatients with borderline personality disorder. *Journal of Nervous and Mental Disease, 186*, 616–622.

Gray, J. A. (1987). *The psychology of fear and stress* (2nd ed.). Cambridge, UK: Cambridge University Press.

Gray, J. A. (1991). Neural systems, emotion, and personality. In J. Madden IV (Ed.), *Neurobiology of learning, emotion, and affect* (pp. 273–306). New York: Hillsdale Press.

Greenberg, L. (2002). *Emotion-focused therapy: Coaching clients to work through their feelings*. Washington, DC: American Psychological Association.

Hardy, G. E., Barkham, M., Shapiro, D. A., Stiles, W. B., Rees, A., & Reynolds, S. (1995). Impact of Cluster C personality disorders on outcomes of contrasting brief psychotherapies for depression. *Journal of Consulting and Clinical Psychology, 63*, 997–1004.

Harkness, A. R., & Lilienfeld, S. O. (1997). Individual differences science for treatment planning: Personality traits. *Psychological Assessment, 9*, 349–360.

Hayes, S. C., Strosahl, K., & Wilson, K. G. (1999). *Acceptance and commitment therapy: An experiential approach to behavior change*. New York: Guilford Press.

Henriques, J. B., & Davidson, R. J. (2000). Decreased responsiveness to reward in depression. *Cognition and Emotion, 14*, 711–724.

Heponiemi, T., Keltikangas-Jaervinen, L., Puttonen, S., & Ravaja, N. (2003). BIS/BAS sensitivity and self-rated affects during experimentally induced stress. *Personality and Individual Differences, 34*, 943–957.

Herman, J. (1992). *Trauma and recovery*. New York: Basic Books.

Herpertz, S. C., Dietrich, T. M., Wenning, B., Krings, T., Erberich, S. G., Willmes, K., et al. (2001). Evidence of abnormal amygdala functioning in borderline personality disorder: A functional MRI study. *Biological Psychiatry, 50*, 292–298.

Herpertz, S. C., Schwenger, U. B., Kunert, H. J., Lukas, G., Gretzer, U., Nutzmann, J., et al. (2000). Emotional responses in patients with borderline as compared with avoidant personality disorder. *Journal of Personality Disorders, 14,* 339–351.

Herpertz, S. C., Werth, U., Lucas, G., Qunaibi, M., Schuerkens, A., Kunert, H.-J., et al. (2001). Emotion in criminal offenders with psychopathy and borderline personality disorders. *Archives of General Psychiatry, 58,* 737–745.

Horvath, A. O., & Bedi, R. P. (2002). The alliance. In J. C. Norcross (Ed.), *Psychotherapy relationships that work* (pp. 37–69). New York: Oxford Press.

Hilsenroth, M. J., Holdwick, D. J., Castlebury, F. D., & Blais, M. A. (1998). The effects of DSM-IV cluster B personality disorder symptoms on the termination and continuation of psychotherapy. *Psychotherapy: Theory, Research, Practice, Training, 35,* 163–176.

Jacobson, N. S., Dobson, K. S., Truax, P. A., Addis, M. E., Koerner, K., Gollan, J. K., et al. (1996). A component analysis of cognitive-behavioral treatment for depression. *Journal of Consulting and Clinical Psychology, 64,* 295–304.

Jang, K. L., & Livesley, W. J. (1999). Why do measures of normal and disordered personality correlate? A study of genetic comorbidity. *Journal of Personality Disorders, 13,* 10–17.

Johnson, S. L., Turner, R. J., & Iwata, N. (2003). BIS/BAS levels and psychiatric disorder: An epidemiological study. *Journal of Psychopathology and Behavioral Assessment, 25,* 25–36.

Joyce A. S., Ogrodniczuk, J. S., Piper, W. E., & McCallum, M. (2003). The alliance as mediator of expectancy effects in short-term individual therapy. *Journal of Consulting and Clinical Psychology, 71,* 672–679.

Kanfer, F. H., & Schefft, B. K. (1988). *Guiding the process of therapeutic change.* Champaign, IL: Research Press.

Kasch, K. L., Rottenberg, J., Arnow, B. A., & Gotlib, I. H. (2002). Behavioral activation and inhibition systems and the severity and course of depression. *Journal of Abnormal Psychology, 111,* 589–597.

Knutson, B., Wolkowitz, O. M., Cole, S. W., Chan, T., Moore, E. A., Johnson, R. C., et al. (1998). Selective alteration of personality and social behavior by serotonergic intervention. *American Journal of Psychiatry, 155,* 373–379.

Kramer, P. D. (1993). *Listening to Prozac: A psychiatrist explores anti-depressant drugs and the remaking of the self.* New York: Viking.

Krueger, R. F., Schmutte, P. S., Caspi, A., Moffitt, T. E., Campbell, K., & Silva, P. A. (1994). Personality traits are linked to crime among men and women: Evidence from a birth cohort. *Journal of Abnormal Psychology, 103,* 328–388.

Krueger, R. F., & Tackett, J. L. (2003). Personality and psychopathology: Working toward the bigger picture. *Journal of Personality Disorders, 17,* 109–128.

Lilienfeld, S. O., Waldman, I. D., & Israel, A. C. (1994). A critical examination of the use of the term and concept of "cormorbidity" in psychopathology research. *Clinical Psychology: Science and Practice, 1,* 71–83.

Linehan, M. M. (1993). *Cognitive-behavioral treatment of borderline personality disorder.* New York: Guilford Press.

Linehan, M. M. (1994). Acceptance and change: The central dialectic in psychotherapy. In S. C. Hayes, N. S. Jacobson, V. M. Follette, & M. J. Dougher (Eds.), *Ac-*

ceptance and change: Content and context in psychotherapy (pp. 73–86). Reno, NV: Context Press.

Livesley, W. J. (2001). A framework for an integrated approach to treatment. In W. J. Livesley (Ed.), *Handbook of personality disorders: Theory, research, and treatment* (pp. 570–600). New York: Guilford Press.

Livesley, W. J., Jang, K. L., & Vernon, P. A. (1998). Phenotypic and genetic structure of traits delineating personality disorder. *Archives of General Psychiatry, 55,* 941–948.

Lyddon, W. J., & Sherry, A. (2001). Developmental personality styles: An attachment theoretical conceptualization of personality disorders. *Journal of Counseling and Developing, 79,* 405–414.

Lynam, D. R., & Widiger, T. A. (2001). Using the five-factor model to represent the DSM-IV personality disorders: An expert consensus approach. *Journal of Abnormal Psychology, 110,* 401–412.

Lyons, M. J., Tyrer, P., Gunderson, J., & Tohen, M. (1997). Heuristic models of comorbidity of Axis I and Axis II disorders. *Journal of Personality Disorders, 11,* 260–269.

Ma, S. H., & Teasdale, J. D. (2004). Mindfulness-based cognitive therapy for depression: Replication and exploration of differential relapse prevention effects. *Journal of Consulting and Clinical Psychology, 72,* 31–40.

Mallinckrodt, B., Gantt, D. L., & Coble, H. M. (1995). Attachment patterns in the psychotherapy relationship: Development of the Patient Attachment to Therapist Scale. *Journal of Counseling Psychology, 42,* 307–317.

Markovitz, P. J. (2004). Recent trends in the pharmacotherapy of personality disorders. *Journal of Personality Disorders, 18,* 90–101.

Martell, C. R., Addis, M. E., & Jacobson, N. S. (2001). *Depression in context: Strategies for guided action.* New York: Norton.

Meyer, B. (2002). Personality and mood correlates of avoidant personality disorder. *Journal of Personality Disorders, 16,* 174–188.

Meyer, B., & Carver, C. S. (2000). Negative childhood accounts, sensitivity, and pessimism: A study of avoidant personality disorder features in college students. *Journal of Personality Disorders, 14,* 233–248.

Meyer, B., Johnson, S. L., & Winters, R. (2001). Responsiveness to threat and incentive in bipolar disorder: Relations of the BIS/BAS scales with symptoms. *Journal of Psychopathology and Behavioral Assessment, 23,* 133–143.

Meyer, B., Olivier, L. E., & Roth, D. (2005). Please don't leave me! BIS/BAS, attachment styles, and responses to a relationship threat. *Personality and Individual Differences, 38,* 151–162.

Meyer, B., & Pilkonis, P. A. (2002). Attachment style. In J. A. Norcross (Ed.), *Psychotherapy relationships that work: Therapists' relational contributions to effective psychotherapy* (pp. 367–382). New York: Oxford University Press.

Meyer, B., & Pilkonis, P. A. (2005). An attachment model of personality disorder. In J. F. Clarkin & M. F. Lenzenweger (Eds.), *Major theories of personality disorder* (2nd ed., pp. 231–281). New York: Guilford Press.

Meyer, B., Pilkonis, P. A., & Beevers, C. G. (2004). What's in a (neutral) face?: Personality disorders, attachment styles, and the appraisal of ambiguous social cues. *Journal of Personality Disorders, 18,* 320–336.

Meyer, B., Pilkonis, P. A., Krupnick, J. L., Egan, M., Simmens, S., & Sotsky, S. (2002). Treatment expectancies, patient alliance, and outcome: Further analyses from the NIMH Treatment of Depression Collaborative Research Program. *Journal of Consulting and Clinical Psychology, 70,* 1051–1055.

Meyer, B., Pilkonis, P. A., Proietti, J., Heape, C., & Egan, M. (2001). Attachment styles, personality disorders, and response to treatment. *Journal of Personality Disorders, 15,* 371–389.

Miller, W. R., & Rollnick, S. (2002). *Motivational interviewing: Preparing people for change* (2nd ed.). New York: Guilford Press.

Millon T., & Davis, R. D. (1996). *Disorders of personality: DSM-IV and beyond.* New York: Wiley.

Mineka, S., Watson, D., & Clark, L. A. (1998). Comorbidity of anxiety and unipolar mood disorders. *Annual Review of Psychology, 49,* 377–412.

Morey, L. C., & Zanarini, M. C. (2000). Borderline personality: Traits and disorder. *Journal of Abnormal Psychology, 109,* 733–737.

Morgenstern, J., Langenbucher, J., Labouvie, E., & Miller, K. J. (1997). The comorbidity of alcoholism and personality disorders in a clinical population: Prevalence rates and relation to alcohol typology variables. *Journal of Abnormal Psychology, 106,* 74–84.

Mulder, R. T. (2002). Personality pathology and treatment outcome in major depression: A review. *American Journal of Psychiatry, 159,* 359–371.

Orlinsky, D. E., Grawe, K., & Parks, B. K. (1994). Process and outcome in psychotherapy—noch einmal. In A. E. Bergin & S. L. Garfield (Eds.), *Handbook of psychotherapy and behavior change* (4th ed., pp. 270–376). New York: Wiley.

Pilkonis, P. A. (2001). Treatment of personality disorders in association with symptom disorders. In W. J. Livesley (Ed.), *Handbook of personality disorders: Theory, research, and treatment* (pp. 541–554). New York: Guilford Press.

Reich, J., & Green, A. I. (1991). Effect of personality disorders on outcome of treatment. *Journal of Nervous and Mental Disease, 179,* 74–82.

Reis, H. T., Sheldon, K. M., Gable, S. L., Roscoe, J., & Ryan, R. M. (2000). Daily well-being: The role of autonomy, competence, and relatedness. *Personality and Social Psychology Bulletin, 26,* 419–435.

Resick, P. A., & Schnicke, M. K. (1993). *Cognitive processing therapy for rape victims: A treatment manual.* Newbury Park, CA: Sage.

Rottenberg, J., Wilhelm, F. H., & Gross, J. J. (2003). Vagal rebound during resolution of fearful crying among depressed and nondepressed individuals. *Psychophysiology, 40,* 1–6.

Rude, S. S., & McCarthy, C. T. (2003). Emotional functioning in depressed and depression-vulnerable college students. *Cognition and Emotion, 17,* 799–806.

Rusting, C. L., & Larsen, R. J. (1998). Diurnal patterns of unpleasant mood: Associations with neuroticism, depression, and anxiety. *Journal of Personality, 66,* 85–103.

Sareen, J., Enns, M. W., & Guertin, J. E. (2000). The impact of clinically diagnosed personality disorders on acute and one-year outcomes of electroconvulsive therapy. *Journal of ECT, 16,* 43–51.

Segal, Z. V., Williams, J. M. G., & Teasdale, J. D. (2002). *Mindfulness-based cognitive therapy for depression: A new approach to preventing relapse.* New York: Guilford Press.

Shea, M. T., Pilkonis, P. A., Beckham, E., Collins, J. F., Elkin, I., Sotsky, S. M., et al. (1990). Personality disorders and treatment outcome in the NIMH Treatment of Depression Collaborative Research Program. *American Journal of Psychiatry, 147,* 711–718.

Sheldon, K. M, Ryan, R., & Reis, H. T. (1996). What makes for a good day? Competence and autonomy in the day and in the person. *Personality and Social Psychology Bulletin, 22,* 1270–1279.

Siever, L. J., & Davis, K. L. (1991). A psychobiological perspective on the personality disorders. *American Journal of Psychiatry, 148,* 1647–1658.

Stiles, W. B., Honos-Webb, L., & Surko, M. (1998). Responsiveness in psychotherapy. *Clinical Psychology: Science and Practice, 5,* 439–458.

Tse, W. S., & Bond, A. J. (2001). Serotonergic involvement in the psychosocial dimension of personality. *Journal of Psychopharmacology, 15,* 195–198.

Tyrer, P., Mitchard, S., Methuen, C., & Ranger, M. (2003). Treatment rejecting and treatment seeking personality disorders: Type R and Type S. *Journal of Personality Disorders, 17,* 263–268.

Vandewater, E. A., Ostrove, J. M., & Stewart, A. J. (1997). Predicting women's well-being in midlife: The importance of personality development and social role involvement. *Journal of Personality and Social Psychology, 72,* 1147–1160.

Veen, G., & Arntz, A. (2000). Multidimensional dichotomous thinking characterizes borderline personality disorder. *Cognitive Therapy and Research, 24,* 23–45.

Viinamäki, H., Tanskanen, A., Koivumaa-Honkanen, H., Haatainen, K., Honkalampi, K., Antikainen, R., et al. (2003). Cluster C personality disorder and recovery from major depression: 24–month prospective follow-up. *Journal of Personality Disorders, 17,* 341–350.

Von Korff, M., Gruman, J., Schaefer, J., Curry, S. J., & Wagner, E. H. (1997). Collaborative management of chronic illness. *Annals of Internal Medicine, 127,* 1097–1102.

Wagner, A. W., & Linehan, M. M. (1999). Facial expression recognition ability among women with borderline personality disorder: Implications for emotion regulation. *Journal of Personality Disorders, 13,* 329–344.

Wagner-Moore, L. E. (2004). Gestalt therapy: Past, present, theory, and research. *Psychotherapy: Theory, Research, Practice, Training, 41,* 179–186.

Wampold, B. E. (2001). *The great psychotherapy debate: Models, methods, and findings.* Mahwah, NJ: Erlbaum.

Wegner, D. M., Schneider, D. J., Carter, S. R., & White, T. L. (1987). Paradoxical effects of thought suppression. *Journal of Personality and Social Psychology, 53,* 5–15.

Weinberger, J. (1995). Common factors aren't so common: The common factors dilemma. *Clinical Psychology: Science and Practice, 2,* 45–69.

Weinfield, N. S., Sroufe, A. L., Egeland, B., & Carlson, E. A. (1999). The nature of individual differences in infant–caregiver attachment. In J. Cassidy & P. R. Shaker (Eds.), *Handbook of attachment: Theory, research, and clinical applications* (pp. 68–88). New York: Guilford Press.

Weissman, M. M., Markowitz, J. C., & Klerman, G. L. (2000). *Comprehensive guide to interpersonal therapy*. New York: Basic Books.

Wenzlaff, R. M., & Wegner, D. M. (2000). Thought suppression. In S. T. Fiske (Ed.), *Annual review of psychology* (Vol. 51, pp. 59–91). Palo Alto, CA: Annual Reviews.

Wenzlaff, R. M., Wegner, D. M., & Roper, D. W. (1988). Depression and mental control: The resurgence of unwanted negative thoughts. *Journal of Personality and Social Psychology, 55,* 882–892.

Winston, A., Rosenthal, R. N., & Muran, J. C. (2001). Supportive psychotherapy. In W. J. Livesley (Ed.), *Handbook of personality disorders: Theory, research, and treatment* (pp. 344–358). New York: Guilford Press.

Yen, S., Sr., Shea, M. T., Battle, C. L., Johnson, D. M., Zlotnick, C., Dolan-Sewell, R., et al. (2002). Traumatic exposure and posttraumatic stress disorder in borderline, schizotypal, avoidant and obsessive–compulsive personality disorders: Findings from the Collaborative Longitudinal Personality Disorders Study. *Journal of Nervous and Mental Disease, 190,* 510–518.

Yeomans, F. E., Gutfreund, J., Selzer, M. A, & Clarkin, J. F. (1994). Factors related to drop-outs by borderline patients: Treatment contract and therapeutic alliance. *Journal of Psychotherapy Practice and Research, 3,* 16–24.

Young, J., Klosko, J. S., & Weishaar, M. (2003). *Schema therapy: A practitioner's guide*. New York: Guilford Press.

Zanarini, M. C., Frankenburg, F. R., Dubo, E. D., Sickel, A. E., Trikha, A., Levin, A., et al. (1998). Axis I comorbidity of borderline personality disorder. *American Journal of Psychiatry, 155,* 1733–1739.

Zanarini, M. C., Williams, A. A., Lewis, R. E., Reich, R. B., Vera, S. C., Marino, M. F., et al. (1997). Reported pathological childhood experiences associated with the development of borderline personality disorders. *American Journal of Psychiatry, 154,* 1101–1106.

Chapter 10

Through the Lens of the Relational Self
Triggering Emotional Suffering in the Social-Cognitive Process of Transference

SUSAN M. ANDERSEN
REGINA MIRANDA

The impact of significant-other relationships on emotional well-being has been of increasing interest in theory and research on psychopathology. The notion that mental representations of important figures from a person's past are held in memory and influence current experience is compelling and spans more than a century of theory. From psychodynamic models (e.g., Freud, 1912/1958, 1912/1963; Kernberg, 1976; Sullivan, 1940, 1953) to attachment theory (Bowlby, 1969, 1973, 1980) and recent research in social cognition (Andersen & Chen, 2002; Andersen & Cole, 1990; Baldwin, 1992) and clinical science (Hammen, 2000; Joiner, Coyne, & Blalock, 1999; Safran & Segal, 1990), these concepts have long been center stage in personality and psychopathology. Yet, research has also focused vastly more on what is individual about human suffering than on what is interpersonal. While valuable, this focus can inadvertently blind researchers to the nexus between the individual and society, and in particular the individual and relationships, and can thus obscure the full range of pathways to suffering and resilience.

In our own theoretical and empirical work, we have examined how past relationships with significant others influence responses to new people, and how the past can thus play out in the present. Based on the process of transference (Andersen & Glassman, 1996; Chen & Andersen, 1999; e.g., Andersen & Cole, 1990), people reexperience their previous interpersonal patterns from specific relationships in the context of new everyday relations. By defining and operationalizing transference in social-cognitive terms, we have been able to generate the first experimental demonstration of this century-old clinical concept, and to show that a central underlying mechanism of much suffering is the process of transference and the relational aspects of the self that it evokes (Andersen & Chen, 2002; Andersen & Saribay, 2005). Mental representations of significant others are triggered by contextual cues (and also by inner ones) that vary in the contemporary situations of a person's life and lead to a wide variety of effects, including specific emotional and motivational dynamics that may at times be maladaptive or may maintain or exacerbate psychopathology.

Beyond this work, we have also developed an independent line of research directed toward understanding the thought processes that may underlie depression (e.g., Andersen, Spielman, & Bargh, 1992). Our focus in this work has been to extend beyond self-schema approaches to depression to take account of how people conceptualize what the future will hold. Understanding how hopelessness may develop or more generally, what role thoughts about the future play in depression is of pressing clinical importance.

Juxtaposing these lines of work, as we do here, brings to light a number of intriguing questions for future research and implications for psychopathology.

OUR MODEL OF THE RELATIONAL
SELF AND TRANSFERENCE

Classical theories have long held that people have a basic need for human connection—for relatedness, attachment, tenderness, and belonging (e.g., Adler, 1927/1957; Bakan, 1966; Batson, 1990; Bowlby, 1969; Deci, 1995; Fairbairn, 1952; J. R. Greenberg & Mitchell, 1983; Guisinger & Blatt, 1994; Helgeson, 1994; Horney, 1939, 1945; McAdams, 1985, 1989; Rogers, 1951; Safran, 1990; Sullivan, 1940, 1953). In social psychology, research suggests consequences of social bonds in cognition, affect, behavior, and overall well-being. For example, the explicit or implicit message that one is accepted or rejected by significant others can have profound effects on subsequent relations (e.g., Ayduk et al., 2000; Bandura, 1986; Baumeister & Leary, 1995; Crocker & Wolfe, 2001; Downey & Feldman, 1996; Higgins, 1989, 1991; Leary, Tambor, Terdal, & Downs, 1995; Markus &

Kitayama, 1991; Smith, Murphy, & Coats, 1999). Likewise, research on attachment processes in infancy (e.g.,Thompson, 1998) and in adulthood (see Simpson & Rholes, 1998) has suggested that mental models of the self and others arise in response to responsive and sensitive interchanges with significant others (or the lack thereof) and that they can have important implications for interpersonal functioning through early experiences with caregivers (Bowlby, 1969, 1973, 1980; see also Ainsworth, Blehar, Waters, & Wall, 1978; Bombar & Littig, 1996; Bretherton, 1985; Hazan & Shaver, 1994; Mikulincer, 1995).

There are, of course, other human needs beyond that for human connection and nurturance—such as the need for felt security (e.g., Epstein, 1973), autonomy (Deci & Ryan, 1985), control or competence (e.g., Bandura, 1977, 1989; Seligman, 1975), and meaning (e.g., Becker, 1971). But at the core of our model of the relational self is this fundamental need for human connection. As such, the relationships people develop with other individuals in their lives occupy a place of great significance. Such significant others can include family members, close friends, relationship partners, and mentors—anyone who has had an impact on the individual, including both people from one's distant past and those who are more current.

Through relationships, one develops knowledge about these others and about the self, that is, people form mental representations of the self. This knowledge is not represented in isolation but, rather, is "entangled" in memory with what one knows about each significant other (Andersen & Chen, 2002; Andersen, Reznik, & Chen, 1997; Andersen & Saribay, 2005; Hinkley & Andersen, 1996). In short, individuals come to develop a range of *relational* selves, each stored in memory and linked to a mental representation of a significant other and relationship, and much research supports this assumption. The assumption that there is a linkage between representations of significant others and the self in memory is also made by relational schema models (Baldwin, 1992). (A compatible but diverging model also emphasizing relevance of significant others to the self goes so far as to assume significant others are incorporated into the self and not simply linked with it in memory, Aron, Aron, Tudor, & Nelson, 1991).

This view of the relational self is largely consistent with Harry Stack Sullivan's (1953) model in which such needs—for satisfaction, including being connected to others while expressing oneself openly, and for felt security—are integral to the "personifications" of the self and other (akin to representations) that are formed, and the "dynamisms" or dynamics that link them. Sullivan also proposed a transference process, "parataxic distortion," in which personifications and dynamisms arise in behavior with persons besides the significant other. By contrast, the process of *transference* originally developed by Freud (1912/1958) involved childhood fantasies and psychosexual conflicts displaced onto an analyst in psychoanalysis (Freud, 1912/1963). Drive-structure assumptions (e.g., Greenberg & Mitchell, 1983) predominated in Freud's view, although he did argue that children also form "imagoes" of early libidinal objects (e.g., parents). Our view of the process thus maps better onto Sullivan's model than onto Freud's, and both assume, as we do, that it occurs both in treatment and in everyday life. In our work, we have focused on how it occurs in everyday interpersonal relations.

Our social-cognitive model assumes that people have mental representations of significant others in memory, just as they have other social constructs and categories, and that these representations lead individuals to "go beyond the information given" (Bruner, 1957; see also Kelly, 1955) about a new person when they are activated and applied to the person. That is, when a significant-other representation is triggered by cues from one's environment, the representation is applied to the new other and used as a kind of lens through which the new person is interpreted. Moreover, the aspects of the self experienced with the significant other become available in working memory. Thus, one's working knowledge of the self shifts in the direction of the self-when-with-the-significant-other (Hinkley & Andersen, 1996). Consequently, past relationships influence one's current experience, even without the actual presence of the significant other. The process guides not only how people relate to others in the varying contexts of their everyday lives but also the nature of self they experience across these varying contexts.

In short, we have shown that it is in this manner that relationships from the past (either with caregivers or important others) and relational selves from past relations arise in present expectancies, feelings, motivations, and patterns of interaction. What is stored in memory and triggered in transference may thus render the person vulnerable to emotional suffering or confer on him or her resilience (Andersen & Chen, 2002; Andersen & Saribay, 2005; see also Ayduk et al., 2000; Downey & Feldman, 1996; Gurung, Sarason, & Sarason, 2001; McGowan, 2002; Murray & Holmes, 1999; Pierce & Lydon, 1998; Shields, Ryan, & Cicchetti, 2001).

Our model is consistent with other social-cognitive views of the relational self. For example, Baldwin's (1992) model of *relational schemas* suggests these are developed through repeated and similar patterns of interactions with various others. These schemas consist of an *interpersonal script*, defined as "a cognitive structure representing a sequence of actions and events that defines a stereotyped relational pattern" (p. 468), along with a self-schema, or representation of the self in the interaction. Relationship schemas thus represent prototypic patterns of interaction between the self and others. By contrast, our model emphasizes idiosyncratic aspects of the self in a given relationship, along with unique characteristics of the relationship with each particular significant other and how this constrains emotions, motives, and self-regulation at any given moment (Hinkley & Andersen, 1996; see Chen & Andersen, 1999). Significant-other representations, in our view, are N-of-one representations or exemplars (Linville & Fischer, 1993; Smith & Zarate, 1992); each designates a unique individual and is associated with a unique experience of the self in that relationship.

Rather than generic styles of responding, we have focused on what is unique to the individual relationship, and have also focused on *if–then* response patterns (see Mischel & Shoda, 1995)—if the significant-other representation is triggered, then the transference response occurs. This accounts for cross-situational variability in how the person responds, such that an individual exhibits different responses (*thens*) across different situations (*ifs*). Because of how commonly used longstanding significant-other responses are, this fact also lends consistency in these response tendencies over time. Overall, we suggest that each significant-other representation is associated with individual patterns of responses, and that different interpersonal situations trigger varying cognitions, affect, and behavior that reflect the psychological situation (Mischel & Shoda, 1995) the individual experiences (Andersen & Chen, 2002; Andersen & Saribay, 2005).

OUR EVIDENCE ON TRANSFERENCE AND THE RELATIONAL SELF

The evidence that demonstrates transference and the notion of the relational self rests on procedures in which significant-other representations are triggered experimentally. In this work, we make use of an idiographic stimulus generation procedure and combine this with a standard (nomothetic) laboratory paradigm. This mixed paradigm has the advantage of enabling us to tap meaningful, idiosyncratic aspects of individuals' significant-other representations while at the same time allowing examination of processes that are generalizable across people.

The Methodology

In this research, participants take part in a two-session research design. In a preliminary session, they are asked to describe positive and negative attributes of two significant others by using a series of sentences that they freely generate. In a second, seemingly unrelated session, participants arrive to a different lab and are led to believe that they will soon be interacting with another person who is seated in a room next door and being interviewed by a trained interviewer. The presumed interviewer, it is said, will soon provide some descriptions of this new person based on the interview. Shortly, participants are then asked to read a series of descriptions "about" the new person and are asked to imagine interacting with the new person.

In the transference condition, the descriptions to which participants are exposed consist of some of the statements (in paraphrased form) that they provided in the prior session to describe their own significant other (along with some filler items). These descriptions are a mix of both positive and negative features so that there is not a preponderance of one valence that might in and of itself drive any subsequent effects. Each participant in the transference condition is also yoked on a one-to-one basis with another person in the control condition who is presented with exactly the same descriptors about the person next door. Thus, in the transference condition, the new person slightly resembles the participant's significant other, and in the control condition this is not the case, even while objective stimulus content is identical across conditions.

After learning about the new person, participants complete various ratings, designed to tap into their evaluations, motives, affect, or expectancies, provide free-form descriptions of "the self at this moment," complete a recognition memory measure, and/or actually engage in an interaction with a stranger. Sometimes their faces are videotaped while they learn about the new person and facial affect assessed by trained judges, or in the case of an actual interaction, their behavior may be assessed by judges. Our main indices of transference tap the extent to which individuals go beyond the information given (Bruner, 1957) about the new person—in terms of ascribing to him or her the same positive or negative evaluation felt toward the significant other and in terms of inferring that he or she has characteristics the significant other has that were not presented about the new person. We typically assess the latter using recognition memory confidence that significant-other features were presented about the person when they were not.

Early Evidence on the Transference Process

Inferences and Memory

One of the earliest forms of evidence arising from this work indicated that individuals who learn about a person who resembles a significant other will show biased inferences and memory about this new person. That is, people tend to report more recognition memory confidence in having learned things about a new person that they did not actually learn when these things describe the significant other—if they were in the resemblance condition rather than the yoked control condition. This occurs whether they have learned about fictional characters with whom they do not expect to interact (Andersen & Cole, 1990; Andersen, Glassman, Chen, & Cole, 1995; Chen, Andersen, & Hinkley, 1999; Glassman & Andersen, 1999b) or have learned about someone presumably next door with whom they do expect to interact (e.g., Andersen & Baum, 1994; Andersen, Reznik, & Manzella, 1996; Berenson & Andersen, 2005; Berk & Andersen, 2000; Hinkley & Andersen, 1996; Reznik & Andersen, 2004). The effect holds whether the new person resembles a positive significant other or a negative one, and also holds across a wide range of significant others. The evidence thus suggests that the transference process does occur and that significant-other representations are powerful inferential devices that are readily triggered and used in perceiving others in a process that appears to arise relatively automatically.

Automatic Activation

Evidence has also shown that similarly biased inferences arise in reference to a new person even when the significant-other-relevant cues are presented entirely nonconsciously (Glassman & Andersen, 1999a). That is, when such features are presented subliminally about one's own significant other (vs. another participant's)—by showing them for about 80 msec in parafoveal vision followed by a pattern mask—participants are more likely to infer that the new person has features of the significant other to which they were never exposed, even subliminally. Mental processes that are relatively effortless, unintentional, and/or uncontrolled are typically considered to be automatic, and those that transpire outside of awareness fit all these criteria (Bargh, 1997). Hence, these data suggest that the transference process is evoked automatically. It can be triggered outside of conscious awareness (see Andersen, Reznik, & Glassman, 2005).

Complementing this work, recently completed research (Andersen, Miranda, & Edwards, 1996) made use of response latency to show automatic activation of the significant-other representation in the transference paradigm. Only if a representation has been activated can it be applied to a new stimulus or person (e.g., Higgins, 1996), and even though evidence suggests that significant-other representations are chronically accessible or active (Andersen et al., 1995), we focus most of our work on the contextual triggering of transference.

Exposure to significant-other-relevant cues in the transference context should thus lead features of this representation to become especially accessible. To test this, after presenting participants with features of a new person (who either did or did not resemble the significant other), we had them complete a lexical decision task. In this task, they indicated as quickly as possible whether or not a series of letter strings were or were not words—with those words either describing the significant other or not. As predicted, participants in the transference condition responded significantly more quickly to words that were highly descriptive versus only minimally descriptive of the significant other, and no such effect occurred in the control condition. Cues known to trigger transference thus lead information associated with the significant other to become more accessible, and this occurs automatically, given that the speed of lexical decision responses has nothing to do with intention or attention concerned with the significant other.

Evaluation and Affect

Research in social cognition shows that individuals automatically evaluate stimuli they encounter as positive or negative (Bargh, Chaiken, Raymond, & Hymes, 1996) and that this occurs even with completely unfamiliar, novel stimuli (see Duckworth, Bargh, Garcia, & Chaiken, 2002). Such automatic evaluation may even represent a kind of "core" affective experience (Russell, 2003), which when combined with degree of arousal or activity is the basis of the experience of discrete emotions. We have found that the same kind of automatic evaluation appears to arise in transference. When a significant-other representation is triggered in transference, people come to evaluate the new person in the same positive or negative way that they evaluate the significant other. If the other is liked or loved, so is the new person; if he or she is disliked, the new person is as well. When people learn of a new person who resembles their own (versus someone else's) significant other, they evaluate the new person more positively when the original significant other was positively rather than negatively evaluated (Andersen et al., 1996; Andersen & Baum, 1994; Berk & Andersen, 2000). Similarly, when the new person resembles the participants' positive significant other, the new person is evaluated more favorably than in a control condition (Baum & Andersen, 1999; Reznik & Andersen, 2005), in accordance with schema-triggered affect (Fiske & Pavelchak, 1986).

We also have more direct evidence of the automatic emergence of affect in transference based on the expression of emotion in people's faces. When reading descriptions of a new person whose features resemble a positive versus a negative significant other, participants' facial expression (recorded by a hidden camera) show more positive facial affect—as coded by independent raters—and no such effect occurred in the absence of transference (Andersen et al. 1996). Indeed, a comparable effect was observed when the significant other in question was a parent, and held even if the parent had physically abused the participant while growing up (Berenson & Andersen, 2005). These changes in facial expression occurred virtually instantaneously, suggesting that they were relatively automatic (see Andersen et al., 2005).

Expectancies

There is evidence that acceptance versus rejection by significant others is particularly important for subsequent relationships (Downey & Feldman, 1996; Shields et al., 2001) and that such expectations may be stored in memory as part of relational schemas involving self and other (Baldwin & Sinclair, 1996). We suggest that when a significant-other representation is triggered in the transference context, one's expectations for acceptance and rejection by that significant other should also be activated, and one should thus expect similar treatment at the hands of the new person. Our research has, in fact, demonstrated just this. When participants expect to interact with someone who resembles a positive versus a negative significant other, they are more likely to expect that the new person will be accepting and not rejecting, which does not occur in the absence of transference (Andersen et al., 1996; Berk & Andersen, 2000). Indeed, even when the significant other in question is a parent who sees the individual as falling far short of the parent's standards, and this leads to painful emotional responses for the individual, these individuals still expect more acceptance from a new person who resembles this parent than from a new person who does not. Such evidence may suggest the deep investment people may have in believing in parental acceptance even in troubled relations.

Behavioral Confirmation

The transference process and the relational self would be far less interesting if there were no evidence that the interpersonal dynamics played themselves out in actual interactions with strangers. Because these representations should involve actual interactional dynamics with the other, triggering the significant-other representation should also trigger these interpersonal patterns, and this prediction is supported by the evidence. In a behavioral confirmation paradigm (see Snyder, Tanke, & Berscheid, 1977), in which a perceiver's expectancies may be confirmed by changes in the actual behavior of a target person (a stranger) (Snyder, 1992; Snyder et al., 1977), this line of research on transference was extended into the realm of an in vivo dyadic interaction with a stranger (Berk & Andersen, 2000). In this work, participants engaged in a brief interaction by telephone with another naive individual after reading phrases that supposedly described this new person, phrases drawn from their own significant other (or not). Individuals in the transference condition somehow elicited conversational behavior from the target person consistent with their overall evaluation of their significant-other representation. That is, independent raters who were blind to the participants' condition detected more positive affect in the target's voice in the positive versus negative transference condition, and no such pattern was observed in the control condition. Hence, transference clearly does emerge in actual interpersonal behavior—in terms of the self-fulfilling prophecy or behavioral confirmation processes that are known to occur outside of conscious awareness (Chen & Bargh, 1997).

Evidence on the Relational Self

Working Self-Concept Change

We have also proposed that people experience themselves differently across the various significant relationships in their lives, and thus that each significant-other representation in memory should be linked with a specific relational self (Andersen & Chen, 2002; Andersen & Saribay, 2005). As a result, when a significant-other representation is activated in transference, the aspects of the self associated with that relationship should become active in working memory—changing how one is construing the self at that moment in the direction of the self-when-with-the-significant-other (see also Ogilvie & Ashmore, 1991). Research examining this proposition (Hinkley & Andersen, 1996) began with a pretest session in which participants first described themselves in their own words, then offered descriptions of two significant others, as usual, and afterward were also asked to describe themselves as they are with each of these significant others, again in their own words. Several weeks later, in the experiment, they learned about a new person who resembled either their positive or their negative significant other and were then asked to describe themselves—again in an open-ended format.

This permitted examination of the features of their self-concept in the experiment for how much they overlapped (were similar to) the self with this significant other as described in the prior session. The evidence showed that participants in the transference condition (vs. the control condition) showed more overlap between their self-concept in the experiment and their description of the self with this significant other, adjusting for such overlap at baseline (between their overall self-concept at pretest and the features of the self-with-this-same-other). This effect, in which people become the self they are with their own significant other when in the context of transference, held across both the positive and negative transference conditions. Moreover, in the positive transference, they classified these particular self-concept changes more positively than they did in the negative transference, showing that in transference the self-with-other features entering into the working self-concept take on the evaluative tone of the relationship with the significant other, an effect that did not occur in the control condition.

Interestingly, this effect has also been demonstrated while holding constant the evaluation of the significant other, i.e., by focusing only on positive significant others—and yet ones with whom the individual tends either to experience a dreaded or a desired sense of self (Reznik & Andersen, 2004). This work replicated the effect that overall changes in the working self-concept occur in transference as people became more like the self they are with the significant other than they would otherwise be. In addition, the self-with-other features entering into working memory were negative in this positive transference when this other was associated with a dreaded self, while being positive when associated with a desired self. Hence, the self-worth implications of these changes do not derive primarily from the valence of the significant-other representation, but also derive from the relational self experienced with the significant other.

Approach–Avoidance Motivation

We assume motives one has toward a significant other are stored in memory along with the representations and that, like goals states, such motives can be activated and thus can energize behavior. Research has shown that goal states can be activated quite automatically through contextual cues associated with the goal (e.g., Aarts & Dijksterhuis, 2000; Bargh, 1990, 1997; Bargh & Gollwitzer, 1994), and this work has recently been extended to the domain of interpersonal relationships (Fitzsimons & Bargh, 2003; Shah, 2003a, 2003b). In the transference domain, research has focused particularly on the motive to feel connection and intimacy with others, and on the assumption that activation of a representation of a significant other whom one likes or loves should activate this motive, leading one to desire more closeness with a new person in a positive transference and less in a negative transference. This is, in fact, what the research has shown. The earliest work on goal states with significant others indicated that activating a representation of a positive versus negative significant other in transference evokes enhanced approach motivation toward a new person (Andersen et al., 1996). When expecting to encounter someone who resembles a positive significant other versus a negative one, people become more motivated to be emotionally close to that person rather than wanting to withdraw from or be distant from him or her. This was replicated in later work (Berk & Andersen, 2000), and this notion of a link between significant-other representations and motives has since been extended to other goals (e.g., competition) in recent research outside of the transference context (Fitzsimons & Bargh, 2003).

Self-Protective Regulatory Responses

Self-regulation entails adjusting the self or one's emotions to attain desired end states (Baumeister, 1998; Carver, 2004; Carver & Scheier, 1990;

Gollwitzer, 1996; Higgins, 1998; Taylor, 1991), and the ability to self-regulate is crucial to well-being (e.g., Carver & Scheier, 2003). Self-regulation ability has also been linked to early attachment and socialization experiences (Calkins, Smith, Gill, & Johnson, 1998; Cassidy, 1994; Eisenberg et al., 1999; Rothbart, Ziaie, & O'Boyle, 1992; Sroufe, 1996) and may often be motivated by interpersonal concerns (see Vohs & Ciarocco, 2004).

The first examination of self-regulation in transference was in the research previously described on the working self-concept in transference (Hinkley & Andersen, 1996). As indicated, activating a negative significant-other representation led to negative changes in the self, accounted for by entry of negative self-with-other features into the working self-concept. In addition, however, a compensatory self-regulatory response was also observed. Those aspects of the working self-concept that did not change in the direction of the self-with-other came, in fact, to be evaluated remarkably positively in the negative transference. This did not occur in the control condition, nor did it occur in the positive transference. Thus, participants appear to have compensated for these negative shifts in the self by self-enhancing—using other self-features. Compensatory self-enhancement is by now well understood (see Greenberg & Pyszczynski, 1985) and has, more recently, been found in a transference involving a positive significant other, as well—when this other is associated with a dreaded self (Reznik & Andersen, 2004).

Considered differently, self-regulation should be triggered in transference to the extent that a particular goal or desired outcome is associated with a significant other. According to *regulatory focus theory*, individuals have different strategies for attaining their goals, depending on whether they wish to approach desired outcomes or to avoid aversive ones (Higgins, 1998). The former is termed *promotion focus* and is related to perceived discrepancies between the self and "ideals" about the self, while the latter is termed *prevention focus* and is related to perceived discrepancies between the self and obligations ("oughts"; see Higgins, 1996).

Other research has shown that activating a significant-other representation involving an ideal or actual self-discrepancy triggered the corresponding regulatory focus (Reznik & Andersen, 2005). That is, participants who learned of a new person resembling a significant other from whose point of view they had an ideal discrepancy were less motivated to avoid the new person when they expected to meet the person, compared to when they no longer expected to, while those learning of someone resembling a significant other associated with an ought discrepancy were more motivated to avoid the new person when they expected to meet the person, compared to when they no longer expected to do so. No such effect was observed in the control condition, suggesting that self-regulatory focus was in fact demonstrated in transference.

Other-Protective Regulatory Responses

There is also evidence that people are motivated to protect how they see their significant others and do so by finding ways to regard their shortcomings in positive terms (e.g., Murray & Holmes, 1993). We have termed this other-protective self-regulation and have suggested that, if this process occurs in transference, it should be limited to positive significant others and should be evoked by exposure to negative information about such others. Research has tended to confirm this assumption that other-protective self-regulation will occur in transference under the right circumstances (Andersen et al., 1996). In particular, when individuals are reading descriptions of someone who resembles a positive significant other and are exposed to some of the negative features of this positive significant other, they should show especially positive facial affect. This is exactly what the evidence shows. When reading negative features of the person that they had designated as a positive significant other in a pretest session, participants nonetheless expressed more positive affect facially when in the positive transference condition than in any other condition or for truly positive features. A negative transference evoked no such effect, and it did not occur in the control condition. This suggests that other-protective regulatory responses do occur in transference. Given evidence that relationship satisfaction and longevity is correlated with such regulatory strategies in close relationships (Murray et al., 1996a, 1996b), it may well be that such processes are quite adaptive. They allow people to hold those they care about in positive regard and to maintain these relationships. At the same time, there may be conditions under which processes of this kind are maladaptive. We now turn our attention to such issues.

The Relational Self and Emotional Suffering

The evidence described thus far highlights the profound importance of significant others for how people experience the self. It shows that interpersonal cues one encounters can trigger a mental representation of a significant other and thus lead one to see a new person "through the lens" of this significant other. This is reflected in biased inferences, evaluations, and expectancies for acceptance or rejection, the latter of which is known to be associated with interpersonal suffering (e.g., Ayduk, Downey, & Kim, 2001; Downey, Feldman, & Ayduk, 2000; Downey, Lebolt, Rincon, & Freitas, 1998; Dutton, Saunders, Staromski, & Bartholomew, 1994; Hammen et al., 1995; Mikulincer, 1998). Indeed, the process even leads relevant behavior to actually be elicited from a new person that confirms one's expectancies, which suggests a still more profound influence on people's interpersonal lives. The process also evokes motives to be close to or to be distant with a new person, and a tendency to engage in self-regulatory processes to try to protect the self or to protect the other, depending on the nature of the threat one experiences and on the nature of the relationship.

What we have yet to consider in detail is the precise manner in which the transference process and relational selves may lead to emotional suffering. We now turn to questions of this kind by reviewing transference research that varies the nature of the significant-other relationship under study and associated individual differences, as well as research that manipulates contextual conditions in ways that may be informative. In short, we now consider some of the ways in which the kind of positive affect typically evoked in a positive transference can in fact be disrupted and likewise the circumstances under which negative affect in general, and discrete mood states in particular, may be evoked. Although we make no claim that the shifts in transient mood states we observe are on par with psychopathology, we assume that the mechanisms by which these states are evoked may be general and have implications for some forms of psychopathology, in particular, the affective disorders. To take another example, when the kinds of self-regulatory processes shown in transference—that work to protect the self or to repair mood among "normal" people—end up breaking down, this process may be an analogue for some of what occurs in more profound forms of emotional suffering and psychopathology.

When Positive Mood is Disrupted in Positive Transference

Triggering the Experience of Role Violation. While we have found that transference involving a positive significant other results in increases in positive affect relative to that involving a negative significant other (e.g., Andersen et al., 1996), there are instances in which positive transference leads to negative affect among nonsymptomatic individuals. One such instance is when a new person who is the subject of a positive transference violates the interpersonal role expectancies that derive from the relational role with the significant other. An interpersonal role involves expectations in the relevant relationship, and role violations can disturb that relationship (e.g., Sheldon & Elliot, 2000). Moreover, knowledge about a significant other and the relational role the other typically occupies should be stored in memory. As such, activation of the significant-other representation should also trigger this interpersonal role and the associated relational expectancies. Indeed, research on transference suggests that when transference that involves an authority figure occurs, the authority role the individual occupies is also activated (Baum & Andersen, 1999). This is suggested by evidence showing that when a significant-other relationship with an authority figure is positive, the positive affect that would otherwise be evoked in a relevant transference involving this other is disrupted when it comes to light that the new person cannot fulfill this role (e.g., because he or she is a novice).

Triggering Chronically Unsatisfied Goals. Another instance in which a positive transference can result in negative affect is when the representation triggered is that of an individual with whom one has experienced chronically unsatisfied goals for affection and acceptance (Berk & Andersen, 2004). Under these conditions, what would otherwise be a positive transference, given that the significant other is one who is liked or loved, actually results in increases in hostility. In fact, when the transference involves a positively regarded member of one's own family (a relationship that is a given rather than having been selected), this increase in hostility in the transference context is actually significantly correlated with overt behaviors aimed toward gaining acceptance from the new person. The more hostile participants felt, the harder they tried to gain the love they chronically failed to obtain from their significant other.

Triggering the Dreaded Self. Yet another instance in which positive mood is disrupted in positive transference involves the case of well-loved significant others around whom one finds oneself behaving in ways one wishes one did not. Some significant others, even if regarded positively, are ones around whom an individual may tend to become a dreaded version of the self, such as by becoming excessively obsequious, oppositional, or manipulative (Reznik & Andersen, 2004). We know that triggering a significant-other representation activates the version of the self one experiences with that significant other (Hinkley & Andersen, 1996), and hence transference involving a significant other with whom one experiences a dreaded sense of self should indirectly activate that dreaded self in the transference. The results of this research suggest that this does in fact occur (Reznik & Andersen, 2004). While activating a representation of a positive significant other leads to positive affective states, especially when associated with a desired sense of self, activation of a comparable significant other associated with a dreaded self leads both to increases in negative mood states and to decreases in positive mood states by comparison.

In short, there are numerous circumstances under which even a positive transference, which is otherwise associated with positive evaluations, expectancies, and the like, can, in fact, disrupt positive affect. Presumably, this can be hurtful and even harmful under some circumstances, as a profound disappointment may seriously compromise how one feels able to proceed interpersonally. At the very least, these data show that a positive transference is not always benign and that its affective qualities will depend on other features of the new person, on other contextual cues, or on problematic elements of the prior (positive) relationship. To the degree that a sense of violation is involved, subsequent affect will not be straightforward.

We now turn to a variety of other studies that speak still more precisely to emotional suffering in terms of highly problematic past relationships and/or specific emotional vulnerabilities.

When Abuse History Evokes Emotional Numbing and Other-Protectiveness

One context in one's early life in which emotions may become confused and self-regulatory strategies problematic is that of exposure to physical and psychological abuse by a parent. Childhood abuse is associated with forming maladaptive relational knowledge that can underlie interpersonal difficulties with peers (Shields et al., 2001). Maltreated children tend to hold parental representations that are more negative, constricted, and incoherent than do children who are not maltreated, and these representations tend to predict peer rejection, aggression, and emotion dysregulation. Evidence also suggests that women sexually abused in childhood appear to hold parental schemas that are more hostile than do women who were never abused in childhood, who tend to view their parents as warm and noncontrolling (Cloitre, Cohen, & Scarvalone, 2002), and such parental schemas may generalize to current relationships (Cloitre et al., 2002). Indeed, among a treatment-seeking sample of adult survivors of childhood sexual abuse, revictimized participants reported more interpersonal problems compared with nonrevictimized participants (Classen, Field, Koopman, Nevill-Manning, & Spiegel, 2001).

In research on this topic in the realm of transference, the assumption was that when individuals abused by a parent in childhood encounter a new person who resembles this parent, activating the parental representation should lead to intense ambivalence and to the various other emotional and regulatory sequelae typically experienced in the relationship (Berenson & Andersen, 2005). In particular, such intense fear and other overwhelming emotions may be addressed through coping efforts that reduce perceptions of threat but also lead to there being little relation between physiological and expressive aspects of emotion (Cloitre, Koenen, Cohen, & Han, 2002; Toth & Cicchetti, 1996) and possibly to a kind of "emotional numbing" or to dissociative phenomena (Liotti, 1999; Lyons-Ruth & Jacobvitz, 1999; Main & Hesse, 1990).

Triggering Mistrust, Disliking, and Indifference. In this research, female college students exposed to physical and psychological abuse by a loved parent (or not) learned about a new person who bore some resemblance to this parent (or did not) and expected to interact with this new person, whom they were told was becoming increasingly tense and irritable while waiting. When the new person resembled their parent, participants abused by this parent indicated that they disliked the new person more, felt more mistrust of him or her (a hypervigilant cautious coping strategy), felt persistent expectations for rejection by him or her, and at the same time indicated being indifferent about the latter (a coping strategy involving emotional disengagement)—as compared to nonabused participants—a pattern that was absent or attenuated in the control condition.

Triggering Automatic Positive Facial Affect. Simultaneously, both abused and nonabused participants showed more positive affect in their facial expressions—while reading the descriptors of the new person—when the new person resembled their parent than they did in the control condition. That is, they showed automatic positive facial affect in transference. Moreover, when exposed to the contextual threat cue—the statement that the new person was becoming increasingly irritable—both abused and nonabused participants responded with positive facial affect to this cue in the context of transference, but not in the control condition, indicating the tendency to give the new person the benefit of the doubt, to dismiss negativity about him or her, protecting the other in this way. Such other-protective regulatory strategies may be quite adaptive in healthy relationships, but may be maladaptive among abused individuals for whom such threat cues should presumably serve as potential signals of impending danger, and yet their immediate automatic affect parallels that of nonabused individuals.

Triggering "Emotional Numbing." Finally, given how problematic these individuals' responses to threat may be, as suggested by the child abuse literature, self-reports of dysphoric mood states were also examined with responses to the threat manipulation in the context of transference. In short, the results showed that abused participants in transference showed an attenuation of dysphoric mood when in the presence of the target irritability cue relative to when it was absent, and showed no such effect in the control condition. That is, in the very context in which there was threat in the transference, they reported the least negative affect. Looked at differently, abused participants showed increases in dysphoric mood in transference relative to the control condition when no target-irritability cue was present, but they showed decreases in dysphoria in transference relative to the control condition when exposed to this target-irritability cue. No such effect was observed for nonabused individuals.

When Anxious Mood and Suppressed Hostility Are Evoked via the Attachment System

Another way in which positive affect associated with a parent may be disturbed in a manner that arises in transference can be found when considering individual differences in attachment (e.g., Bowlby, 1969). The attachment system is assumed to be intimately bound up with parents or caretakers, with internal working models of self and other defined in early interactions reflecting the complex affective dynamics in the relationship. Individual differences in attachment have been examined both in infancy (Thompson, 1998) and in adulthood (e.g., Hazan & Shaver, 1994), and the assumption is that individuals who are securely attached are comfortable in their relationships and able to venture out as needed, while those who are insecurely attached are not and instead suffer a variety of emotional conflicts. While attachment style is typically assessed as a generic individual difference, research has recently shown that differing attachment styles can coexist in the same person and that people vary in the attachment style they experience across their various relationships, with the specific nature of the attachment in the specific relationship making a difference both cognitively and affectively (Baldwin, Keelan, Fehr, Enns, & Koh-Rangarajoo, 1996; Pierce & Lydon, 2001). Moreover, contextual cues can also activate the attachment system under the right circumstances (e.g., Mikulincer, Gillath, & Shaver, 2002).

This suggests that activating a parental representation in transference may well activate the attachment system and the specific emotions typically experienced in the relationship. In research on this topic in the transference domain (Andersen, Keczkemethy, & Klinger, 2003), participants were preselected on the basis of their attachment style with one of their parents rather than in terms of generic attachment style, enabling the specific emotional sequelae in this relationship to be the focus. Although there are measurement debates about whether or not attachment style with parents can be assessed by using questionnaires or by other noninterview procedures among adults (see Shaver & Mikulincer, 2002), the present research ventures into this territory. If the evidence were to show that the attachment system is in fact activated in transference, it would be of importance because it would suggest that transference could be an underlying mechanism by which attachment processes arise in everyday relations, a hypothesis that has otherwise gone unexamined.

Triggering Global Positive Affect. The simplest proposition this research examined is the notion that activating a mental representation of a parent in transference should result in increases in positive affect among people with a secure attachment to this parent as compared with those who are insecurely attached to this parent (i.e., classified as avoidant, anxious-ambivalent, or fearful), who should not. The research largely supported this hypothesis, yielding more positive affect among those securely versus insecurely attached, whereas no such effect was apparent in the control condition. Moreover, among those securely attached to the parent, the activation of this parental representation in transference led to increases in global positive mood state as compared with the control condition. Hence, the emotional comfort and ease thought to be part of the attachment system of securely attached individuals is in fact contextually cued in transference, suggesting that transference may be one mechanism by which the attachment system is activated and evoked in daily interactions.

Triggering Anxious Mood in a Preoccupied Attachment. If the attachment system is activated in transference when a parental representation is activated, this should also evoke the discrete emotional responses thought to be associated with the attachment style one has with that parent. That is, individuals with a preoccupied (or anxious–ambivalent) attachment style with the parent should show increases in anxiety in the context of transference as the hallmark of the emotional vulnerability in this relationship associated with this attachment style. When the representation of this parent is activated in transference among individuals with a preoccupied attachment to the parent, it should lead to increases in anxious mood. This is in fact exactly what the evidence shows. Preoccupied (or anxious–ambivalent) individuals showed increases in anxious mood in transference relative to the control condition, and this did not occur for avoidant, fearful, or secure individuals. Considered differently, in the absence of transference, there were no differences between preoccupied individuals and avoidant, fearful, and secure individuals, but in transference the differences in emotional vulnerability were crystal clear.

Triggering Suppression of Hostility in an Avoidant Attachment. On another level, one of the hallmarks of avoidant (or dismissive) attachment style is the lack of affective expressiveness, and especially a lack of negative emotion. If the attachment system is activated when transference is activated, then this should lead avoidant individuals to experience constriction or suppression in negative emotions involving the significant other. The emotion most threatening to relationships and hence this affective state should be particularly likely to be suppressed by avoidant individuals in the context of transference, meaning they should show larger decreases in hostility and resentment in transference than in the control condition as compared with other individuals (i.e., those who are preoccupied, fearful, or secure). The evidence suggests that this is what in fact occurred. The pattern of data for avoidant individuals stood out relative to the pattern for other groups. Avoidants appeared to suppress their hostility in transference as compared with the control condition, in part given the very high degree of hostility they experienced in the absence of transference, higher than any other group. Indeed, other evidence has shown that avoidants may also suppress the accessibility of attachment figures, overall, in response to attachment-related threat, given their motivation to avoid and not to be expressive around them (Mikulincer et al., 2002).

In sum, the transference process appears to evoke the attachment system as reflected both in global positive affect and in specific negative moods (anxiety and hostility), depending on individual differences in attachment dynamics with a loved parent. This is the first evidence we know of to show that transference may be a mechanism by which the attachment system is evoked in everyday life. Given longstanding assumptions that internal working models involving caretakers are integral to the attachment system and evidence that the transference process is evoked by activating a parental representation and associated self-knowledge, assessing these processes in tandem fills a gap in the literature of special theoretical relevance. It is of considerable importance theoretically, given half a century of theorizing on attachment processes and a full century of theory on transference, that both processes are grounded in science as never before and in fact have been shown to co-occur.

ON BEING VULNERABLE TO DEPRESSION: CONCEIVING SIGNIFICANT OTHERS AND PREDICTING THE FUTURE

We now turn to a consideration of some of the processes underlying depression and, specifically, depressive mood states. We take up this question not only within the framework of the relational self and transference, consistent with the work already described, but also from the point of view of an approach to conceptualizing hopelessness in depression and its implications for maladaptive ways of thinking about the future.

First, it is worth noting that several cognitive theories of depression propose that faulty cognitive structures are at the heart of depression. For example, Beck's (1967) theory argues that depression results from dysfunctional mental representations, or *schemas*, that organize information in memory and guide new information processing. The argument is that these *schemas* are acquired in childhood and adolescence as a result of stressful or traumatic events and interpersonal interactions, and are ultimately reflected in a cognitive triad of biased thought processes—involving negative views of the self, the world, and the future. Much research over the past few decades has examined negative views of the self in depression, that is, depressive self-schemas, and although the causal role of self-schemas in precipitating depression has been questioned (e.g., Coyne, 1994), they have also been implicated in the development of depression (see Ingram, Miranda, & Segal, 1998). But in spite of frequent reference to Beck's cognitive triad, relatively little research has examined the degree to which depressives engage in biased or maladaptive processing about the world beyond the self or biased processing about the future. In our work, we have explored each of these domains.

In terms of how people make sense of the world around them, as it pertains to depression, we have given particular emphasis of late to the interpersonal world that people inhabit and how representations of this world may be linked to depressive experiences. Of course, considerable research has examined interpersonal processes in depression (see Hammen, 2000; Joiner et al., 1999; Katz & Joiner, 2001), but from our point of view relatively little work has explicitly targeted mental representations of the interpersonal world in depressive mood states. In our work, the focus is significant others, and we turn to this work now.

When Depressed Mood or Agitated States Are Evoked Stemming from Others' Standards

Broadly speaking, interpersonal models of depression tend to assume that depression results from "a disruption of the social space in which the person obtains support and validation for his experience" (Coyne, 1976, p. 33). Depressed individuals interact with others in ways that actually lead these others to become depressed themselves (Strack & Coyne, 1983). They also do so in ways designed to elicit assurance of support and acceptance but that are ineffective and lead to negative reactions and that increase feelings of rejection and needs for reassurance. Some support for this proposition was obtained in a naturalistic study showing that depressed people, more than those not depressed, cope with stressful events by seeking emotional support in their social environment, perhaps to resolve uncertainty about how they can achieve desired outcomes in their lives (Coyne, Aldwin, & Lazarus, 1981). Other research has also shown that excessive reassurance seeking specifically predicts the development of symptoms of depression (Joiner, 1994; Joiner & Metalsky, 2001; Joiner, Metalsky, Gencoz, & Gencoz, 2001; Joiner & Schmidt, 1998; see also Davila, 2001). Still other work has shown that dysfunctional interpersonal attachment beliefs—about one's inability to depend on others—predict the onset of depression following interpersonal stressors (Hammen et al., 1995).

All told, the evidence that predominates in the literature focuses on the interpersonal dynamics that precipitate or maintain depression. In part because of our interest in addressing beliefs about the world, as in Beck's cognitive triad, we have focused more on mental representations, and in particular those about significant others and standards.

Some emotional vulnerabilities can arise that are based on the standards that significant others hold. The behavior of significant others and the standards that they hold can be sufficiently extreme or out of step with "reality" that one may come to believe one has fallen far short of these standards in the eyes of a given significant other—that living up to these standards is out of reach. One framework for conceptualizing vulnerability to depression in these terms is self-discrepancy theory (Higgins, 1987), which suggests that a discrepancy between one set of standards held in memory and the actual self as one is will create an emotional vulnerability. Moreover, such a discrepancy can be held from the point of view of a significant other or from one's own point of view. Regardless, however, the model suggests that when the actual self is discrepant from hopes and aspirations ("ideals") or from duties and obligations ("oughts"), respectively, it will constitute a distinct emotional vulnerability. A discrepancy between ideal standards and the actual self leaves one vulnerable to experiencing dejection-related affect, while a discrepancy between ought standards and the actual self evokes agitation-related affect. The framework also assumes that mental representations of one's parents are linked by memory to representations of the parent's standards and of self-discrepancies.

Hence, the research on transference examining these issues (Reznik & Andersen, 2005) has suggested that triggering a parental representation among people with such a discrepancy should activate the discrepancy the parent holds, along with the associated emotional vulnerability. In short, in the context of transference when a significant-other representation is activated and one thus comes to see the new person through this lens, one should not only transfer positive expectancies about the significant other to a new person but also sink into despair or become greatly agitated, depending on the standards the parent holds.

Triggering Dejection-Related Affect

In particular, individuals with an ideal self-discrepancy from their parent's standpoint came to experience significant increases in depressed mood when the parental representation was activated in transference as compared to the control condition when the representation was not activated. No such effect occurred among individuals with an ought self-discrepancy. Hence, ideal self-discrepancies can in fact be activated indirectly among ideal-discrepant individuals on the basis of activation of a mental representation when one perceives oneself as falling short of the parent's ideals, and it is this that results in exacerbated depressed mood (Reznik & Andersen,

2005; see Andersen & Chen, 2002; Andersen et al., 2005; Andersen & Saribay, 2005).

Triggering Agitation-Related Affect

Likewise, when a new person resembled their own parent, individuals with ought self-discrepancies (from their parent's standpoint) showed more agitation-related affect—specifically, increases in resentful and hostile mood, and decreases in relaxation and calm—than did comparable participants in the control condition (see also Strauman & Higgins, 1988). Individuals with an ideal self-discrepancy showed no such effect. This evidence demonstrates, again, that self-discrepancies can be activated entirely indirectly by means of the activation of a parental representation in transference—when the self-discrepancy is held from the parent's perspective.

In short, specific negative emotions deriving from individual differences in emotional vulnerabilities associated with a parent can be evoked in transference. This evidence forges a theoretical and empirical link between the relational self, transference, and self-discrepancy theory, and offers more evidence as to the processes that may predict the emergence of discrete affective states in transference—that is, when the content of linkages between the significant other and the self specify such vulnerability. These data also offer some evidence that the way people conceptualize the world around them (beyond the self and the future per se) contributes to depressive mood states, much as would be assumed on the basis of Beck's (1967) cognitive triad.

When Dysphoria in Depressives Is Exacerbated Due to the Imagined Responses of Others

Perhaps because of the special relevance of the social world in people's lives, a relevance that may have particular primacy for some people, Beck (1983, 1987) ultimately refined his theory to distinguish two modes of thinking that presumably predispose people to depression. The tendency to overly value positive interchange with others and to wish for intimacy, acceptance, understanding, and support is known as *sociotropy*, while the tendency to overly value independence and achievement is known as *autonomy*. Although research on these constructs has produced mixed results, evidence has shown that the interaction between high levels of sociotropy and negative interpersonal events is in fact associated with depression (Little & Garber, 2000; Robins, 1990; Robins & Block, 1988; Rude & Burnham, 1993).

One illustration of the ubiquitous importance of the interpersonal world across a wide variety of people is suggested by research on what happens when early relationships are profoundly impaired. For example, research indicates that offspring of depressed mothers tend to have a higher risk for developing depression than do offspring of nondepressed mothers (Weissman, Warner, Wickramaratne, Moreau, & Olfson, 1997), and it has been suggested that an interpersonal impairment hypothesis may explain this risk (Hammen & Brennan, 2001; see also Hammen, 2000). That is, the offspring of depressed women may end up developing social vulnerabilities to depression through the acquisition of maladaptive schemas about other people (and about the self), and thus deficiencies in interpersonal skills, that derive from relationships with these caregivers. Data from a large community sample indicated that offspring of depressed women showed poorer social (though not academic) functioning, reported experiencing more stressful interpersonal life events, and had a more negative view of their capacity to form close friendships (Hammen & Brennan, 2001). In a related vein, longitudinal research has shown that perceptions of interpersonal rejection were found to predict the onset of symptoms of depression among adolescents, while initial levels of depression did not predict subsequent rejection (Nolan, Flynn, & Garber, 2003), suggesting a potentially pivotal role for rejection in depression.

On the basis of evidence of this kind, we assumed in our work that depressed individuals are more likely to have experienced disrupted, problematic personal relationships than are nondepressed individuals (see also Aneshensel, 1985; Barnett & Gotlib, 1988; Benazon & Coyne, 2000; Billings & Moos, 1985; Coyne, 1976; Davila, Bradbury, Cohan, & Tochluk, 1997; Davila, Hammen, Burge, Paley, & Daley, 1995; Hammen, Shih, & Brennan, 2004; Joiner & Coyne, 2000; Oatley & Bolton, 1985; Rao, Hammen, & Daley, 1999). Likewise, their significant-other relationships should be more likely to be ones in which they failed to receive the levels of support and acceptance that they would have preferred and in which they experienced more suffering. Given the mood disturbance inherent in depressive syndromes, depression should also involve a breakdown of self-regulatory responses to negative thoughts and painful moods (e.g., Nolen-Hoeksema, 1991; Teasdale, 1983; Teasdale et al., 2002). This suggests that the transference process should be more likely to evoke mood disturbances among depressed individuals, because the relational self with the significant other is more problematic and the regulatory and mood-repair capacities of depressed individuals are compromised.

As a result, when depressed individuals encounter a new person who resembles a loved significant other from whom they have experienced a sense of rejection, this should evoke in them a painful vulnerability and lead to exacerbation of an already dysphoric mood—as compared with nondepressed individuals in a comparable transference (concerning a loved but rejecting significant other). No such pattern should be observed in the absence of transference.

We examined this hypothesis among a college student sample with moderately significant symptoms of depression that were shown to be stable over three separate assessments (over a period ranging from 1½ months to 3 months) using the Beck Depression Inventory (BDI; Beck, Rush, Shaw, & Emery, 1979). The control sample of nondepressed individuals was also stable over time in their scores on this instrument. In the usual preexperimental session we use in the transference paradigm, participants identified a positive and a negative family member from whom they had not experienced the level of acceptance that they would have preferred (i.e., who had rejected them) at some point in their lives, and then listed both positive and negative descriptions of each. In the later experiment, as usual, some of these positive and negative features were presented to them in paraphrased form as part of a description of a new person whom they were told they would later meet (Andersen et al., in preparation).

On a general level, the results supported prior theory and evidence by showing that moderately depressed participants indicated that they were less motivated to approach and more motivated to avoid the new person, regardless of whether or not the new person resembled a loved but rejecting significant other. Also in line with prior work, they indicated that they expected to be evaluated more negatively by the new person and to be less likely accepted by the new person than did nondepressives. In addition, independently of the experimental manipulations, they reported higher overall levels of sensitivity to rejection (see Downey & Feldman, 1996) and lower levels of state self-esteem (see Heatherton & Polivy, 1991) than did nondepressed individuals, which offers further support for our preselection criteria.

More important, and as predicted, depressed individuals who learned about the new person resembling their loved but rejecting family member showed more exacerbation in their dysphoric mood (controlling for baseline mood at the start of the session) than comparably depressed individuals in the control condition. No such effect occurred among those individuals who were not depressed, suggesting that nondepressed individuals may have had more self-regulatory capacity to protect against the dysphoric mood on the basis of the transference. We know from prior research, as indicated, that activating a significant-other representation in transference activates the relational self typically experienced with this other, and these findings extend this evidence into the realm of depression, at least to individuals suffering subclinical or analogue levels of depression. Triggering a representation of a rejecting family member for whom participants still felt love and regard led to greater increases in depressed mood. Interestingly, no such effect occurred when the rejecting family member was not well loved and in fact was regarded negatively, suggesting that it may be the continuing investment in a rejecting significant-other relationship that is responsible for increases in depressive mood among the depressed individuals in transference.

In this research, beyond assessing self-reported mood states, we also asked participants, shortly after they were exposed to the information about the new person, to describe their own qualities by freely listing a series of sentence completions. We then had independent judges (who were blind to condition) rate the entire description in terms of the degree to which the individual appeared to feel rejected by close others. Judges' ratings showed adequate reliability and were averaged before they were analyzed. As we anticipated, the results showed that depressed individuals in the positive transference with the rejecting significant other, as contrasted with depressives in the control condition, offered characterizations of themselves suggesting (to objective raters) that they felt more rejected, adjusting for their baseline tendency to describe themselves this way, as assessed in the preliminary session. This pattern did not arise for nondepressed individuals. In short, depressed individuals were uniquely responsive to a positive transference involving a rejecting significant other, both in terms of coming to experience and describe themselves as more rejected and in terms of sinking further into dysphoria.

These findings show that depressed individuals are vulnerable to transient changes in their mood states and in their very sense of self, such that their dysphoria and perception of the self as rejected by others are both exacerbated. The fact that this occurs in the context of transference is important in its own right because it demonstrates the relevance of the transference phenomenon to this important clinical domain and suggests that transference may well have implications for the maintenance or exacerbation of depression among individuals experiencing a depressive episode. Moreover, the fact that the transference effect holds only when the significant-other representation involves a rejecting other who is nonetheless loved, and does not extend to negative significant others, is intriguing because it implies that it is the continued engagement in the relationship that makes the loss and lack of acceptance so palpable and painful. This evidence is also quite consistent with research suggesting that rejection sensitivity not only is associated with hypervigilance to cues indicating disapproval and with chronically accessible rejection expectancies (Baldwin & Meunier, 1999; Baldwin & Sinclair, 1996; Downey & Feldman, 1996) but also can result in symptoms of depression when there is a serious interpersonal loss that also communicates rejection (Ayduk et al., 2001).

When Certainty in Future Suffering and Future-Event Schemas May Set In

Our work on depression discussed thus far has examined how conceptualizations of the world—specifically, of significant others and new people—

can constitute a vulnerability to increased depressive affect. Other research we have conducted has taken the different but complementary approach of examining how conceptualizations of the future are associated with depression and can precipitate depressive affect and depressive thought patterns among otherwise not depressed individuals. This program of research arose independently from that on significant others and transference, and developed on the heels of critiques of learned helplessness theory in its original form (e.g., Hollon & Garber, 1980). In particular, in spite of the inadequacies of the learned helplessness model in explaining depression in humans, the attributional reformulation of learned helplessness that emerged to correct this led investigators to focus primarily on how people interpret their pasts—that is, explain outcomes that have already occurred. This led away from expectancies and thus eschewed the problem of the future, which was both conceptually problematic in terms of the original model and in terms of Beck's model and the third element of his proposed triad of negative beliefs—that is, the future.

The conceptual rationale for early work conducted along these lines (Andersen & Lyon, 1987) was that in the etiology of depression it may matter a great deal whether or not one is certain about the continuation or onset of future suffering. If undesired events are merely quite likely but not certain, it may not be pleasant, but it leaves room for hope that the future will not actually transpire in that manner. On the other hand, if dreaded events are seen as inevitable, then future suffering is inevitable and there is no room for hope, and this is what should precipitate the slide into depression. In the tradition of experimental psychopathology, the paradigm testing this hypothesis involved normal college students and an experimental design in which depressive affect was assessed as a function of whether a dreaded outcome was 0%, 25%, 50%, 75%, or 100% likely to occur. The results showed that depressive affect increased precipitously and dichotomously in the 100% (certainty) condition and not as a linear function of incremental increases in probability. This was true both for the manipulated outcome probabilities and the subjective outcome probabilities that research participants perceived (Andersen & Lyon, 1987).

In subsequent research (Andersen, 1990) that built on this work and was emboldened by the hopelessness model of depression (Abramson, Metalsky, & Alloy, 1989), the aim was to demonstrate that naturally occurring depressive symptoms (at subclinical levels) are positively correlated with the perceived inevitability of future suffering—that is, with *depressive predictive certainty*—when controlling for continuous ratings of pessimism about the future. That is, the aim was again to conceptualize hopelessness in dichotomous terms and, in this case, in terms of the certainty both that desired outcomes would not occur and that dreaded outcomes would. The results showed, in a cross-sectional design, that moderately depressed individuals (as assessed by the BDI) made more pessimistic predictions about the future—rating negative events as more likely and positive events as less likely—and also made more of these predictions with certainty, even controlling for pessimism and for generalized hopelessness, both assessed continuously. In a follow-up, again cross-sectional, study, the purported vulnerability factor of depressive attributional style was, when in interaction with stressful life events, associated with predictive certainty and with depression, and certainty appeared to partially mediate this relationship (Andersen, 1990). In later work, a mini-longitudinal design and a different vulnerability factor were examined among college students (Andersen & Schwartz, 1992), and the evidence showed that ambiguity intolerance at the beginning of the semester interacted with stressful life events occurring in the interim to predict both certainty and depression at the end of the semester, and that certainty again appeared to partially mediate the prediction of depression.

On this basis, one might reason that if depressed individuals are certain about the pessimistic predictions they make about the future, it could be because they have developed negatively biased future-event schemas through which they have come to make snap judgments about the future (Andersen et al., 1992). This would imply that depressed individuals make future-event predictions automatically, that is, with little effort. Research examining this question engaged college students who were moderately, mildly, or not depressed in an experimental design in which they predicted whether positive or negative events would happen to them (or to an average person) sometime in the future and did so as quickly as possible while under an attentional load (remembering random digit strings) or while under no such load. Results indicated that moderately depressed individuals made more negatively biased future-event predictions and made their predictions with automaticity, while nondepressed and mildly depressed individuals did not. That is, the attention-demanding task interfered far less with the speed with which they made their predictions than it did for mildly or nondepressed individuals (Andersen et al., 1992), suggesting effortlessness in these responses and supporting the notion that depressives develop well-elaborated future-event schemas. Recent work has replicated these findings with clinically depressed individuals—that is, with college students qualifying for a diagnosis of major depression (Andersen & Limpert, 2001)—and has also shown that future-event schemas seem to co-occur with rumination about the future. Our most recent research has examined the potential relationship between these two processes.

In this most recent work (Miranda & Andersen, 2006), we conceptualized rumination as a kind of extended mental rehearsal in which one tries repeatedly to predict whether or not positive and negative events will happen—to oneself and to others. By this definition, rumination about the future consists of mental operations that can repeatedly be practiced and, as with any other well-practiced mental operation, might become increasingly efficient over time, requiring little mental effort—a heightened efficiency that might be treated as indicative of the "truth" value of the prediction and thus result in *depressive predictive certainty*.

To test this hypothesis, we conducted an experiment in which nondepressed college students took part in a computer-guided session in which they were led repeatedly to make pessimistic predictions about their future (i.e., to predict that negative events would occur and that positive events would not) or to do a completely different task involving the same stimuli (i.e., a lexical decision task, indicating whether or not the phrase included an adjective). Following numerous practice trials of this kind, in which participants were led to make pessimistic, mixed, or optimistic predictions, they completed a final block of test trials in which their predictions were in no way constrained and concerned either the self and another person. Compared to individuals who did the control task using the same stimuli, those who were induced to engage in the mental rehearsal of repeatedly making pessimistic future-event predictions ended up making these predictions increasingly quickly and easily—that is, with increased efficiency—both about the self and about another person. Furthermore, individuals who were induced to practice making pessimistic future-event forecasts also came to show greater depressive predictive certainty. This work suggests that one process through which depressive certainty, or hopelessness, may be acquired is practice, or mental rehearsal, in trying to predict the future. When one repeatedly attempts to decide what the future will hold and tends to come to decisions that are pessimistic in nature—that is, that positive outcomes will not occur and that negative outcomes will—this can produce the kinds of efficiency in thinking about the future shown in the future-event schemas that depressives appear to hold. Given that repetitive thought is known to characterize rumination (Martin & Tesser, 1996; Segerstrom, Stanton, Alden, & Shortridge, 2003) and that it clearly plays an important role in depression (Nolen-Hoeksema, 1991), these findings are of some importance.

In sum, there is accumulating evidence to support the notion that the way people think about the world around them (specifically, significant others and new people) and, moreover, think about what the future will hold may play an important role in the emotional suffering that is part and parcel of depression.

LIMITATIONS OF THIS RESEARCH AND FUTURE DIRECTIONS

Some limitations of the present research should be noted. First, it was conducted with college students, and this could call into question its generalizability to clinical populations and phenomena. Depression in college students, one could argue, does not represent an appropriate analogue for clinical depression (see Coyne, 1994). On the other hand, there is some support for the idea that studies utilizing college student samples often yield similar results to studies that use clinical samples (see Vredenburg, Flett, & Krames, 1993). Furthermore, examining normal processes among nonclinical samples may provide information about how "normal" processes might become maladaptive or pathological. Nevertheless, in order to draw more definitive conclusions about the relevance of normal transference processes to clinical phenomena, it is important to conduct research with clinical samples and/or to assess maladaptive self-regulatory responses in transference prospectively in predicting later psychopathology.

A second limitation might be found in the fact that we examined transference in a laboratory setting in this research—in the face of an anticipated interaction with a new person. Although these processes have been shown to transpire in vivo in actual behavior in a dyadic interaction with a stranger (Berk & Andersen, 2000), we have not examined transference naturalistically in face-to-face interactions with the significant-other representation triggered by means of the interaction, and this is a limitation. Learning about a new person in advance could perhaps lead to different responses than learning about a new person through direct interaction.

Most intriguing from our point of view, little research we know of has directly examined the potential confluence between mental representations of significant others and how people conceptualize the future (although there is one important exception, Oatley & Bolton, 1985). We regard it as quite feasible that conceptions of one's interpersonal life and conceptions of the future are intimately intertwined. That is, we believe it is likely that thoughts about the world and the future, as denoted in Beck's cognitive triad (Beck, 1967), are intertwined. We assume these aspects of thought, along with thoughts about the self, may have a reciprocal influence on one another. As a simple example, we know from our own work that practice in making pessimistic predictions about the self can lead to depressive predictive certainty (concerned with others). We suspect it is also likely that activation of a mental representation of a significant other with whom an individual has experienced high degrees of uncertainty, for example, would activate not only generalized certainty needs but also the tendency to ruminate about whether or not negative and positive future events will occur, which might ultimately result in developing depressive certainty, or hopelessness, about such a future. Alternatively, the experience of loss in a relationship with a loved significant other should set the stage for experiencing a positive transference with a minimally similar other and to selectively attend to signals of loss in this new relationship, which may well lead to maladaptive interactions in the relationship and, in turn, may lead more generalized future-event expectancies to emerge, a fruitful area for future work.

CONCLUDING COMMENTS

In sum, we have shown that relationships with significant people in one's life define not only the nature of the self experienced in other interpersonal contexts but also the precise nature of the emotional suffering being experienced. Painful shifts in free-floating mood states arise on the basis of interpersonal dynamics when they evoke a mental representation of a prior significant other from one's past that happens to be associated with problematic aspects of self or relationship patterns, or with standards that one continually fails to meet. The phenomenon is well supported by a systematic program of empirical research, and the evidence suggests that it is embedded in a social-cognitive process of transference. The relational nature of the self is activated by means of this social-cognitive mechanism in ways that have relevance for emotional suffering and resilience, broadly defined, and, we would argue, for psychopathology as well.

When it comes to mood and anxiety disorders, the work has specific implications for processes involved in psychopathology and potentially also for those involved in psychotherapy (Andersen & Berk, 1998). With respect to depression in particular, which we have considered at some extended length, the evidence on significant others and transference suggests that there is more to depressive mood than how the individual self is conceived. While this has long been known (Coyne, 1976; Joiner, Coyne, & Blalock, 1999), the near exclusive focus on self-schema approaches to depression among the cognitive researchers in the field until quite recently (e.g., Hammen, 2000) has made it particularly critical that empirical work more thoroughly and systematically examine how the way people make sense of the world around them—including the immediate world of their significant others and interpersonal lives writ large—may be related to the emergence of depressive symptoms.

In our view, this comports well with Beck's (1967) cognitive model of depression, in which negative beliefs about the self, the world, and the future may each coalesce into schemas that facilitate the emergence of rapid, automatic thought processes. We regard significant others as part of the overall "world" that people inhabit and thus well positioned within this characterization of the domains of thought relevant to depression. In this spirit, because there is also so little work, relatively speaking, on the question of how depressed individuals in fact conceptualize the future—and whether or not there is a future they can envision that they could stand living in—we have focused as well on research that examines these matters.

That is, we have presented evidence showing that depressed individuals see future suffering as inevitable and tend to make snap judgments about the future. In particular, the people suffering from depression appear to hold well-elaborated future-event schemas in memory that they use quite automatically (i.e., without effort) to decide what the future will hold—namely, that it will involve continued suffering, of which they are certain. Using a complex experimental paradigm, we have also shown that one pathway by which future-event schemas may develop is through continuous mental rehearsal, or practice, in attempting to predict the future, particularly if one ends up making relatively pessimistic predictions. In the tradition of experimental psychopathology, the work suggests one process by which the mental processes associated with depression may arise.

It is our hope that future research will examine and reveal the precise interrelation between interpersonal processes in depression based on the activation and use of significant-other representations and the particular ways in which people ponder future prospects and attempt to know the unknown—that is, what the future will hold. In the meantime, our research thus far suggests that representations of significant others and also of the future can contribute in myriad ways to describing the variability in human suffering and resilience.

ACKNOWLEDGMENTS

This research was funded in part by Grant No. R01-MH48789 from the National Institute of Mental Health.

REFERENCES

Abramson, L. Y., Metalsky, G. I., & Alloy, L. B. (1989). Hopelessness depression: A theory-based subtype of depression. *Psychological Review, 96*, 358–372.

Abramson, L. Y., Seligman, M. E. P., & Teasdale, J. D. (1978). Learned helplessness in humans: Critique and reformation. *Journal of Abnormal Psychology, 87*, 49–74.

Adler, A. (1957). *Understanding human nature.* New York: Fawcett Premier. (Original work published 1927)

Ainsworth, M. D. S., Blehar, M. C., Walters, E., & Wall, S. (1978). *Patterns of attachment: A psychological study of the strange situation.* Hillsdale, NJ: Erlbaum.

Andersen, S. M. (1990). The inevitability of future suffering: The role of depressive predictive certainty in depression. *Social Cognition, 8*, 203–228.

Andersen, S. M., & Baum, A. (1994). Transference in interpersonal relations: Inferences and affect based on significant-other representations. *Journal of Personality, 62*, 459–498.

Andersen, S. M., & Berk, M. S. (1998). Transference in everyday experience: Implications of experimental research for relevant clinical phenomena. *Review of General Psychology, 2,* 81–120.

Andersen, S. M., & Chen, S. (2002). The relational self: An interpersonal social-cognitive theory. *Psychological Review, 109,* 619–645.

Andersen, S. M., & Cole, S. W. (1990). "Do I know you?": The role of significant others in general social perception. *Journal of Personality and Social Psychology, 59,* 383–399.

Andersen, S. M., & Glassman, N. S. (1996). Responding to significant others when they are not there: Effects on interpersonal inference, motivation, and affect. In R. M. Sorrentino & E. T. Higgins (Eds.), *Handbook of motivation and cognition* (Vol. 3, pp. 262–321). New York: Guilford Press.

Andersen, S. M., Glassman, N. S., Chen, S., & Cole, S. W. (1995). Transference in social perception: The role of chronic accessibility in significant-other representations. *Journal of Personality and Social Psychology, 69,* 41–57.

Andersen, S. M., Keczkemethy, C., & Klinger, A. (2003). *Triggering the attachment system in transference: Evoking specific emotions through transiently activating a parental representation.* Unpublished manuscript, New York University.

Andersen, S. M., & Limpert, C. (2001). Future-event schemas: Automaticity and rumination in Major Depression. *Cognitive Therapy and Research, 25,* 311–333.

Andersen, S. M., & Lyon, J. E. (1987). Anticipating undesired outcomes: The role of outcome uncertainty in the onset of depressive affect. *Journal of Experimental Social Psychology, 23,* 428–443.

Andersen, S. M., Miranda, R., & Edwards, T. (1996). *The walking wounded: Worsening dysphoria among depressed individuals through indirect activation of rejection expectancies in transference.* Manuscript in preparation.

Andersen, S. M., Reznik, I., & Chen, S. (1997). The self in relation to others: Motivational and cognitive underpinnings. In J. G. Snodgrass & R. L. Thompson (Eds.), *The self across psychology: Self-recognition, self awareness, and the self-concept* (pp. 233–275). New York: New York Academy of Science.

Andersen, S. M., Reznik, I., & Glassman, N. S. (2005). The unconscious relational self. In R. Hassin, J. S. Uleman, & J. A. Bargh (Eds.), *The new unconscious.* New York: Oxford University Press.

Andersen, S. M., Reznik, I., & Manzella, L. M. (1996). Eliciting facial affect, motivation, and expectancies in transference: Significant-other representations in social relations. *Journal of Personality and Social Psychology, 71,* 1108–1129.

Andersen, S. M., & Saribay, S. A. (2005). The relational self and transference: Evoking motives, self-regulation, and emotions through activation of mental representations of significant others. In M. Baldwin (Ed.), *The interpersonal self* (pp. 1–32). New York: Guilford Press.

Andersen, S. M., & Schwartz, A. H. (1992). Intolerance of ambiguity and depression: A cognitive vulnerability factor linked to hopelessness. *Social Cognition, 10,* 271–298.

Andersen, S. M., Spielman, L. A., & Bargh, J. A. (1992). Future-event schemas and certainty about the future: Automaticity in depressives' future-event predictions. *Journal of Personality and Social Psychology, 63,* 711–723.

Aneshensel, C. S. (1985). The natural history of depressive symptoms: Implications for psychiatric epidemiology. *Research in Community and Mental Health, 5,* 45–75.

Aron, A., & Aron, E. N. (1996). Self and self-expansion in relationships. In G. J. O. Fletcher & J. Fitness (Eds.), *Knowledge structures in close relationships: A social psychology approach* (pp. 325–344). Mahwah, NJ: Erlbaum.

Aron, A., Aron, E. N., Tudor, M., & Nelson, G. (1991). Close relationships as including other in the self. *Journal of Personality and Social Psychology, 60,* 241–253.

Aron, A., & Fraley, B. (1999). Relationship closeness as including other in the self: Cognitive underpinnings and measures. *Social Cognition, 17,* 140–160.

Ayduk, O., Downey, G., & Kim, M. (2001). Rejection sensitivity and depressive symptoms in women. *Personality and Social Psychology Bulletin, 27,* 868–877.

Ayduk, O., Mendoza-Denton, R., Mischel, W., Downey, G., Peake, P. K., & Rodriguez, M. (2000). Regulating the interpersonal self: Strategic self-regulation for coping with rejection sensitivity. *Journal of Personality and Social Psychology, 79,* 776–792.

Bakan, D. (1966). *The duality of human existence.* Chicago: Rand McNally.

Baldwin, M. W. (1992). Relational schemas and the processing of information. *Psychological Bulletin, 112,* 461–484.

Baldwin, M. W., Fehr, B., Keedian, E., Seidel, M., & Thompson, D. W. (1993). An exploration of the relational schemata underlying attachment styles: Self-report and lexical decision approaches. *Personality and Social Psychology Bulletin, 19,* 746–754.

Baldwin, M. W., Keelan, J. P. R., Fehr, B., Enns, V., & Koh-Rangarajoo, E. (1996). Social-cognitive conceptualization of attachment working models: Availability and accessibility effects. *Journal of Personality and Social Psychology, 71,* 94–109.

Baldwin, M. W., & Meunier, J. (1999). The cued activation of attachment relational schemas. *Social Cognition, 17,* 209–227.

Baldwin, M. W., & Sinclair, L. (1996). Self-esteem and "if. . . then" contingencies of interpersonal acceptance. *Journal of Personality and Social Psychology, 71,* 1130–1141.

Bandura, A. (1977). Self-efficacy: Toward a unifying theory of behavioral change. *Psychological Review, 84,* 191–215.

Bandura, A. (1986). *Social foundations of thought and action: A social cognitive theory.* Englewood Cliffs, NJ: Prentice Hall.

Bandura, A. (1989). Human agency in social–cognitive theory. *American Psychologist, 44,* 1175–1184.

Bargh, J. A. (1990). Auto-motives: Preconscious determinants of social interaction. In E. T. Higgins & R. M. Sorrentino (Eds.), *Handbook of motivation and cognition: Foundations of social behavior* (Vol. 2, pp. 93–130). New York: Guilford Press.

Bargh, J. A. (1997). The automaticity of everyday life. In R. S. Wyer, Jr. (Ed.), *Advances in social cognition* (Vol. 10, pp. 1–61). Mahwah, NJ: Erlbaum.

Bargh, J. A., Chaiken, S., Raymond, P., & Hymes, C. (1996). The automatic evaluation effect: Unconditionally automatic attitude activation with a pronunciation task. *Journal of Experimental Social Psychology, 32,* 185–210.

Bargh, J. A., & Gollwitzer, P. M. (1994). Environmental control of goal-directed action: Automatic and strategic contingencies between situations and behavior. *Nebraska Symposium on Motivation, 41,* 71–124.

Barnett, P. A., & Gotlib, I. H. (1988). Psychosocial functioning and depression: Distinguishing among antecedents, concomitants, and consequences. *Psychological Bulletin, 104,* 97–126.

Batson, C. D. (1990). How social an animal? The human capacity for caring. *American Psychologist, 45,* 336–346.

Baum, A., & Andersen, S. M. (1999). Interpersonal roles in transference: Transient mood states under the condition of significant-other activation. *Social Cognition, 17,* 161–185.

Baumeister, R. F. (1998). The self. In D. T. Gilbert, S. T. Fiske, & G. Lindzey (Eds.), *Handbook of social psychology* (4th ed., pp. 680–740). New York: McGraw-Hill.

Baumeister, R. F., & Leary, M. R. (1995). The need to belong: Desire for interpersonal attachments as a fundamental human motivation. *Psychological Bulletin, 117,* 497–529.

Beck, A. T. (1967). *Depression: Causes and treatment.* Philadelphia: University of Pennsylvania Press.

Beck, A. T. (1987). Cognitive model of depression. *Journal of Cognitive Psychotherapy, 1,* 2–27.

Beck, A. T., Epstein, N., & Harrison, R. (1983). Cognitions, attitudes and personality dimensions in depression. *British Journal of Cognitive Psychotherapy, 1,* 1–16.

Beck, A. T., Rush, A. J., Shaw, B. F., & Emery, G. (1979). *Cognitive therapy of depression.* New York: Guilford Press.

Becker, E. (1971). *The birth and death of meaning* (2nd ed.). New York: Free Press.

Benazon, N. R., & Coyne, J. C. (2000). Living with a depressed spouse. *Journal of Family Psychology, 14,* 71–79

Berenson, K. R., & Andersen, S. M. (2005). *Childhood physical and emotional abuse by a parent: Transference-based manifestations in adult interpersonal relations.* Manuscript under review, New York University.

Berk, M. S., & Andersen, S. M. (2000). The impact of past relationships on interpersonal behavior: Behavioral confirmation in the social–cognitive process of transference. *Journal of Personality and Social Psychology, 79,* 546–562.

Berk, M. S., & Andersen, S. M. (2004). *Chronically unsatisfied goals with significant others: Triggering unfulfilled needs for love and acceptance in transference.* Unpublished manuscript, New York University.

Billings, A. G., & Moos, R. H. (1985). Psychosocial processes of remission in unipolar depression: Comparing depressed patients with matched community controls. *Journal of Consulting and Clinical Psychology, 53,* 314–325.

Bombar, M., & Littig, L., Jr. (1996). Babytalk as a communication of intimate attachment: An initial study in adult romances and friendships. *Personal Relationships, 3,* 137–158.

Bowlby, J. (1969). *Attachment and loss: Vol. 1. Attachment.* New York: Basic Books.

Bowlby, J. (1973). *Attachment and loss: Vol. 2. Separation: Anxiety and anger.* New York: Basic Books.

Bowlby, J. (1980). *Attachment and loss: Vol. 3. Loss: Sadness and depression.* New York: Basic Books.

Bretherton, I. (1985). Attachment theory: Retrospect and prospect. *Monographs for the Society for Research in Child Development, 50,* 3–35.

Bruner, J. S. (1957). Going beyond the information given. In H. E. Gruber, K. R. Hammond, & R. Jessor (Eds.), *Contemporary approaches to cognition* (pp. 41–69). Cambridge, MA: Harvard University Press.

Calkins, S. D., Smith, C. L., Gill, K. L., & Johnson, M. C. (1998). Maternal interactive style across contexts: Relations to emotional, behavioral, and physiological regulation during toddlerhood. *Social Development, 7,* 350–369.

Carver, C. S. (2004). Action and affect. In R. F. Baumeister & K. D. Vohs (Eds.), *Handbook of self-regulation: Research, theory, and applications* (pp. 13–39). New York: Guilford Press.

Carver, C. S., & Scheier, M. F. (1990). Principles of self-regulation: Action and emotion. In E. T. Higgins & R. M. Sorrentino (Eds.), *Handbook of motivation and cognition: Foundations of social behavior* (Vol. 2, pp. 3–52). New York: Guilford Press.

Carver, C. S., & Scheier, M. F. (2003). Self-regulatory processes and responses to health threats: Effects of optimism on well-being. In J. Suls & K. A. Wallston (Eds.), *Social psychological foundations of health and illness: Blackwell series in health psychology and behavioral medicine* (pp. 395–428). Malden, MA: Blackwell.

Cassidy, J. (1994). Emotion regulation: Influences of attachment relationships. Emotion regulation: Behavioral and biological considerations. *Monographs of the Society for Research in Child Development, 59,* 228–249.

Chen, M., & Bargh, J. A. (1997). Nonconscious behavioral confirmation processes: The self-fulfilling consequences of automatic stereotype activation. *Journal of Experimental Social Psychology, 33,* 541–560.

Chen, S., & Andersen, S. M. (1999). Relationships from the past in the present: Significant-other representations and transference in interpersonal life. In M. P. Zanna (Ed.), *Advances in experimental social psychology* (Vol. 31, pp. 123–190). San Diego, CA: Academic Press.

Chen, S., Andersen, S. M., & Hinkley, K. (1999). Triggering transference: Examining the role of applicability and use of significant-other representations in social perception. *Social Cognition, 17,* 332–365.

Classen, C., Field, N. P., Koopman, C., Nevill-Manning, K., & Spiegel, D. (2001). Interpersonal problems and their relationship to sexual revictimization among women sexually abused in childhood. *Journal of Interpersonal Violence, 16,* 495–509.

Cloitre, M., Cohen, L. R., & Scarvalone, P. (2002). Understanding revictimization among childhood sexual abuse survivors: An interpersonal schema approach. *Journal of Cognitive Psychotherapy, 16,* 91–112.

Cloitre, M., Koenen, K. C., Cohen, L. R., & Han, H. (2002). Skills training in affective and interpersonal regulation followed by exposure: A phase-based treatment for PTSD related to childhood abuse. *Journal of Consulting and Clinical Psychology, 70,* 1067–1074.

Coyne, J. C. (1976). Toward an interactional description of depression. *Psychiatry, 39,* 28–40.

Coyne, J. C. (1994). Self-reported distress: Analog or ersatz depression? *Psychological Bulletin, 116,* 29–45.

Coyne, J. C., Aldwin, C., & Lazarus, R. S. (1981). Depression and coping in stressful episodes. *Journal of Abnormal Psychology, 90*, 439–447.

Crocker, J., & Wolfe, C. T. (2001). Contingencies of worth. *Psychological Review, 108*, 593–623.

Davila, J. (2001). Refining the association between excessive reassurance seeking and depressive symptoms: The role of related interpersonal constructs. *Journal of Social and Clinical Psychology, 20*, 538–559.

Davila, J., Bradbury, T. N., Cohan, C. L., & Tochluk, S. (1997). Marital functioning and depressive symptoms: Evidence for a stress-generation model. *Journal of Personality and Social Psychology, 73*, 849–861.

Davila, J., Hammen, C., Burge, D., Paley, B., & Daley, S. (1995). Poor interpersonal problem-solving as a mechanism of stress generation in depression among adolescent women. *Journal of Abnormal Psychology, 104*, 592–600.

Deci, E. L. (1995). *Why we do what we do.* New York: Putnam.

Deci, E. L., & Ryan, R. M. (1985). *Intrinsic motivation and self-determination in human behavior.* New York: Plenum Press.

Downey, G., & Feldman, S. I. (1996). Implications of rejection sensitivity for intimate relationships. *Journal of Personality and Social Psychology, 70*, 1327–1343.

Downey, G., Feldman, S., & Ayduk, O. (2000). Rejection sensitivity and male violence in romantic relationships. *Personal Relationships, 7*, 45–61.

Downey, G., Lebolt, A., Rincon, C., & Freitas, A. L. (1998). Rejection sensitivity and children's interpersonal difficulties. *Child Development, 69*, 1072–1089.

Duckworth, K. L., Bargh, J. A., Garcia, M., & Chaiken, S. (2002). The automatic evaluation of novel stimuli. *Psychological Science, 13*, 513–519.

Dutton, D. G., Saunders, K., Staromski, A., & Bartholomew, K. (1994). Intimacy anger and insecure attachment as precursors of abuse in intimate relationships. *Journal of Applied Social Psychology, 24*, 145–156.

Eisenberg, N., Fabes, R. A., Shepard, S. A., Guthrie, I. K., Murphy, B. C., & Reiser, M. (1999). Parental reactions to children's negative emotions: Longitudinal relations to quality of children's social functioning. *Child Development, 70*, 513–534.

Epstein, S. (1973). The self-concept revisited or a theory of a theory. *American Psychologist, 28*, 405–416.

Fairbairn, W. R. D. (1952). *Psychoanalytic studies of personality.* London: Tavistock.

Fiske, S. T., & Pavelchak, M. (1986). Category-based versus piecemeal-based affective responses: Developments in schema-triggered affect. In R. M. Sorrentino & E. T. Higgins (Eds.), *Handbook of motivation and cognition* (pp. 167–203). New York: Guilford Press.

Fitzsimons, G. M., & Bargh, J. A. (2003). Thinking of you: Nonconscious pursuit of interpersonal goals associated with relationship partners. *Journal of Personality and Social Psychology, 84*, 148–164.

Freud, S. (1958). The dynamics of transference. In J. Strachey (Ed., & Trans.), *The standard edition of the complete psychological works of Sigmund Freud* (Vol. 12, pp. 97–108). London: Hogarth. (Original work published 1912)

Freud, S. (1963). The *dynamics of transference: Therapy and technique.* New York: Macmillan. (Original work published 1912)

Glassman, N. S., & Andersen, S. M. (1999a). Activating transference without consciousness: Using significant-other representations to go beyond what is subliminally given *Journal of Personality and Social Psychology, 77,* 1146–1162.

Glassman, N. S., & Andersen, S. M. (1999b). Transference in social cognition: Persistence and exacerbation of significant-other based inferences over time. *Cognitive Therapy and Research, 23,* 75–91.

Gollwitzer, P. M. (1996). The volitional benefits of planning. In P. M. Gollwitzer & J. A. Bargh (Eds.), *The psychology of action: Linking cognition and motivation to behavior* (pp. 287–312). New York: Guilford Press.

Greenberg, J., & Pyszczynski, T. (1985). Compensatory self-inflation: A response to the threat to self-regard of public failure. *Journal of Personality and Social Psychology, 49,* 273–280.

Greenberg, J. R., & Mitchell, S. A. (1983). *Object relations in psychoanalytic theory.* Cambridge, MA: Harvard University Press.

Guisinger, S., & Blatt, S. J. (1994). Individuality and relatedness: Evolution of a fundamental dialectic. *American Psychologist, 49,* 104–111.

Gurung, R. A. R., Sarason, B. R., & Sarason, I. G. (2001). Predicting relationship quality and emotional reactions to stress from significant-other-concept clarity. *Personality and Social Psychology Bulletin, 27,* 1267–1276.

Hammen, C. (2000). Interpersonal factors in an emerging developmental model of depression. In S. L. Johnson, & A. M. Hayes (Eds.), *Stress, coping, and depression* (pp. 71–88). Mahwah, NJ: Erlbaum.

Hammen, C., & Brennan, P. A. (2001). Depressed adolescents of depressed and nondepressed mothers: Tests of an interpersonal impairment hypothesis. *Journal of Consulting and Clinical Psychology, 69,* 284–294.

Hammen, C. L., Burge, D., Daley, S. E., Davila, J., Paley, B., & Rudolph, K. D. (1995). Interpersonal attachment cognitions and prediction of symptomatic responses to interpersonal stress. *Journal of Abnormal Psychology, 104,* 436–443.

Hammen, C., Shih, J. H., & Brennan, P. A. (2004). Intergenerational transmission of depression test of an interpersonal stress model in a community sample. *Journal of Consulting and Clinical Psychology, 72,* 512–522.

Hazan, C., & Shaver, P. (1994). Attachment as an organizational framework for research on close relationships. *Psychological Inquiry, 5,* 1–22.

Heatherton, T. F., & Polivy, J. (1991). Development and validation of a scale for measuring state self-esteem. *Journal of Personality and Social Psychology, 60,* 895–910.

Helgeson, V. S. (1994). Relation of agency and communion to well-being: Evidence and potential explanations. *Psychological Review, 116,* 412–428.

Higgins, E. T. (1987). Self discrepancy: A theory relating self and affect. *Psychological Review, 94,* 319–340.

Higgins, E. T. (1989). Knowledge accessibility and activation: Subjectivity and suffering from unconscious sources. In J. S. Uleman & J. A. Bargh (Eds.), *Unintended thought* (pp. 75–123). New York: Guilford Press.

Higgins, E. T. (1991). Development of self-regulatory and self-evaluative processes: Costs, benefits, and tradeoffs. In M. R. Gunnar & L. A. Stroufe (Eds.), *Self processes and development: The Minnesota Symposia on Child Development* (Vol. 23, pp. 125–165). Hillsdale, NJ: Erlbaum.

Higgins, E. T. (1996). Ideals, oughts, and regulatory focus: Affect and motivation from distinct pains and pleasures. In P. M. Gollwitzer & J. A. Bargh (Eds.), *The psychology of action* (pp. 91–114). New York: Guilford Press.

Higgins, E. T. (1998). Promotion and prevention: Regulatory focus as a motivational principle. In M. P. Zanna (Ed.), *Advances in experimental social psychology* (Vol. 30, pp. 1–46). New York: Academic Press.

Hinkley, K., & Andersen, S. M. (1996). The working self-concept in transference: Significant-other activation and self change. *Journal of Personality and Social Psychology, 71,* 1279–1295.

Hollon, S. D., & Garber, J. (1980). A cognitive-expectancy theory for helplessness and depression. In J. Garber & M. E. P. Seligman (Eds.), *Human helplessness: Theory and applications.* New York: Academic Press.

Horney, K. (1939). *New ways in psychoanalysis.* New York: Norton.

Horney, K. (1945). *Our inner conflicts.* New York: Norton.

Ingram, R. E., Miranda, J., & Segal, Z. V. (1998). *Cognitive vulnerability to depression.* New York: Guilford Press.

Joiner, T. E. (1994). Contagious depression: Existence, specificity, to depressed symptoms, and the role of reassurance seeking. *Journal of Personality and Social Psychology, 67,* 287–296.

Joiner, T., & Coyne, J. C. (Ed.). (1999). *The interpersonal nature of depression: Advances in interpersonal approaches.* Washington, DC: American Psychological Association.

Joiner, T., Coyne, J. C., & Blalock, J. (1999). On the interpersonal nature of depression: Overview and synthesis. In T. E. Joiner & J. C. Coyne (Eds.), *The interactional nature of depression: Advances in interpersonal approaches* (pp. 3–19). Washington, DC: American Psychological Association.

Joiner, T. E., & Metalsky, G. I. (2001). Excessive reassurance seeking: Delineating a risk factor involved in the development of depressive symptoms. *Psychological Science, 12,* 371–378.

Joiner, T. E., Metalsky, G. I., Gencoz, F., & Gencoz, T. (2001). The relative specificity of excessive reassurance-seeking to depressive symptoms and diagnoses among clinical samples of adults and youth. *Journal of Psychopathology and Behavioral Assessment, 23,* 35–41.

Joiner, T. E., & Schmidt, N. B. (1998). Excessive reassurance-seeking predicts depressive but not anxious reactions to acute stress. *Journal of Abnormal Psychology, 107,* 533–537.

Katz, J., & Joiner, T. E., Jr. (2001). The aversive interpersonal context of depression: Emerging perspectives on depressotypic behavior. In R. M. Kowalski (Ed.), *Behaving badly: Aversive behaviors in interpersonal relationships* (pp. 117–147). Washington, DC: American Psychological Association.

Kelly, G. A. (1955). *The psychology of personal constructs.* New York: Norton.

Kernberg, O. (1976). *Object relations theory and clinical psychoanalysis.* New York: Aronson.

Leary, M. R., Tambor, E. S., Terdal, S. K., & Downs, D. L. (1995). Self-esteem as an interpersonal monitor: The sociometer hypothesis. *Journal of Personality and Social Psychology, 68,* 518–530.

Linville, P. W., & Fischer, G. W. (1993). Exemplar and abstraction models of perceived group variability and stereotypicality. *Social Cognition, 11,* 92–125.

Liotti, G. (1999). Disorganization of attachment as a model for understanding dissociative psychopathology. In J. Solomon & C. George (Eds.), *Attachment disorganization* (pp. 291–317). New York: Guilford Press.

Little, S. A., & Garber, J. (2000). Interpersonal and achievement orientations and specific stressors predicting depressive and aggressive symptoms in children. *Cognitive Therapy and Research, 24*, 651–670.

Lyons-Ruth, K., & Jacobvitz, D. (1999). Attachment disorganization: Unresolved loss, relational violence, and lapses in behavioral and attentional strategies. In J. Cassidy & P. R. Shaver (Eds.), *Handbook of attachment: Theory, research, and clinical applications* (pp. 520–554). New York: Guilford Press.

Main, M., & Hesse, E. (1990). Parents' unresolved traumatic experiences are related to infant disorganized attachment status: Is frightened and/or frightening parental behavior the linking mechanism? In M. T. Greenberg & D. Cicchetti (Eds.), *Attachment in the preschool years: Theory, research, and intervention* (pp. 161–182). Chicago: University of Chicago Press.

Markus, H., & Kitayama, S. (1991). Culture and the self: Implications for cognition, emotion, and motivation. *Psychological Review, 98*, 224–253.

Martin, L. L., & Tesser, A. (1996). Some ruminative thoughts. In R. S. Wyer, Jr. (Ed.), *Advances in social cognition* (pp. 1–47). Hillsdale, NJ: Erlbaum.

McAdams, D. P. (1985). *Power, intimacy. and the life story: Personological inquiries into identity.* New York: Guilford Press.

McAdams, D. P. (1989). *Intimacy: The need to be close.* New York: Doubleday.

McGowan, S. (2002). Mental representations in stressful situations: The calming and distressing effects of significant others. *Journal of Experimental Social Psychology, 38*, 152–161.

Mikulincer, M. (1995). Attachment style and the mental representation of the self. *Journal of Personality and Social Psychology, 69*, 1203–1215.

Mikulincer, M. (1998). Adult attachment style and individual differences in functional versus dysfunctional experiences of anger. *Journal of Personality and Social Psychology, 74*, 513–524.

Mikulincer, M., Gillath, O., & Shaver, P. R. (2002). Activation of the attachment system in adulthood: Threat-related primes increase the accessibility of mental representations of attachment figures. *Journal of Personality and Social Psychology, 83*, 881–895.

Mills, J., & Clark, M. S. (1994). Communal and exchange relationships: Controversies and research. In R. Erber & R. Gilmour (Eds.), *Theoretical frameworks for personal relationships* (pp. 29–42). Hillsdale, NJ: Erlbaum.

Miranda, R., & Andersen, S. M. (2006). *On acquiring hopelessness: Rehearsal of pessimistic predictions about the future induces processing efficiency and depressive certainty.* Manuscript in preparation.

Mischel, W., & Shoda, Y. (1995). A cognitive-affective system theory of personality: Reconceptualizing situations, dispositions, dynamics, and invariance in personality structure. *Psychological Review, 102*, 246–268.

Murray, S. L., & Holmes, J. G. (1993). Seeing virtues in faults: Negativity and the transformation of interpersonal narratives in close relationships. *Journal of Personality and Social Psychology, 65*, 707–722.

Murray, S. L., & Holmes, J. G. (1999). The (mental) ties that bind: Cognitive structures that predict relationship resilience. *Journal of Personality and Social Psychology, 77,* 1228–1244.

Murray, S. L., Holmes, J. G., & Griffin, D. W. (1996a). The benefits of positive illusions: Idealization and the construction of satisfaction in close relationships. *Journal of Personality and Social Psychology, 70,* 79–98.

Murray, S. L., Holmes, J. G., & Griffin, D. W. (1996b). The self-fulfilling nature of positive illusions in romantic relationships: Love is not blind, but prescient. *Journal of Personality and Social Psychology, 71,* 1155–1180.

Nolen-Hoeksema, S. (1991). Responses to depression and their effects on the duration of depressive episodes. *Journal of Abnormal Psychology, 100,* 569–582.

Nolan, S. A., Flynn, C., & Garber, J. (2003). Prospective relations between rejection and depression in young adolescents. *Journal of Personality and Social Psychology, 85,* 745–755.

Oatley, K., & Bolton, W. (1985). A social-cognitive theory of depression in reaction to life events. *Psychological Review, 92,* 372–388.

Ogilvie, D. M., & Ashmore, R. D. (1991). Self-with-other representation as a unit of analysis in self-concept research. In R. C. Curtis (Ed.), *The relational self: Theoretical convergencies in psychoanalysis and social psychology* (pp. 282–314). New York: Guilford Press.

Pierce, T., & Lydon, J. (1998). Priming relational schemas: Effects of contextually activated and chronically accessible interpersonal expectations on responses to a stressful event. *Journal of Personality and Social Psychology, 75,* 1441–1448.

Pierce, T., & Lydon, J. E. (2001). Global and specific relational models in the experience of social interactions. *Journal of Personality and Social Psychology, 80,* 613–631.

Rao, U., Hammen, C., & Daley, S. (1999). Continuity of depression during the transition to adulthood: A 5–year longitudinal study of young women. *Journal of the American Academy of Child and Adolescent Psychiatry, 38,* 908–915.

Reznik, I., & Andersen, S. M. (2004). *Being one's dreaded self: Painful self-experience concerning positive significant others in transference.* Unpublished manuscript, New York University.

Reznik, I., & Andersen, S. M. (2005). *Agitation and despair in relation to parents: Activating emotional suffering in transference.* Manuscript under review. New York University.

Robins, C. J. (1990). Congruence of personality and life events in depression. *Journal of Abnormal Psychology, 99,* 393–397.

Robins, C. J., & Block, P. (1988). Personal vulnerability, life events, and depressive symptoms: A test of a specific interactional model. *Journal of Personality and Social Psychology, 54,* 847–852.

Rogers, C. (1951). *Client-centered therapy.* Boston: Houghton-Mifflin.

Rothbart, M. K., Ziaie, H., & O'Boyle, C. G. (1992). Self-regulation and emotion in infancy. *New Directions for Child Development, 55,* 7–23.

Rude, S. S., & Burnham, B. L. (1993). Do interpersonal and achievement vulnerabilities interact with congruent events to predict depression? Comparison of DEQ, SAS, DAS, and combined scales. *Cognitive Therapy and Research, 17,* 531–548.

Russell, J. A. (2003). Core affect and the psychological construction of emotion. *Psychological Review, 110,* 145–172.

Safran, J. D. (1990). Toward a refinement of cognitive therapy in light of interpersonal theory: I. Theory. *Clinical Psychology Review, 10,* 87–105.

Safran, J. D., & Segal, Z. V. (1990). *Interpersonal process in cognitive therapy.* Northvale, NJ: Jason Aronson.

Segerstrom, S. C., Stanton, A. L., Alden, L. E., & Shortridge, B. E. (2003). A multidimensional structure for repetitive thought: What's on your mind, and how, and how much? *Journal of Personality and Social Psychology, 85,* 909–921.

Seligman, M. E. P. (1975). *Helplessness: On depression, development, and death.* San Francisco: Freeman.

Shah, J. (2003a). Automatic for the people: How representations of significant others implicitly affect goal pursuit. *Journal of Personality and Social Psychology, 84,* 661–681.

Shah, J. (2003b). The motivational looking glass: How significant others implicitly affect goal appraisals. *Journal of Personality and Social Psychology, 85,* 424–439.

Shaver, P. R., & Mikulincer, M. (2002). Attachment-related psychodynamics. *Attachment and Human Development, 4,* 133–161.

Shields, A., Ryan, R. M., & Cicchetti, D. (2001). Narrative representations of caregivers and emotion dysregulation as predictors of maltreated children's rejection by peers. *Developmental Psychology, 37,* 321–337.

Sheldon, K. M., & Elliot, A. J. (2000). Personal goals in social roles: Divergences and convergences across roles and levels of analysis. *Journal of Personality, 68,* 51–84.

Simpson, J. A., & Rholes, W. S. (1998). *Attachment theory and close relationships.* New York: Guilford Press.

Smith, E. R., Murphy, J., & Coats, S. (1999). Attachment to groups: Theory and management. *Journal of Personality and Social Psychology, 77,* 94–110.

Smith, E. R., & Zarate, M. A. (1992). Exemplar-based model of social judgment. *Psychological Review, 99,* 3–21.

Snyder, M. (1992). Motivational foundations of behavioral confirmation. In M. P. Zanna (Ed.), *Advances in experimental social psychology* (Vol. 25, pp. 67–114). New York: Academy Press.

Snyder, M., Tanke, E. D., & Berscheid, E. (1977). Social perception and interpersonal behavior: On the self-fulfilling nature of social stereotypes. *Journal of Personality and Social Psychology, 35,* 656–666.

Sroufe, A. L. (1996). *Emotional development: The organization of emotional life in the early years.* New York: Cambridge University Press.

Strack, S., & Coyne, J. C. (1983). Social confirmation of dysphoria: Shared and private reactions to depression. *Journal of Personality and Social Psychology, 44,* 798–806.

Strauman, T. J., & Higgins, E. T. (1988). Self-discrepancies as predictors of vulnerability to distinct syndromes of chronic emotional distress. *Journal of Personality, 56,* 685–707.

Sullivan, H. S. (1940). *Conceptions in modern psychiatry.* New York: Norton.

Sullivan, H. S. (1953). *The interpersonal theory of psychiatry.* New York: Norton.

Taylor, S. E. (1991). Asymmetrical effects of positive and negative events: The mobilization minimization hypothesis. *Psychological Bulletin, 110*, 67–85.

Teasdale, J. D. (1983). Negative thinking in depression: Cause, effect, or reciprocal relationship. *Advances in Behaviour Research and Therapy, 5*, 3–25.

Teasdale, J. D., Moore, R. G., Hayhurst, H., Pope, M., Williams, S., & Segal, Z. V. (2002). Metacognitive awareness and prevention of relapse in depression: Empirical evidence. *Journal of Consulting and Clinical Psychology, 70*, 275–287.

Thompson, R. A. (1998). Early sociopersonality development. In W. Damon (Series Ed.) & N. Eisenberg (Vol. Ed.), *Handbook of child psychology: Vol. 3. Social, emotional, and personality development* (5th ed., pp. 25–104). New York: Wiley.

Toth, S. L., & Cicchetti, D. (1996). Patterns of relatedness, depressive symptomatology, and perceived competence in maltreated children. *Journal of Consulting and Clinical Psychology, 64*, 32–41.

Vohs, K. D., & Ciarocco, N. J. (2004). Interpersonal functioning requires self-regulation. In R. F. Baumeister & K. D. Vohs (Eds.), *Handbook of self-regulation: Research, theory, and applications* (pp. 392–407). New York: Guilford Press.

Vredenberg, K., Flett, G. L., & Krames, L. (1993). Analogue versus clinical depression: A critical reappraisal. *Psychological Bulletin, 113*, 327–344.

Weissman, M., Warner, V., Wickramaratne, P., Moreau, D., & Olfson, M. (1997). Offspring of depressed parents: 10 years later. *Archives of General Psychiatry, 54*, 932–940.

Chapter 11

Back to the Future

Personality Structure as a
Context for Psychopathology

DREW WESTEN
GLEN O. GABBARD
PAVEL BLAGOV

The past decade has seen what may well turn out to be a watershed in the understanding of psychopathology. DSM-III (American Psychiatric Association, 1980) standardized and operationalized diagnosis in a way that allowed researchers for the first time to generate replicable data for a wide range of disorders. Almost immediately, what became apparent was that psychopathology was not the offspring of an obsessive–compulsive god who created depression on one day, anxiety on the next, and rested on the seventh day once he was certain that his disorders were cleanly separated. Instead, comorbidity among Axis I disorders, among Axis II disorders, and between the axes was the norm rather than the exception. The result was a veritable cottage industry on comorbidity, with thousands of articles exploring the associations between one disorder and its cousins, including cousins with little obvious family resemblance. And despite the best efforts of multiple DSM work groups and task forces to maximize the distinctness of diagnoses, comorbidity continues to be the wicked stepchild of psychiatric taxonomy.

Over the past decade, what has become clear is that we cannot readily rid our nosology of comorbidity because virtually all nonpsychotic syndromes share common factors with other syndromes, and these factors comprise what we traditionally understand as aspects of personality—that is, enduring ways of thinking, feeling, regulating emotion, regulating impulses, and behaving that manifest across time or situation. The work of Watson and Clark (1984, 1992), Brown, Chorpita, and Barlow (1998), and Krueger (1999) has documented that negative affectivity or internalizing spectrum personality pathology is a common factor shared by virtually all the Axis I mood and anxiety disorders and accounts for much of their co-occurrence. Krueger and colleagues (2002) similarly suggest that a broad-band externalizing factor underlies many other DSM-IV disorders, notably substance use and antisocial personality disorders. The implication is clear: if we want to understand symptoms, we have to know something about the person who hosts them.

This insight is both exciting and eerily familiar. In the late 19th and early 20th centuries, Sigmund Freud formulated a theory of psychopathology intended to explain (and help ameliorate) a range of anxiety, mood, and other "neurotic" symptoms, most of which are now coded on Axis I of DSM-IV. He began with a model of discrete syndromes but ultimately came to believe that he could not understand his patients' symptoms in isolation from what came to be called their character or personality structure.[1] In many respects, the last century of psychoanalytic theory has been about the nature, structure, and dysfunction of character and how patients' character structure provides the foundation for their symptoms—including the way two very different forms of personality organization can predispose patients toward a common symptom (final common pathway). Correspondingly, the length of psychoanalytic treatments has expanded dramatically from the 3- to 6-month treatments characteristic of Freud's early encounters with his patients to long-term therapies aimed at characterological change.

Our goal in this chapter is to explore the relevance of the clinical understanding of personality that first emerged from psychoanalytic theory and observation for current questions about the relation between personality and psychopathology. We suggest that there is an important message in the fact that, a century ago, clinically trained observers, immersed in the lives of their patients, blazed trails where we now have the technology to bulldoze but until relatively recently did not recognize the importance of exploring. The issues with which clinical theorists have struggled over the past 100 years, we believe, are of tremendous relevance to our efforts to forge ahead in the next century of theory and research on psychopathology, and data from the clinic provide an important source of hypotheses, causal conjecture, and observation that is complementary to the sources of data on which empirical psychopathologists generally rely (see Westen & Weinberger, 2004, 2005).

We begin by briefly exploring the historical path from symptom neurosis to character neurosis in psychoanalytic theory (that is, from a view of symptoms as relatively independent of personality to a view of symptoms as emanations or expressions of personality). We then examine clinically informed conceptions of personality structure and relevant empirical data that challenge us to know history as well as, perhaps, to repeat it. We conclude with the question of whether and in what ways clinically derived and empirically derived views of personality structure can be integrated and how each might guide the clinical understanding of psychopathology and treatment.

Before beginning, we briefly address two meanings of *personality structure*. The concept of "structure" in psychoanalytic theory refers to repetitively activated, functionally defined processes, such as psychological processes involved in motivation, regulation of mood, and regulation of impulses. When Freud wrote about the "superego," he was referring to a set of functions often activated concurrently that allow a comparison of one's own actions, thoughts, or feelings with ideal standards and internalized values. Freud actually never used the mechanistic Latin terms for the structures that came to be labeled id, ego, and superego (Bettelheim, 1983). The original German for what became an (often reified) construct of *super ego* simply meant "above me," meaning a part of one's mind that stands apart and judges one's actions, as if from above. The "id" referred to wishes, feelings, impulses or symptoms that seemed like "not me" even though they were mine—that is, they felt like "an it" (id) instead of "me" (ego).

Psychoanalytic theorists today are much less likely to talk about the id, ego, and superego. However, when they talk about structure, what they have in mind is the dynamic interplay of repetitively activated processes that normally serve adaptive functions but can become dysfunctional, either on their own or in interaction. For example, conscience is an essential personality function that allows humans to interact relatively peaceably with conspecifics, but it can lead to psychopathology if it is overly severe on the one hand or hypoactive on the other. Thus, Freud (1933) described patients with a harsh, punitive superego, who mercilessly attack themselves and are vulnerable to mood disorders. Subsequent research on "introjective," "self-critical," or "autonomous" depression suggests that, indeed, harsh moral or other standards can predispose vulnerable individuals to depression (Blatt, 2004; Blatt, Quinlan, Chevron, McDonald, & Zuroff, 1982; Whisman, 1993). Nor would Freud the neurologist have been surprised to find that damage to the frontal lobes can cause irreversible moral pathology (Anderson, Bechara, Damasio, Tranel, & Damasio, 1999; Ishikawa & Raine, 2003).

Psychopathology can also reflect the *interaction* of enduring personality structures or functions, as when a patient develops a symptom that constitutes a compromise among competing affective–motivational "pulls" (for empirical data, see Westen, Blagov, Feit, Arkowitz, & Thagard, 2005). For example, a patient whose father brutalized her as a child developed both the wish that he would die and a harsh, self-hating way of judging herself. The symptom with which she presented—an obsessional "thought" that her father would die, which she could not seem to "erase" from her mind—appeared to represent a compromise between her wish that something terrible would befall him in retribution for what he had done to her and her desire to avoid the guilt of attributing the wish to herself (hence, its repetitive appearance in her consciousness without attribution to its author, herself).

This concept of personality structure is very different from the corresponding psychometric concept of structure. From the point of view of trait theory, personality structure generally connotes a factor structure deemed to fit the data well, that is, a way of identifying patterns of covariation among items that provides insight into latent variables common to several of them. Part of the difference lies in the fact that this latter concept of structure is nomothetic rather than idiographic, describing patterns of covariation that emerge across individuals rather than covariation or coactivation of processes within individuals. However, as we shall see, nomothetic models of personality structure used to guide case formulation (idiographic analysis) in clinical practice also differ substantially from the psychometric concept of personality structure in their emphasis on functional domains. To what extent psychometric (factor) structure can be uncovered from data on personality structure functionally defined is unclear.[2]

RETRACING STEPS: THE EVOLUTION FROM SYMPTOM TO CHARACTER IN PSYCHOANALYTIC THEORY

Contemporary thinking about the distinction between Axis I and Axis II in many respects mirrors a transformation that occurred in psychoanalysis in its early years of development. Tracing the evolution from symptomatic neurosis to character neurosis, and more broadly from a view that views symptoms as relatively discrete to one that places symptoms in characterological context, may be useful in laying a historical foundation for issues confronted by contemporary taxonomists.

From Symptom Neurosis to Character Neurosis

In the late 1890s, in his early work with Breuer, Freud (Freud & Breuer, 1895/1957) used hysterical symptoms as a prototype for the symptomatic neuroses upon which he founded psychoanalysis. According to his early theoretical views, a symptom arises in the form of a compromise between the expression of a wish and defenses against it (because acknowledging the wish would lead to anxiety, guilt, or other unpleasant emotions). Hence, a young man might develop paralysis of the arm that simultaneously expresses a wish to strike his father and a defense against that wish. The defense is expressed by being unable to use his arm, and the aggression is indirectly expressed by his inability to do any work in the yard or around the house that his father demands of him. His father then ends up feeling infuriated by this passive expression of aggression in his son. According to this model, a symptom is a compromise formation—that is, a compromise among competing motivational "pulls" or dynamics.

This understanding of symptom formation informed Freud's early forays into treatment. Heavily influenced by Charcot and Janet, Freud relied on hypnosis and suggestion to do a great deal of the work. By placing his hand on the forehead of the patient and insisting that she fully remember the repressed memory, he thought he could de-repress an instinctually or emotionally charged memory and cure the patient of the symptom.

Freud soon found that his method led to short-lived results. He could not simply plow through these defenses using hypnosis and suggestion. Treatment was complicated. Freud's increasing understanding of the complexity and depth of what he later called "ego" functions—notably, the ways people chronically protect themselves from emotionally threatening information—led him to rethink the role of symptoms in psychopathology. Rather than viewing symptoms as isolated psychic "boils" that needed to be lanced to clean out a psychological infection, he gradually came to realize that his patients' symptoms emerged in the context not only of their enduring motives and conflicts but of a psychological "immune system" that was constantly surveying the landscape and sending out its killer cells when it detected threatening psychological material. (Interestingly, social psychologists have recently recast what Freud called defenses in terms of a psychological "immune system"; see Gilbert, 1998). Wilhelm Reich (1931) subsequently elaborated a view of entrenched, characterological defenses of this sort, arguing that people develop "character armor," habitual ways of defending that become automatic and inflexible over time. Paradoxically, while protecting them from confronting unpleasant aspects of themselves, this armor ultimately limits their psychological freedom of action.

For example, a patient with obsessive–compulsive personality dynamics, who was chronically quietly angry but would not allow himself to express or acknowledge it, came to his analyst's office 5 minutes early for every session. He dutifully entered the office and nodded obsequiously to his analyst each day. He paid his bill on the first day after receiving it, and he dutifully arranged his vacations to coincide with those of his analyst. He tried to be the perfect patient in every way, including an avoidance of any expression of disagreement or anger toward his analyst. On the few occasions when his analyst was late, the patient immediately forgave him and denied any feelings whatsoever about the inconvenience. During the sessions, he kept an eye on his watch and always ended right on time. He bid adieu to his analyst in the same way each day: "Thank you, and I'll see you tomorrow."

The conflicts and "character armor" the analyst observed in the consulting room appeared to restrict any spontaneity in the patient's life and led to a range of work inhibitions in which he feared being too aggressive or too ambitious. He worried that his boss would think of him as someone who wanted to replace him. He worried that his analyst might think of him as someone who could have angry or aggressive feelings toward him or who might doubt his "interpretations" (which of course any sensible patient would). In understanding this patient, one would be hard-pressed to identify specific symptoms of a neurosis. His character was his neurosis. He lived an orderly existence, designed to avoid aggression and conflict, but he had little pleasure in his life. He also denied himself the success of which he was capable.

Freud never abandoned the concept of compromise formation, which is probably one of the most useful of all psychoanalytic constructs (Brenner, 1982, 1994; Gabbard, 1998; for research, see Westen, 1998b; Westen, Blagov et al., 2005; Westen & Gabbard, 2002). However, his recognition of the pervasive role of maladaptive as well as adaptive defenses gradually led him to move from a symptom-focused theory of psychopathology to a view that recognizes the importance of character in the development of psychological symptoms. This shift can be seen, for example, in his early work on the "anal character" (Freud, 1908). Freud noted that certain people could be characterized by a triad of personality traits: obstinacy, parsimony, and orderliness. Factor-analytic work supports the covariation of these personality traits (as well as several relatively specific hypotheses about "anal" dynamics that have proven surprisingly robust empirically; Fisher & Greenberg, 1996), which are today often described as obsessive–compulsive personality traits or extreme conscientiousness.

Freud believed that such traits were precipitates of the anal phase of development, when children are learning about self-control, authority (and resistance to it), and, more concretely, potty training. Setting aside his etiological theories, which in this case likely underemphasize genetic contributions to personality, Freud made some trenchant observations about the covariation of certain personality traits and dynamics and of the types of symptoms that seemed to beset individuals with what we now call, in less scatological language, an obsessive–compulsive personality style (see, e.g., Shapiro, 1965; Westen, 1999a, 1999b). Freud observed that patients who fit his description of the "anal" character, like the obsessional patient described above, tend to be "tight" (i.e., overly constrained), self-righteous (insistent on certain forms of authority and moral perfection), self-critical, critical of others, and uncomfortable with affect. Beneath their demands for order, control, and "appropriate" behavior from others was often a simmering anger. Perhaps not surprisingly, when they became symptomatic, they often developed obsessional symptoms, compulsions, and somatic complaints reflecting a relatively high "ambient" level of stress that often accompanies an unwillingness to acknowledge emotions such as anger (Shedler, Mayman, & Manis, 1993). Further, unlike the "oral" character, who was likely to become depressed when her dependency needs were not met, the anal character was most likely to become depressed because of failure to meet rigid internal standards. In different language, Blatt (e.g., Blatt & Zuroff, 1992) and Beck (Bieling, Beck, & Brown, 2004) have offered similar descriptions of characterological diatheses for depression.

Ego Psychology

A major step forward in understanding the relation between character and psychopathology emerged in the years before Freud's death, in the body of literature known as psychoanalytic ego psychology (Blanck & Blanck, 1974, 1979). Anna Freud (1936) delineated various mechanisms of defense and suggested that they may be hierarchically organized, from relatively immature and problematic to more mature and adaptive. Vaillant (Vaillant, 1977, 1992; Vaillant & McCullough, 1998) elaborated the concept of hierarchically organized defenses and developed a body of longitudinal empirical work examining the relation between defenses in young adulthood and later outcomes. At the bottom level of the hierarchy are psychologically primitive defenses, such as projection, in which the person cannot acknowledge his own wishes or attributes and instead sees them in others and attacks them there. Supporting this theory as applied to homophobia, Adams and colleagues (Adams, Wright, & Lohr, 1996) (who were, interestingly, not themselves psychoanalytically inclined) found that when homophobic men viewed gay porn, they showed stronger arousal as assessed by genital plethysmography than nonhomophobes. Baumeister (Baumeister, Dale, & Sommer, 1998; Newman, Duff, Schnopp-Wyatt, Brock, & Hoffman, 1997) has similarly examined some of the cognitive mechanisms involved in projection, and Westen and Shedler (1999a; Shedler & Westen, 2004b) have documented empirically its centrality to paranoid personality disorder. At the top of Vaillant's hierarchy are psychological processes that can transform conflict and distress into more socially appropriate and adaptive forms, such as humor and sublimation.

Vaillant has linked characterological ways of defending against unwanted thoughts or feelings to different forms of psychopathology and life outcomes in several longitudinal studies (e.g., Vaillant, 1977). For example, in a longitudinal study of 306 inner-city men, Vaillant and McCullough (1998) identified five groups of men based on observer ratings of defenses from transcripts of 2-hour semistructured interviews. The group of men who used the fewest mature and the greatest number of immature defenses (such as acting out, passive aggression, hypochondriasis, and dissociation) evidenced the greatest severity on measures of global mental health as well as life problems such as antisocial behavior, unemployment, and alcohol use problems at the time of assessment. In addition, they were more likely to show downward social mobility and had the worst psychosocial functioning approximately 15 years later (at about age 50). The men in the groups defined as having the least mature defenses also had the most marital instability over time. In contrast, men who used mature defenses (e.g., altruism, suppression, and sublimation) scored the highest on most domains of functioning, lending support to the evidence for a hierarchy of characterological defense styles.

More generally, ego psychologists argued that the way people chronically defend is of substantial consequence to the way they are likely to fall ill psychologically. Someone who deals with adversity by blaming him- or herself is likely to be vulnerable to depression; someone who rigidly defends against painful memories of abuse is likely to develop posttraumatic stress symptoms, often alternating between unbidden images that come "out of the blue" and numbness, dissociation, or lack of memory; someone who regulates anxiety by binge eating may leave him- or herself vulnerable to developing bulimia nervosa. Recent cognitive-behavioral theories of generalized anxiety disorder propose a similar mechanism, whereby rumination begins as a way of regulating anxiety but backfires by exacerbating it (Borkovec, Shadick, & Hopkins, 1991; Borkovec & Sharpless, 2004). Common to these views is the notion that people develop ways of regulating their emotions that become habitual and unconscious, rendering them less able to confront situations or information in the long run, so that "the solution becomes the problem."

Along with its focus on defense, or what today we might call implicit forms of emotion regulation (Westen, 1985, 1994; Westen, Muderrisoglu, Fowler, Shedler, & Koren, 1997), ego psychology focused on other psychological functions that foster adaptation. Guided by evolutionary theory and the cognitive-developmental theories of the time (particularly Werner and Piaget), Heinz Hartmann (1939/1958) and his colleagues (see Hartmann, Kris, & Loewenstein, 1946) attempted to delineate a range of processes involved in cognition and self-regulation, with an eye to understanding what happens when these functions go awry. For example, Redl and Wineman (1951) observed a large group of delinquent adolescents and delineated a range of deficits that appeared to inhibit their ability to regulate their impulses. Bellak, Chassan, Gediman, and Hurvich (1973) developed a taxonomy of ego functions that they operationalized for systematic empirical investigation, and Loevinger (Loevinger, 1979; Loevinger & Wessler, 1970) developed a model and measure of ego development that generated thousands of empirical studies (see Cohn & Westenberg, 2004; Westenberg, Jonckheer, Treffers, & Drewes, 1998). From an ego–psychological standpoint, we cannot understand a symptom such as depression without understanding its characterological "scaffolding." A person who has a strong need for connection to others but minimal capacity for regulating affects or impulses is going to have tumultuous, short-lived relationships, and is hence going to be vulnerable to depression.

Object Relations Theory

Although psychoanalysis is often seen as quintessentially impractical (e.g., four or five times a week on the couch), theoretical developments in psychoanalysis have often been nothing if not pragmatic. Ego psychology was an attempt to understand repetitive, counterproductive ways of thinking and behaving and deficits in functioning in character-disordered patients that could not be readily understood in terms of specific conflicts. The same was true of object relations theories, which emerged to explain the behavior of patients with severe personality disorders, whose difficulties seemed more entrenched, wide-ranging, and systemic than the encapsulated psychological "infections" of early Freudian theory.

   Object relations refers to interpersonal behavior in intimate relationships and to the cognitive, affective, and motivational processes that mediate that behavior (particularly representations of self, others, and relationships) (Westen, 1991b). What psychoanalysts call "internalized object relations," or internalized patterns of thinking, feeling, and behaving in relationships, are hypothesized by most contemporary psychoanalytic theorists to be implicated in many if not most forms of psychopathology (Aron, 1996; Aron & Harris, 2005; Gabbard, 2005; Mitchell & Aron, 1999). Considerable research supports a broad role for such dynamics in psychopathology; indeed, object relations theory (and its offshoot, attachment theory; see, e.g., Shaver & Mikulincer, 2005) has been the most generative area of psychoanalytically oriented research in the past two decades (Huprich & Greenberg, 2003; Stricker & Healey, 1990). For example, patients with specific Axis II disorders can be distinguished in terms of the complexity with which they view themselves and others, the extent to which they attribute benevolence or malevolence to others' actions, their capacity to invest emotionally in another person (i.e., their ability to show genuine caring and concern vs. viewing others as objects to gratify their needs or desires), and their ability to understand why people behave as they do (Ackerman, Clemence, Weatherill, & Hilsenroth, 1999; Blais, Hilsenroth, Fowler, & Conboy, 1999; Blatt, 1974; Nigg, Lohr, Westen, Gold, & Silk, 1992; Nigg et al., 1991; Westen, 1990b, 1991b; Westen, Ludolph, Lerner, Ruffins, & Wiss, 1990).

From an object relations standpoint, a symptom or syndrome such as depression can be the product of many different kinds of object relational dynamics, and appropriate treatment requires attention to these dynamics (Benjamin, 1996a, 1996b; Blatt, 2004; Masterson, 1976; McWilliams, 1998; Scharff, 2004). A patient could be depressed because he or she has internalized attitudes of hostile, abusive, critical, or neglectful parents. As a result, he or she may be vulnerable to fears of abandonment, self-hatred, feelings of emptiness, or chronic self-criticism. These are very different vulnerabilities, reflecting very different development histories in the context of genetic endowments.

Problematic internalizations of the attitudes or behaviors of significant others can lead to depression in a different, and often complementary, way as the patient unknowingly creates situations that would make anyone depressed, even if he or she had no specific liability toward depression. For example, one patient with a highly critical father continually chose work environments that were "safe," in which he could not fail. As a result, he constantly felt bored, unchallenged, demeaned by his station in life, and as if he were sleepwalking through his job 8 hours a day. Another patient, who had been the victim of severe physical abuse in childhood, was constantly vigilant for signs of mistreatment by authority figures and, not surprisingly, frequently lost jobs during altercations with superiors. As a result, she often found herself both financially and socially destitute. She brought malevolent expectations into her romantic relationships as well, which similarly led her to experience a constant series of losses, as one relationship after another would crash and burn. Yet another patient, a professor, could never produce enough to make himself feel worthy, despite an objectively impressive career. Although these patients have similar Axis I diagnoses (dysthymic disorder, with periodic major depressive episodes), from a psychoanalytic point of view, it is difficult to see how one could understand who they are, why they chronically feel dysphoric, why they periodically become deeply depressed, and how to help them without thoroughly understanding these object-relational processes.

From an object relations standpoint, patients with severe personality pathology tend to have difficulty forming mature, constant, multifaceted representations of the self and others. This may leave them vulnerable to emotional swings when significant others are momentarily disappointing, particularly given their difficulty understanding or imagining what might be in the minds of the people with whom they interact (Fonagy, Steele, & Steele, 1991; Fonagy & Target, 1997; Fonagy, Target, Gergely, Allen, &

Bateman, 2003). Research has linked these "mentalization" deficits (difficulties forming complex representations of others' mental states, involving relatively accurate perspective taking) with early maltreatment (Cicchetti, Rogosch, Maughan, Toth, & Bruce, 2003; Cicchetti & Toth, 2003; Toth, Cicchetti, & Kim, 2002; Toth, Cicchetti, Macfie, Maughan, & Vanmeenen, 2000), although they appear to have multiple causes. Similarly, attachment research has linked difficulties forming coherent expectations about others' behavior, and particularly about contingencies between one's own behavior and that of attachment figures, with attachment relationships with primary caregivers who have unresolved loss and trauma from their own past (Agrawal, Gunderson, Holmes, & Lyons-Ruth, 2004; Goldberg et al., 2003; Koos & Gergely, 2001; Lyons-Ruth & Jacobvitz, 1999; Lyons-Ruth, Melnick, Bronfman, Sherry, & Llanas, 2004; Main, Kaplan, & Cassidy, 1985; Ward, Lee, & Lipper, 2000). Clinical theorists have repeatedly observed the difficulty severely personality disordered patients often have in forming realistic, balanced views of the self that can help them weather momentary failures, criticisms, or ruptures in relationships. A substantial body of research supports many of these propositions, particularly vis-à-vis borderline personality disorder, the most extensively studied personality disorder (Baker, Silk, Westen, Nigg, & Lohr, 1992; Gunderson, 2001; Westen, 1990a, 1991a).

Two recent clinical trials of psychodynamically based treatments for borderline personality disorder have in fact focused on precisely these kinds of deficits in mental representations and are achieving promising initial results in randomized controlled clinical trials. Fonagy and Bateman (Bateman & Fonagy, 2003, 2004; Fonagy, 2002) have developed a mentalization therapy aimed at helping patients with borderline personality disorder imagine others' minds. Kernberg and colleagues (Yeomans, Clarkin, & Kernberg, 2002) have developed a therapy aimed at helping patients form complex, multifaceted representations of self and others that integrate positive and negative feelings. What will be of particular interest over the long run is the extent to which these treatments can alter the risk of future episodes of Axis I symptoms such as depression, anxiety, and bulimic binge purging, all of which are common in patients with borderline personality disorder, and whether they are able to maintain their effects over time.

To summarize, psychoanalysis began with a focus on discrete symptoms but evolved over time into an approach to psychopathology and treatment that places symptoms in their characterological context. This does not mean that all symptoms are emanations of character, that personality is not shaped substantially by biology, that no one ever becomes phobic after a dog bite, or that addressing personality will erase symptoms that have developed functional autonomy over time or burned neural tracks through repeated activation (Westen, 2000). What it does suggest, however, is a very different conception of symptoms and treatment than has become the norm during the past decade with the empirically supported therapies (EST) movement, which assumes discrete syndromes, each of which requires its own treatment manual (Westen, Novotny, & Thompson-Brenner, 2004). Psychoanalytic theorists have long argued that one cannot separate the symptom from the person in treatment—and the amassing data on the relation between psychopathology and personality described in this volume support that view.

CLINICAL CONCEPTUALIZATIONS OF PERSONALITY STRUCTURE

We move now from history to contemporary clinical understanding of personality structure informed by empirical research. Although cognitive-behavioral theorists have recently begun to offer accounts of personality functioning in patients with personality disorder (Beck, Freeman, & Davis, 2004; Linehan, 1993; Young, 1990), we focus here primarily on psychodynamic models of personality structure, which provide a clinically grounded complement and counterpoint to models of personality structure that have evolved outside of the clinic (Kernberg, 1984; McWilliams, 1994; McWilliams, 1999; Westen, 1998a; Westen & Gabbard, 1999).

As Max Weber noted years ago (Weber, 1949), the way we classify depends not only on the nature of the phenomenon we are classifying but also on our purposes in classifying it. One of the major differences between models of personality structure that emerged from clinical practice and trait models that emerged from research on normal personality is that the former reflect the demands of clinical practice, particularly the need to make systematic case formulations that can guide practice. Dynamic clinical models of personality structure address three distinct but related aspects of personality organization: functional domains, levels of disturbance, and personality configurations.

Functional Domains

From a clinical perspective, a useful assessment of personality is a *functional assessment*, that is, an assessment of how the individual tends to function cognitively, affectively, and behaviorally under conditions relevant to psychological and social adaptation. A functional assessment presupposes a model of domains of function and dysfunction. It also focuses, by necessity, on areas of health as well as maladaptation because helping a patient requires knowledge of his or her adaptive capacities as well as limitations. A comprehensive functional assessment will thus address personality characteristics in the normal range as well as those that are more or less problematic.

For years Freud's structural model provided the primary model of personality for clinical case formulation. In contemporary practice, however, no single model predominates, although theorists such as Kernberg (1983) and McWilliams (1999) have offered compelling accounts. Gabbard (2005) proposes a contemporary psychoanalytic perspective on character that includes a set of internalized object relations, a specific constellation of defense mechanisms (often associated with a characteristic cognitive style), a biologically based temperament, and an enduring sense of self (Gabbard, 2005).

For heuristic purposes, we focus here on a model of functional domains designed to integrate dynamic concepts of personality structure with empirical research in personality, developmental, clinical, cognitive, and social psychology (Heim & Westen, 2005; Westen, 1995, 1996, 1998a). The model suggests that three sets of variables, defined by three questions, provide a relatively comprehensive roadmap of personality:

1. What does the person wish for, fear, and value, and to what extent are these motives conscious and mutually compatible?
2. What are the individual's psychological resources for adapting to internal and external demands?
3. What is the person's capacity for engaging in intimate relationships, and how does the individual experience the self, others, and relationships?

Each of these questions comprises multiple specific variables, elaborated below, that together describe the way the person tends to respond cognitively, affectively, motivationally, and behaviorally over time or circumstance (Table 11.1).

This view of personality is dynamic, in two senses. First, it views personality as the interaction of psychological processes activated under specific conditions, not as the possession of particular traits to particular degrees. Indeed, as described below, the same trait could reflect different interactions of processes. Second, although delineation of these variables drew extensively from research across several subfields of psychology, the questions address, respectively, the concerns of classical psychoanalytic theory (motivation and conflict); ego psychology (adaptation); and object relations theory, self psychology, and more recent relational approaches (experience of self, others, and relationships). This model was designed both to reflect and to systematize the kind of judgments most skilled clinicians intuitively make in a way that is both clinically and empirically sound.

TABLE 11.1. Outline of a Clinical Model of Personality Structure

I. What does the person wish for, fear, and value, and to what extent are these motives conscious or conflicting?
   a. Fears
   b. Wishes
   c. Values
   d. Conflicts among fears, wishes, and values
   e. Conscious awareness of motives
   f. Notable compromise formations

II. What psychological resources (affective, cognitive, and self-regulatory) does the person have to deal with reality and attain his/her goals?
   a. Cognitive functions
      i.   Intellectual functioning
      ii. Coherence or disorder of thought processes
      iii. Cognitive style
   b. Affective experience
      i.   Positive and negative affect
      ii. Tendency to experience particular affects
      iii. Intensity of affective experience
      iv. Lability of affect
      v.   Affect recognition and tolerance
      vi. Capacity for experiencing ambivalent emotions
   c. Affect regulation
      i.   Coping strategies
      ii. Defenses
      iii. Affect-regulatory behavior
   d. Impulse regulation

III. How does the person experience the self, others, and relationships, and to what extent is s/he capable of mature, intimate relationships?
   a. Cognitive structure of representations of self and others
      i.   Complexity of representations
      ii. Integration of diverse elements
      iii. Differentiation of different representations from each other
   b. Affective quality of representations
   c. Capacity for emotional investment in relationships
      i.   Developmental level (from need-gratifying approach to mature interdependence)
      ii. Style (e.g., attachment status)
   d. Capacity for emotional investment in values and moral standards
   e. Understanding of social causality
   f. Identification and disidentifications
   g. Dominant interpersonal concerns (chronically activated wishes, fears, and constructs)
   h. Social skills
   i. Self-structure
      i.   Sense of self-continuity or coherence; sense of self as thinker, feeler, and agent; experience of self as continuous over time
      ii. Implicit and explicit self-representations
      iii. Self-with-other representations
      iv. Self-esteem
      v.   Feared, wished-for, ought, and ideal self-representations
      vi. Self-presentation (how the person wants to be perceived)
      vii. Identity

• *Question 1: What does the person wish for, fear, and value, and to what extent are these motives conscious and mutually compatible?* The first question regards motivation: What does the individual wish, fear, and value? To put it another way, what representations of desired, feared, and valued states has the patient come to associate with affect such that these representations guide behavior as goal states? Contemporary views of motivation, rooted in research with both human and nonhuman animals, emphasize approach and avoidance systems motivated by positive and negative affect (Carver, 2001; Davidson, Jackson, & Kalin, 2000; Gray, 1990). For decades clinical supervisors have exhorted young psychotherapists to "go where the affect is" (or where it should be but does not seem to be), reflecting the recognition that the quality and intensity of emotion attached to various representations is what tends to drive both healthy striving and problematic motives and conflicts.

These affectively imbued representations can be conscious, unconscious, or somewhere in between from a dynamic standpoint (e.g., acknowledged but only in alternation or recognized with considerable clinical probing and support, such as wishes for revenge, or unpleasant memories). They can also be organized at varying hierarchical levels, such as a strong need to be liked, to be liked by authority figures, or to be liked by male authority figures (Westen, 1997). Central to psychodynamic formulations is that wishes, fears, and values, including emotionally invested ideals and standards (see Higgins, 1990; Strauman, 1992) can be in conflict, and that the resolutions to these conflicts (compromise formations) can be adaptive or maladaptive (see Brenner, 1982). Whereas these postulates were once based exclusively on clinical data, today a considerably body of empirical evidence supports them (McClelland, Koestner, & Weinberger, 1989; Weinberger, in press; Westen, 1998b; Westen, Blagov, et al., 2005; Westen & Gabbard, 1999; Westen, Weinberger, & Bradley, in press).

From a psychoanalytic standpoint, knowing a person requires understanding the structure of his or her motivation. People with very different constellations of motives could show similar overt behavior or self-report similar personality characteristics. From the surface, the obsessional patient described above might be described (and describe himself) as relatively low in aggression or hostility. In fact, however, he may be quite hostile or angry but overregulate his aggression. In so doing, he may inadvertently keep himself angry and focused on other people's flaws, slights, or insults (on the paradoxical effects of suppression, see Wegner & Bargh, 1998). From a clinical point of view, this combination of angry criticism of others and defenses against it is not readily described as either hostile or not hostile; it is both, depending on which level of consciousness one is describing.

• *Question 2: What psychological resources—cognitive, affective, and behavioral dispositions—does the individual have at his or her disposal?* The second question regards adaptive functioning. It comprises several subdimensions, largely focusing on patterns of cognition, emotion, and self-regulation. The first set of dimensions pertains to the cognitive resources at the individual's disposal. One such dimension (or set of dimensions) is intellectual functioning in multiple domains, particularly as it reflects on the capacity to problem solve (Gardner, 1999). A second cognitive variable, first studied by psychoanalytic ego psychologists, is the degree to which a person's thought processes are intact or disordered (Coleman, Levy, Lenzenweger, & Holzman, 1996; Johnston & Holzman, 1979; Perry, Minassian, Cadenhead, Sprock, & Braff, 2003; Rapaport, Gill, & Schafer, 1945). Research from our laboratory suggests that "subclinical" (i.e., not overtly psychotic) disturbances in thinking have diverse etiologies, some reflecting a genetic liability for schizophrenic spectrum pathology (Walker & Gale, 1995; Walker, Logan, & Walder, 1999) and others reflecting adverse developmental experiences, notably childhood separations and sexual abuse (Heim, Thomas, & Westen, unpublished data). Another cognitive variable is cognitive style (Shapiro, 1965) (e.g., such as the global, impressionistic, hysterical style that usually co-occurs with defenses such as pseudonaiveté or denial of obvious but unpleasant ideas).

A second domain of psychological resources regards the person's emotional experience. Individuals differ on a number of affective dimensions, many of which have been studied empirically, including affective lability (the extent to which their emotions fluctuate from one emotional state to another) (Koenigsberg et al., 2002; Mitropoulou, New, Koenigsberg, Silverman, & Siever, 2001; Tolpin, Gunthert, Cohen, & O'Neill, 2004), affect intensity (the extent to which emotions are strong; Larsen, Billings, & Cutler, 1996; Schimmack & Diener, 1997), the extent to which they chronically experience positive and negative (i.e., pleasant and unpleasant) affects (Watson & Clark, 1992), the extent to which they experience specific affects such as shame and guilt (Tangney, 1994; Watson & Tellegen, 1985; Westen, 1994), their comfort with conscious awareness of affect (Pennebaker, 1997; Shedler et al., 1993), and, as emphasized by Kernberg (1975), their ability to recognize and experience conflicting affective states and appraisals simultaneously (that is, capacity for ambivalence; for empirical work on the capacity for ambivalence; see Baker et al., 1992; Harter, 1999; Whitesell & Harter, 1989)

A third domain of psychological resources is emotion regulation, which refers to the conscious and unconscious procedures used to maximize pleasant and minimize unpleasant emotions (see Gross, 1998; Westen, 1985; Westen, 1994; Westen et al., 1997). Emotion regulation strategies that are explicit (i.e., under conscious control) are usually referred to as coping strategies (e.g., anticipation, cognitive reframing, self-distraction, suppression). Emotion regulation strategies that are implicit or unconscious are usually referred to as defenses. People also use overt behavior to try to alter reality to eliminate an aversive situation or to alter the affect directly (e.g., by ingesting drugs or alcohol). The lines among explicit, implicit, and behavioral emotion regulation strategies are, of course, somewhat arbitrary (see Haan, 1977; Plutchik, 1980).

A fourth and related domain of psychological resources involves the regulation of impulses. Block (1971) has described empirically the dangers that can beset people who either overcontrol or undercontrol their impulses. Impulsivity appears to be a multidimensional construct (Barratt, 1993; Webster & Jackson, 1997) that plays a significant part in many forms of psychopathology. For example, as described below, a substantial percentage of patients with eating disorders have a tendency to over-regulate their impulses, whereas others show the opposite pattern; and these personality patterns are associated with a range of variables including but not limited to their eating symptoms (Thompson-Brenner & Westen, 2005; Westen & Harnden-Fischer, 2001).

• *Question 3: How does the person experience the self and others, and to what extent can the individual enter into intimate relationships?* The third question, regarding interpersonal functioning, has been the focus on object relations theory, self psychology, and relational theories in psychoanalysis (Aron, 1996; Aron & Harris, 2005; Greenberg & Mitchell, 1983; Mitchell, 1988; Mitchell & Aron, 1999; Westen, 1991b). Several dimensions of object relations are empirically distinguishable and have been examined in studies using samples of normal and clinical children, adolescents, and adults (Blatt & Lerner, 1983; Huprich & Greenberg, 2003; Stricker & Healey, 1990; Westen, 1991b; Westen, Huebner, Lifton, Silverman, & Boekamp, 1991; Westen, Klepser, et al., 1991; Westen, Lohr, Silk, Gold, & Kerber, 1990; Westen, Ludolph, Lerner, et al., 1990; Westen, Ludolph, Silk, et al., 1990). As described earlier, people differ in not only the content but the cognitive structure of their representations of people and relationships. People's representations of significant others differ in their complexity and integration (particularly of elements with contrasting affective valences). Patients with severe personality pathology often have difficulty forming complex multidimensional representations of people, and instead tend to think about others in simplistic or black-and-white ways. People also differ in the affective quality of their representations of people, that is, on the extent to which they tend to expect relationships to be destructive or enriching.

The capacity for emotional investment in relationships—the ability to care about another person for more than what that person can give or what desires that person can gratify—is another central aspect of object relations, as is the capacity for emotional investment in moral values and standards (e.g., the capacity to feel or anticipate guilt, rather than primarily concern, about punishment when committing or thinking of committing a moral infraction). The understanding of social causality (i.e., why people do what they do) is another central dimension of object relations that has received empirical attention. In different terms, social causality has also been a focus of attachment research, which has linked the experience of unpredictable caregiving to the inability to development coherent expectations and internal working models of relationships that allow the growing child to predict, understand, and hence adapt optimally to significant others (Cassidy & Mohr, 2001; Lyons-Ruth & Jacobvitz, 1999; Main et al., 1985). Other dimensions of object relations include identifications and disidentifications (e.g., fears of becoming like one's mother; Benjamin, 1996a; McWilliams, 1998); dominant interpersonal concerns (fears, wishes, and cognitive constructions) that repetitively emerge in the person's relationships and are manifest in narratives of interpersonal encounters (e.g., in psychotherapy hours; Baldwin, Fehr, Keedian, Seidel, & Thomson, 1993; Horowitz, 1999; Luborsky & Crits-Christoph, 1990); and social skills, which are often deficient in patients with Axis II Cluster A pathology (paranoid, schizoid, and schizotypal) but can be seen in more attenuated forms in people who have difficulty reading other people's emotions, do not maintain culturally appropriate physical proximity from others while talking, and so forth (Lancelot & Nowicki, 1997; McClure & Nowicki, 2001; Nowicki & Duke, 2002).

A final set of variables related to interpersonal functioning and of obvious relevance to many forms of psychopathology involves aspects of self (see Gabbard, 2005). Although the term "self" is often used to refer to multiple different phenomena (see Westen, 1992), clinically relevant aspects of self include the coherence of the person's sense of self (i.e., sense of agency and continuity through time); the nature of chronically recurring implicit and explicit self-representations; self-esteem (implicit and explicit) and self-esteem regulation; feared, wished-for, and ideal self-representations that serve as standards or guides for behavior (Higgins, 1990; Strauman & Higgins, 1993); and what Erikson (1986) referred to as identity, which includes the sense of self, representations of self, the recognition of one's selfhood by the social milieu, and an emotional weighting of elements of self (such as roles) the person experiences as self-defining.

From a clinical perspective, these domains of functioning are essential in case formulation because they describe what the person is characterologically able or unable to do—and hence provide targets for intervention. They are also crucially important in understanding the ways people become symptomatic. A person with rigid values regarding his feelings and impulses, who believes (consciously or unconsciously) that he is culpable for his thoughts as well as his deeds, may be vulnerable to alternations of compulsive rigidity and breakthroughs of impulsive actions (as appeared to be the case with the televangelists who fell from grace in the 1980s, who preached by day against the evils of sex and practiced by night one or another colorful, illicit, or perverse version of it). A person with an avoidant or dismissing adult attachment style who regulates emotion by denying or suppressing it may become vulnerable to panic attacks or generalized anxiety disorder precisely because he is working so hard to avoid feeling (and hence responding adaptively) to his emotions. A person with low intelligence is, empirically, more likely to succumb to posttraumatic stress disorder in wartime (Macklin et al., 1998; McNally & Shin, 1995). A person whose enduring attitude toward herself, or view of herself under particular circumstances, is characterized by self-loathing is likely to be vulnerable to mood, anxiety, and substance use disorders. Below we explore the question of how well these functional domains and their implications for psychopathology map on to prominent trait models of personality.

Level of Pathology

Nancy McWilliams (1999) tells the charming story of a not terribly psychologically minded friend who did not understand how someone could spend her days listening to other people's problems. To him, people could be grouped into two large classes: nuts and not nuts. McWilliams suggests that a psychoanalytic view places everyone in the first class (nuts) but asks two questions about their character: how nuts, and what kind of nuts? In this section, we address the issue of *how* nuts (levels of personality pathology). In the next, we address the issue of *what kind*.

Freud inherited from Kraepelin the distinction between patients with neurotic and psychotic pathology (see McWilliams, 1999). As we have seen, over time, Freud and other psychoanalysts began to differentiate "neurosis" into symptom neuroses (relatively isolated pockets of pathology) and character neuroses (pathology widely dispersed throughout the person's personality). Over time, however, what became clear was that in the characterological realm patients varied from relatively functional to relatively dysfunctional. As early as the 1920s, clinicians and clinical theorists began to write about patients who were not psychotic but who were too sick to consider merely neurotic (what today we call severe personality pathology). Menninger, Mayman, and Pruyser (1962) proposed that patients could be described on a continuum of functioning in terms of their capacity for coping and adaptation.

The concept of a general health–sickness continuum that emerged from the Menninger Clinic ultimately led to the development of the Global Assessment Scale (Endicott, Spitzer, Fleiss, & Cohen, 1976), later renamed Global Assessment of Functioning (GAF), which is now Axis V of the DSM and can be coded with high reliability (Hilsenroth et al., 2000). Although useful as a rough index of pathology, however, the GAF mixes severity of current symptoms, degree of medical risk (e.g., severity of suicidality), and level of personality functioning at each of its levels, rendering it a somewhat rough index of personality health–sickness.

Kernberg (1975) systematized the notion of levels of personality health/sickness in distinguishing three levels of character organization, which he called neurotic, borderline, and psychotic.[3] The gist of the notion of levels of pathology in Kernberg's work, which is shared now by most psychodynamic theorists, is as follows. Personality pathology lies on a continuum reflecting the extent to which the individual is able to love, work, and enjoy life. Patients at a *neurotic* to normal level are capable of forming meaningful relationships, finding and maintaining steady employment, and generally attending to the demands normally placed on adults in their society. They may, nevertheless, have substantial neurotic conflicts, symptoms, and defensive and relational patterns that decrease their life satisfaction (e.g., rigid obsessional defenses, high levels of anxiety, a tendency to get into repetitive patterns in relationships that interfere with their happiness). At the lower (more troubled) end of the neurotic range (often called a *low-functioning neurotic*), the person may be seriously compromised in love, work, or play (e.g., working far below his abilities because of inhibitions, unable to commit to an enduring love relationship without repetitive affairs) but is typically able to adjust to the demands of reality (e.g., meeting rent payments, keeping a job, having some friends).

Empirically, much of personality pathology encountered in clinical practice is in this range. For example, Westen and Arkowitz-Westen (1998) asked 238 experienced clinicians to describe 714 nonpsychotic patients in treatment for personality patterns that were dysfunctional or led to significant distress regardless of whether or not they met PD criteria. Clinicians completed checklists for all DSM-IV personality disorders, Axis I categories, and problems that did not necessarily meet the criteria for any personality disorder (e.g., problems with intimacy, self-esteem, emotional constriction, impulsivity). Roughly 60% of patients had personality difficulties deserving clinical attention and yet could not be diagnosed by the DSM-IV because they were not of sufficient severity to merit a diagnosis of personality disorder.

Other research has documented the consequences of subthreshold personality pathology, or "neurotic-level" character disturbances. Daley et al. (1999) used dimensional measures of personality disorder symptomatology based on a diagnostic questionnaire and the SCID-II (First, Spitzer, Gibbon, & Williams, 1997) with a sample of 155 girls in late adolescence to predict Axis I problems prospectively. Only about 6% qualified for a formal personality disorder diagnosis; however, subthreshold endorsement predicted depression at 2- to 3-year follow-up, holding initial depression constant. In another longitudinal study (Daley, Burge, & Hammen, 2000), the investigators found that subthreshold levels of nearly all personality disorders predicted romantic stress, interpersonal conflicts, and dysfunction (e.g., unwanted pregnancy) at 4-year follow-up. Similar findings emerge from studies of adult attachment status. In prospective and longitudinal studies, insecure attachment predicts difficulty at work and in the family (Vasquez, Durik, & Hyde, 2002), interpersonal aggression (Crowell, Treboux, & Waters, 2002), and later psychopathology (Carlson, 1998). Retrospective studies (e.g., Klohnen & Bera, 1998) have found avoidant attachment to predict increasingly unhappy relationships over the lifespan. Although most people with personality disorders have attachment problems, most people with insecure attachment styles do not have personality disorders (Brennan & Shaver, 1998).

Patients at a personality disordered level (what Kernberg calls borderline personality organization) can generally distinguish reality from their own thoughts (i.e., they do not have hallucinations or fixed delusions), but their capacity to love and work is seriously compromised. From a descriptive point of view, they may have difficulty holding a job, may have few or tumultuous relationships, or may find themselves in and out of psychiatric hospitals. From a more dynamic standpoint, Kernberg suggests that what they share are immature or maladaptive defenses and difficulty forming complex, multifaceted, integrated representations of the self and others (Kernberg, 1975, 1984). Patients with paranoid personality disorder, for example, tend to project and externalize, and their representations of others are rigidly malevolent and one-dimensional. Patients with borderline personality disorder, have difficulty regulating powerful affect states, turning instead to behaviors such as cutting and suicide attempts, and their representations of others tend to be highly state-dependent (e.g., unidimensional and malevolent when confronted with turbulence in an emotionally significant relationship). Empirically, these long-held clinical beliefs have stood the test of time (Shedler & Westen, 2004b; Westen & Shedler, 1999a).

Within the broad range of disorders defined as personality disorders in DSM-IV, however, is considerable variability in level of pathology in Kernberg's sense. Although the criteria for DSM-IV obsessive–compulsive personality disorder describe a severely disturbed personality, empirically many patients who meet criteria for this disorder actually have reasonably high GAF scores (because they are capable of working, often with a high level of productivity) and can maintain relationships over time (even if compromised by their lack of emotional connection; e.g., Gunderson et al., 2000; Westen & Shedler, 1999a). Patients with borderline personality disorder range from those who can encapsulate their work so that they retain some degree of functionality, or can maintain relatively stable relationships with friends over time, to patients often described as just "north of the border" (of psychosis), whose reality testing can become extremely compromised. Interestingly, in our research, we have repeatedly found that clinicians of all theoretical orientations are able to make a simple 5-point rating of level of personality health–sickness based loosely on Kernberg's model of levels of functioning that is more predictive of dimensional measures of personality disorders than is the GAF, and these single-item ratings show surprisingly high interjudge reliability (see Westen & Muderrisoglu, 2003).

Forms of Personality Organization (Personality Disorders and Personality Styles)

The concept of personality styles or constellations should be familiar to readers because it formed the basis of Axis II of DSM-IV. The current personality disorders were largely derived from the clinical observations of psychoanalytically and biologically oriented taxonomists. As noted above, the concept of personality disorder emerged from psychoanalytic clinical observation and led to the development of diagnoses such as borderline and narcissistic personality disorder. Pioneering psychiatric taxonomists of the early 20th century noted that many first-degree relatives of patients with severe mental illness themselves appeared a bit "touched," ultimately leading to constructs such as schizotypal personality disorder.

In classifying personality pathology, Kernberg (1967, 1984, 1996) proposed a severity axis (described earlier) that is orthogonal to an axis of personality styles or types such as the personality disorders on Axis II of DSM-IV. For example, a patient could have a narcissistic personality style organized at a neurotic level, a high-functioning personality disorder level, or a low-functioning personality disorder level. Individuals with a narcissistic character style organized at a neurotic level tend to be self-absorbed and overly sanguine about their abilities and accomplishments, but they are still capable of forming long-lasting love relationships and friendships, and they are often highly productive. Narcissistic patients organized at a more severely disturbed level tend to have little capacity for empathy, little interest in others except for what they can provide, and few if any close relationships. They may even undo themselves occupationally by virtue of their difficulty in regulating angry outbursts or their inability to let the obstacles most people encounter on their way up in an organization "roll off their back."

Drawing on Kernberg's work, McWilliams (1994) offered a diagnostic grid in which columns represent personality styles, each distinguished by its complaints, affects, relational problems, primary defenses, strengths, and so forth, and rows represent levels of severity. As in Kernberg's model, different personality styles may present at neurotic, borderline, psychotic, or intermediate levels of disturbance. Based on clinical experience and available empirical data, McWilliams describes psychopathic, narcissistic, schizoid, depressive and/or manic, obsessive and/or compulsive, masochistic (self-defeating), hysterical (histrionic), and dissociative personality styles.

Kernberg has offered a similar typology. Both suggest that, although different personality styles can occur at different levels of personality organization (severity), not all sectors of McWilliams's grid are equally populated. People with genuinely schizoid dynamics, for example, are less likely to be well adapted to social life and hence are more likely to fall into the lower ranges of personality pathology. However, many individuals who are introverted—but who do not show the tendency toward either concrete representations of self and others or the overly elaborated fantasy life often attributed to schizoid characters—function in the normal to neurotic range.

Kernberg, McWilliams, and virtually all psychoanalytically oriented taxonomists of character have drawn on Shapiro's (1965) classic work on "neurotic styles." These styles include characteristic conflicts, defensive strategies, and cognitive styles. For example, the hysterical style is characterized by an impressionistic, overly glib and global cognitive style and a tendency to rely on repressive defenses. Individuals with a hysterical style may seem polyannish, overly optimistic, and naive, and they tend not to think deeply about information that might be threatening. They tend to be conflicted about their sexual impulses and to sexualize interactions with others without acting on their desires, often leading others to feel confused, disappointed, or "led on." People often perceive them as naively romantic, immature, flighty, or shallow.

At a neurotic level, an individual with a hysterical style is likely to be extroverted, to have multiple friends and acquaintances, to be flirtatious (but generally not to "mean it"), to disavow negative affect, and to be valued by others for his or her positive outlook (e.g., the classic high school cheerleader). The same character style, when organized at a borderline level of personality organization, often manifests as histrionic personality disorder and is characterized by substantially greater egocentrism, self-centeredness, powerful affects that seem to come and go by the moment, and a level of seductiveness that can be socially inappropriate. The notion of a hysterical style organized at different levels of pathology was first described in some detail by Zetzel (1968), who distinguished between the "good hysteric" and the "bad hysteric." The latter would today be diagnosed with borderline or histrionic personality disorder, or both.

Although personality disorders now constitute an axis of the diagnostic manual (lumped unceremoniously with mental retardation), neurotic styles did not make their way into the official diagnostic nomenclature for historical reasons (Bayer & Spitzer, 1985). Personality pathology received minimal research attention until DSM-III instituted a multiaxial diagnostic system (American Psychiatric Association, 1980). The personality disturbances in DSM-I (American Psychiatric Association, 1952) and DSM-II (American Psychiatric Association, 1968) were never operationalized, and were mixed in with syndromes such as depression and schizophrenia. The move toward operationalization that began with the Research Diagnostic Criteria (Spitzer, Endicott, & Robins, 1978), and ultimately DSM-III, introduced high diagnostic thresholds defined by relatively arbitrary cutoffs (Widiger, 1993). Whereas the descriptions of personality categories in DSM-I and DSM-II were phrased in ways that allowed clinicians to use them to describe higher or lower levels of dysfunction (but to do so unreliably), DSM-III and its descendants maximized reliability by limiting personality diagnoses to relatively severe forms of personality disturbance. Thus, paradoxically, by emphasizing the importance of diagnosing personality pathology (placing it on its own axis), DSM-III passed over the less severe and probably more common forms of personality disturbance.

Not surprisingly, because of their absence from the diagnostic manual, neurotic styles have received minimal empirical attention (except in terms of subthreshold personality disorders). Blagov and Westen (in preparation) have recently attempted to derive diagnostic prototypes of naturally occurring personality styles at a neurotic level. The investigators asked a random sample of 168 clinicians to describe a randomly selected patient in their care for personality difficulties that did not meet DSM-IV cutoffs for a PD. Clinicians described the patients using the Shedler–Westen Assessment Procedure—200 (SWAP-200; Westen & Shedler, 1999a), a 200-item personality pathology Q-sort instrument. The investigators then used Q-factor analysis (also called inverted factor analysis, a procedure for grouping together individuals based on shared characteristics) to try to identify neurotic styles empirically. Aside from the high-functioning obsessional character style identified in their prior work (in contradistinction to the DSM-IV obsessive–compulsive personality disorder, which describes someone much more severely ill; see Westen & Shedler, 1999b), Q-factor analysis identified three additional neurotic styles: a high-functioning depressive style (similar to a prototype previously identified as a depressive or dysphoric personality disorder subtype); a hostile/competitive style, characterized by strong needs for power, dominance, and success, coupled with acknowledged and unacknowledged anger; and a hysterical personality style resembling Shapiro's (1965) description. Whether a typological approach (or in this case, dimensional typology, or prototype approach) or trait approach to personality pathology (or some combination) will prove more useful in prediction is, however, an open question.

Integrating the Three Components of the Clinical Model of Personality Structure: Functional Domains, Levels of Pathology, and Personality Styles or Constellations

Clinical theorists have been relatively clear in their writing about the relation between levels and types of personality pathology. Patients with similar personality styles can be organized at different levels of pathology, depending on the extent to which their pathology is severe, rigid, ubiquitous across roles and relationships, and destructive of the capacity to love, work, and enjoy life. Different theorists have offered particular criteria for linking functional domains to levels of pathology. For example, Kernberg emphasizes maturity of defense and integrity of representations of self and others in distinguishing patients at different levels of pathology. Using the model of functional domains described here, disturbances in motivation (e.g., lack of a well-developed conscience), deficits in adaptive psychological resources (e.g., inability to regulate affects and impulses in mature ways), and difficulties in understanding and interacting with people in mature, mutually pleasurable, and socially competent ways are all of relevance in assessing levels of pathology.

With respect to the relation between functional domains and personality styles (or, as we suggest below, personality traits), we would argue that descriptive diagnosis (whether of personality disorders in the DSM tradition or traits in the tradition of personality psychology) can and should be derivative of a functional assessment. Indeed, the goal of clinical work is to alter functioning in dysfunctional domains; hence, functional diagnosis and descriptive diagnosis must be closely related if descriptive diagnosis is to be clinically useful.

Case Illustration

To illustrate how functional diagnosis can be translated into descriptive diagnosis, and equally important, how a nomothetic approach using a standardized psychometric instrument designed for clinically experienced observers can be used for idiographic personality assessment, we briefly describe a quantified case study. The case was taken from a study using the SWAP-200 Q-sort, in which a random national sample of 530 clinicians was asked to describe a patient with a personality disorder. Our description of this patient, whom we shall call Ms. Z, reflects only the data provided by the treating clinician.

Ms. Z is a 36-year-old woman who has been in treatment for 2 years. Despite a college education, she works as a semiskilled worker. The reporting psychiatrist gave her an Axis I diagnosis of major depressive disorder, recurrent. The clinician reported that the patient described a history of severe physical abuse beginning at age 7 and a history of repeated sexual abuse by a neighbor for slightly less than 1 year at age 13. The clinician also reported a family history of substance abuse and depression in first-degree biological relatives.

An Idiographic Narrative Description. The following narrative was obtained by listing the SWAP-200 items the clinician assigned to the three highest (most descriptive) categories (categories 5, 6, and 7) of the Q-sort. The items are reprinted verbatim, except for minor grammatical changes to aid the flow of the narrative.

Ms. Z lacks close friendships and relationships. She lacks social skills, tending to be socially awkward or inappropriate. She tends to feel like an outcast or outsider, and avoids confiding in others for fear of betrayal, expecting that the things she says will be used against her. She tends to believe she can only be appreciated by, or should only associate with, people who are high-status, superior, or otherwise "special." Her relationships tend to be unstable, chaotic, and rapidly changing.

Ms. Z is exclusively homosexual in her sexual orientation. She tends to choose sexual or romantic partners who seem inappropriate in terms of age, status (e.g., social, economic, intellectual), and so on. She tends to get drawn into or remain in relationships in which she is emotionally or physically abused, and she has difficulty directing both tender feelings and sexual feelings toward the same person (e.g., she sees people as respectable and virtuous, or sexy and exciting, but not both). She has a sexual perversion or fetish, a rigidly scripted or highly idiosyncratic condition that must be met before she can experience sexual gratification.

Ms. Z tends to use her psychological or medical problems to avoid work or responsibility (whether consciously or unconsciously). She tends to develop somatic symptoms in response to stress or conflict (e.g., headache, backache, abdominal pain, asthma, etc.). She is hypochondriacal, tending to have unfounded fears of contracting medical illness, and interpreting normal aches and pains as symptomatic of illness. She tends to be preoccupied with food and diet. She also tends to be preoccupied with death and dying.

Ms. Z tends to enter altered, dissociated states of consciousness when distressed (e.g., the self or the world feels strange, unfamiliar, or unreal). She tends to be superstitious or believe in magical or supernatural phenomena (e.g., astrology, tarot, crystals, ESP, "auras," etc.). Her reasoning processes or perceptual experiences seem odd and idiosyncratic (e.g., she may make seemingly arbitrary inferences; may see hidden messages or special meanings in ordinary events), and her speech tends to be circumstantial, vague, rambling, digressive, and so on. Her verbal statements often seem incongruous with her accompanying affect, or incongruous with accompanying nonverbal messages.

Ms. Z tends to think in abstract and intellectualized terms, even in matters of personal import. She tends to describe experiences in generalities and is unwilling or unable to offer specific details. She has difficulty acknowledging or expressing anger and appears, more generally, to have a limited or constricted range of emotions. She has difficulty allowing herself to experience strong pleasurable emotions (e.g., excitement, joy, pride). She tends to feel unhappy, depressed, or despondent.

Ms. Z tends to be passive and unassertive. She appears inhibited about pursuing goals or successes; her aspirations or achievements tend to be below her potential. She tends to be conflicted about authority (e.g., may feel she must submit, rebel against, win over, defeat, etc.), although she is conscientious and responsible. She tends to be suggestible or easily influenced.

Clinical Formulation. Research assessing the relation between SWAP-200 data obtained from treating clinicians and from independent observers using a systematic clinical interview finds interobserver correlations on dimensional Axis II diagnoses and on trait dimensions derived factor-analytically between $r = .70$ and $.80$ (Westen & Muderrisoglu, 2003, in press). Thus, the description of Ms. Z above is likely to be very similar to the description that would be generated by any competent, experienced clinician using the SWAP-200.

Based on this description, we can offer a tentative case formulation, or set of clinical hypotheses. Ms. Z has difficulty forming meaningful relationships because her past experiences have engendered deep distrust. She attempts to protect herself by keeping others at a distance, and her social skills deficits likely interfere with her capacity to form and maintain relationships. She feels like an outsider and attempts to compensate through fantasies of superiority, but at some level she probably feels deeply defective socially.

Unwittingly, Ms. Z re-creates her abusive childhood world by forming inappropriate relationships in which she feels abused or mistreated. Sexual relationships are particularly problematic, perhaps because she has learned to associate love with abuse. Her sexual perversion most likely contains sadomasochistic elements.

Like many abuse survivors, Ms. Z is numb to her emotions. She employs a range of defensive processes to avoid affect-laden memories, including intellectualization, thinking in generalities, and ultimately dissociation. Along with chronic depression, the language she uses to express her pain is the language of the body: she turns her anger, fear, and sadness into somatic complaints and hypochondriacal concerns. She has little awareness of her anger, and likely learned to inhibit anger that might provoke her physically abusive parents.

Cognitively, Ms. Z is prone to disorganization, digression, "empty" generalizations without the accompanying memories and feelings, and idiosyncratic and superstitious thinking, which are also likely sequelae of her severe abuse history. In many ways her behavior appears peculiar to others, both because of the way she thinks and speaks but also because of the incongruities between what she expresses verbally and nonverbally (e.g., in her behavior). She probably has difficult telling a coherent life narrative, or even coherent "stories" about relatively circumscribed events, because of her inability to think in a clear, linear way and to take the perspective of the listener.

Ms. Z's social and cognitive idiosyncrasies, as well as her tendency to somatize and hence to miss work frequently, probably contribute to her inability to maintain employment commensurate with her level of education. Although she is diligent and conscientious, she is passive, unassertive, and inhibited in asking for, and taking the necessary steps to achieve, what she wants. She has problems with authority figures and may see her bosses as unfair or abusive, like her parents. At the same time, she handles anger by being compliant and self-effacing, and doing what is asked. In her occupational life, as in her personal life, her inability to use her feelings as guides leaves her rudderless.

SWAP-200 DSM-IV PD and Factor (Trait) Profiles. Figure 11.1 shows Ms. Z's dimensional Axis II profile, using the SWAP-200. For ease of interpretation the scores are converted to T-scores (mean = 50, *SD* = 10), similar to a Minnesota Multiphasic Personality Inventory—2 (MMPI-2) profile. Because the normative sample for the SWAP-200 comprised only patients with personality disorders, a T-score of 60 would typically translate to a DSM-IV categorical diagnosis, and a T-score of 55 would translate to "features." (We are currently norming the latest version of the instrument, the SWAP-II, using a sample and procedures that will allow more ready translation to a DSM-IV diagnosis, although the instrument is intended primarily for dimensional diagnosis.) As can be seen from the figure, Ms. Z would receive a diagnosis of schizotypal PD. As can be seen from her score on the high-functioning or health index, she is below the mean on personality health–sickness even for a PD sample.

Figure 11.2 shows Ms. Z's profile on the 12 SWAP-200 factors (traits) derived by factor analysis (Shedler & Westen, 2004b). Once again for ease of interpretation, the factor scores have been converted to T-scores. Ms. Z shows a marked elevation on dissociated consciousness (more than two standard deviations above the mean), indicating disconnected thoughts, feelings, and memories, gaps in memory, and a tendency to enter altered, dissociated states (common in survivors of childhood sexual abuse). Her profile also reveals an elevation on thought disorder, indicating gaps in reality testing and peculiar and idiosyncratic reasoning (hence the schizotypal diagnosis). (As described above, we have identified what appear to be at least two pathways to schizotypy, one related to schizophrenia spectrum pathology and the other to a history of childhood trauma; this patient's pathology appears to reflect the latter pathway.) A marked elevation on histrionic sexualization (which includes a tendency to choose inappropriate or unavailable partners) plus some elevation on sexual conflict indicates disturbed sexual functioning and problematic romantic relationships. Ms. Z is

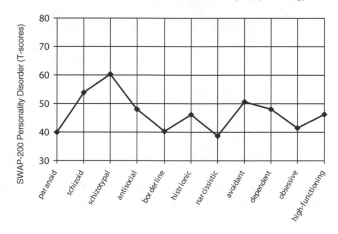

FIGURE 11.1. SWAP-200 personality disorder profile of Ms. Z.

more than a standard deviation below the mean on hostility and emotional dysregulation, suggesting constricted affect and difficulty in expressing anger.

We describe this case as an example of how a model of personality structure that emerged from clinical practice and was designed to meet the needs of clinical work could be operationalized in a rigorous quantitative way. Although items from the SWAP-200 were derived from multiple

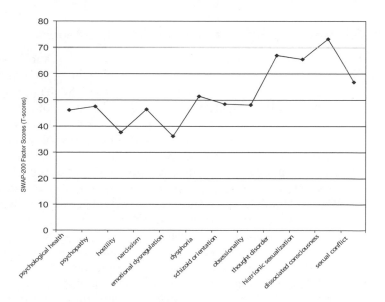

FIGURE 11.2. SWAP-200 trait profile of Ms. Z.

sources (including the diagnostic criteria for the personality disorders listed on Axis II from DSM-III through DSM-IV, and clinical writing and research on neurotic-range personality pathology), we used the model of functional domains described above to maximize content validity, that is, to ensure that the item set comprehensively sampled the domains central to the clinical assessment of personality. What we hope to have shown with this example is that one need not choose between clinical "thick description" and empirical rigor.

INTEGRATING CLINICAL AND PSYCHOMETRIC PERSPECTIVES ON PERSONALITY STRUCTURE

We conclude with some reflections on the question of whether, and in what ways, the models of personality structure that emerged from psychoanalytic clinical observation over the past century may be integrable with contemporary trait approaches to personality that have breathed new life into the marriage of personality and psychopathology following a period of prolonged estrangement. We briefly address two issues: the relation between traits generated by self-reports and clinician reports (as in the SWAP); and the extent to which trait models of personality structure can provide adequate models for clinical practice, notwithstanding their obvious merits for research purposes.

Traits Generated by Self-Reports and Clinician-Reports

Although much of the taxonomic work using the SWAP-200 (and its latest version, the SWAP-II) has focused on identifying personality *configurations* as a way of revising Axis II personality disorder diagnoses and diagnostic criteria, as should be clear from Figure 11.2, nothing in the nature of the instrument prevents the derivation of traits by conventional factor analysis. Westen, Shedler, and colleagues have derived traits in both adult and adolescent samples using the SWAP-200 (Shedler & Westen, 2004; Westen, Dutra, & Shedler, 2005). The traits identified using the SWAP and the "Big Four" traits identified in recent research with psychopathological samples (see Markon, Krueger, & Watson, 2005; Trull & Durrett, 2005; Widiger & Simonsen, in press) have substantial overlap. For example, both the adolescent and adult versions of the SWAP-200 include dimensions relevant to negative affectivity or neuroticism (dysphoria, anxious obsessionality); introversion or low positive affectivity (schizoid orientation, peer rejection); antagonism or low agreeableness (hostility, malignant narcissism); and impulsivity, low constraint, or low conscientiousness (psychopathy, delinquent behavior).

Some traits identified using the SWAP-200, however, are not easily understood in terms of the Big Four or Big Five. For example, emotional dysregulation refers to the tendency for emotions to spiral out of control and appears to be empirically distinct from neuroticism or negative affectivity. The difference between the two constructs is perhaps best exemplified by the difference between patients who are stably depressed or anxious (e.g., patients with dysthymic disorder or generalized anxiety disorder) and patients with borderline personality disorder, whose emotional dysregulation may or may not be superimposed on stable characterological depression or anxiety. The distinction between emotional dysregulation and negative affect has now emerged in several samples using multiple instruments (Shedler & Westen, 2004a; Westen et al., 1997; Westen et al., 2005). We suspect it has largely been overlooked because emotional dysregulation is a relatively low base rate phenomenon in the normal samples from which most trait constructs were derived. (Interestingly, emotional dysregulation has emerged as a factor, though not distinct from negative affect, on self-report instruments intended to assess personality pathology and derived from clinicians' ratings of items prototypic of different personality disorders; see Larstone, Jang, Livesley, Vernon, & Wolf, 2002; Wang, Du, Wang, Livesley, & Jang, 2004).

Westen, Jenei, Walsh, and Bradley (2005) recently used factor analysis to "decompose" each DSM-IV personality disorder into its component traits or endophenotypes, using the SWAP-200 to identify item sets of 20–25 items per disorder. The procedure generated 3–6 factors per disorder. By way of illustration, Table 11.2 presents the trait structure of schizotypal personality disorder (including any secondary factor loadings ≥ .30). As can be seen, the factor structure captures three central features of the disorder but may also help explain its overlap with other disorders. For example, social avoidance is characteristic not only of schizotypal personality disorder but of paranoid, schizoid, and avoidant personality disorder; and schizotypy is characteristic of patients with paranoid personality disorder.

Of particular relevance to the present discussion, once the investigators identified the factor structure of each personality disorder in isolation, they conducted a second-order factor analysis of the 31 traits identified across disorders. This higher-order factor analysis yielded six factors: negative affect, schizotypy, hostility, constraint, emotional dysregulation, and attachment pathology. Convergence with the Big Four is clear. However, schizotypy was a broader and somewhat different construct than extreme introversion, as it also included peculiar thinking. Emotional dysregulation and attachment pathology also have no obvious representation among the Big Four. To what extent they predict incremental variance on relevant criterion variables is as yet unknown.

Moving from personality traits to personality patterns or prototypes (i.e., constellations of traits or relatively specific attributes that empirically

TABLE 11.2. Trait Structure of Schizotypal Personality Disorder

SWAP-200 item	Social avoidance	Schizotypy	Impoverished thought/affect
Tends to avoid social situations because of fear of embarrassment or humiliation.	.76		
Tends to be shy or reserved in social situations.	.75		
Tends to feel like an outcast or outsider; feels as if s/he does not truly belong.	.66		
Lacks social skills; tends to be socially awkward or inappropriate.	.57		
Lacks close friendships and relationships.	.55		
Tends to avoid confiding in others for fear of betrayal; expects things s/he says or does will be used against him/her.	.42		
Appears to have little need for human company or contact; is genuinely indifferent to the presence of others.	.41		
Reasoning processes or perceptual experiences seem odd and idiosyncratic (e.g., may make seemingly arbitrary inferences; may see hidden messages or special meanings in ordinary events).		.95	
Tends to be superstitious or believe in magical or supernatural phenomena (e.g., astrology, tarot, crystals, ESP, "auras," etc.).		.72	
Perception of reality can become grossly impaired under stress (e.g., may become delusional).		.64	
Appearance or manner seems odd or peculiar (e.g., grooming, hygiene, posture, eye contact, speech rhythms, etc. seem somehow strange or "off").		.61	
Feels some important other has a special, almost magical ability to understand his/her innermost thoughts and feelings (e.g., may imagine rapport is so perfect that ordinary efforts at communication are superfluous).		.53	
Speech tends to be circumstantial, vague, rambling, digressive, etc.		.52	
Tends to become irrational when strong emotions are stirred up; may show a noticeable decline from customary level of functioning.		.38	
Appears unable to describe important others in a way that conveys a sense of who they are as people; descriptions of others come across as two-dimensional and lacking in richness.			.72
Tends to think in concrete terms and interpret things in overly literal ways; has limited ability to appreciate metaphor, analogy, or nuance.			.60
Has little psychological insight into own motives, behavior, etc.; is unable to consider alternate interpretations of his/her experiences.			.54
Has difficulty making sense of other people's behavior; often misunderstands, misinterprets, or is confused by others' actions and reactions.			.45
Appears to have a limited or constricted range of emotions.	.39		.43
Verbal statements seem incongruous with accompanying affect, or incongruous with accompanying nonverbal messages.			.41

tend to covary, reflecting broader personality "styles"), our most recent efforts to derive such constellations empirically using large, relatively unselected samples of adults (N = 1,201) and adolescents (N = 950) with personality pathology have led to substantial concordance with trait models developed by Krueger and colleagues (Krueger, 1999; Krueger, Markon, Patrick, & Iacono, in press; Krueger & Piasecki, 2002). Applying Q (person-centered, rather than variable-centered) factor analysis, we are obtaining a hierarchical structure in both adult and adolescent samples with superordinate configurational dimensions of internalizing, externalizing, and borderline spectrum pathology. We have just begun analyzing these data, but nested within the internalizing and externalizing spectra are highly recognizable personality disorders. For example, in preliminary analyses, the adult internalizing spectrum appears to include depressive, anxious, dependent, and schizoid personality disorders. The externalizing dimension includes paranoid, narcissistic, and psychopathic personality disorders. What is potentially exciting about this hierarchical structure is its relation both to trait dimensions identified by Krueger and others and more traditional personality disorder diagnoses, although it suggests what may be a more empirically grounded hierarchical structure than the personality disorder "clusters" in DSM-IV.

Applying Trait Models of Personality Structure to Clinical Practice

Although we have suggested that trait models can be derived from factor analysis of clinician reports just as they can from self- or other lay informant-report measures, to what extent trait models alone can provide adequate guidance for clinical work is unclear. Clinicians do not find Axis II of DSM-IV particularly helpful clinically, but recent data suggest that they find trait models such as the FFM and Cloninger's (Cloninger & Svrakic, 1994) seven-factor model even less clinically informative (First, Spitzer, & Skodal, 2005). From a clinical perspective, neither traditional DSM diagnosis nor traditional trait description appears adequate to guide clinical practice. Clinicians do not tend to find it useful to ask questions of the form "Does the patient cross the threshold for avoidant personality disorder?" or "How high is the patient on neuroticism?" Rather, clinicians tend to ask questions of the form "Under what circumstances do which cognitive, affective, motivational, and behavioral patterns and their interactions get triggered in ways that lead to distress for the patient or those around him?"

As argued above, this is a functional question, and questions of function tend to be the focus of clinical work. Both the DSM and trait traditions share the problem for which Mischel (1968) years ago criticized trait theories and has articulated more accurately since (e.g., Mischel & Shoda,

1995), namely, the failure to specify the eliciting conditions for personality processes (Westen, 1995, 1996, in press). Consider the following item from the SWAP-II: "When distressed, perception of reality can become grossly impaired (e.g., thinking may seem delusional)." Thought disorder is not well represented in five-factor space, and even Axis II is limited in addressing disordered thinking that emerges only under certain circumstances. We suspect, for example, that much of the "comorbidity" found between borderline and paranoid personality disorders reflects the failure to distinguish the chronic suspiciousness of the paranoid patient (well indexed by the Big Four or Big Five facet of *mistrust*) from the contingent malevolent expectations of the borderline patient (which has no counterpart in any trait model). The contingency of malevolence in patients with borderline personality disorder has been documented empirically by its differential elicitation by stimuli with different affective "pulls" (Westen, Lohr, et al., 1990).

There is no inherent reason item sets used to derive trait structures cannot include eliciting conditions (e.g., the item from the SWAP-200, cited earlier, that includes the qualifier "when distressed"). Such qualifiers are not, however, consistent with a lexical approach to deriving items from everyday language, if the goal is to represent traits adjectivally, because single-word descriptors (adjectives) by definition cannot easily express context or qualification. Regardless of the item set, however, an important challenge ahead for taxonomists using factor analysis to derive clinically useful trait constructs will be to find ways to avoid the loss of resolution vis-à-vis eliciting conditions and qualifiers that comes with factor-analytic aggregation. For example, factor analysis is likely to group together aggression differentially expressed toward one sex or the other, subordinates, peers, and authority figures under the broader rubric of "hostility" or "aggression," but this loses precisely the distinctions that are likely to be clinically useful.[4] Trait descriptions using the SWAP are not immune to this criticism, which we have attempted to address, as in the case study above, by providing a narrative description using items written in everyday clinical language along with a trait profile. However, a more elegant mathematical way of preserving some of the complexity of idiographic description that does not wash out the activating conditions as systematically as factor analysis tends to do would certainly be a welcome development.

Aside from their relative inattention to context or activating conditions, widely used trait models generally fail to addresses internal psychological *processes* in a way that clinicians find useful. Many psychological processes (mental states and their conditional transformations) that can be captured by an instrument such as the SWAP (designed for clinically experienced observers) are difficult to represent using more common self-report trait measures. Consider the following psychological processes and the SWAP-II items designed to assess them:

- *Cognitive style*: "Tends to perceive things in global and impression-istic ways (e.g., misses details, glosses over inconsistencies, mispro-nounces names)."
- *Affect regulation*: "Attempts to avoid feeling helpless or depressed by becoming angry instead."
- *Complexity of representations of people*: "Appears unable to de-scribe important others in a way that conveys a sense of who they are as people; descriptions of others come across as two-dimen-sional and lacking in richness."
- *Capacity for self-reflection*: "Has the capacity to recognize alterna-tive viewpoints, even in matters that stir up strong feelings."
- *Beliefs and feelings toward the self*: "Has a deep sense of inner bad-ness; sees self as damaged, evil, or rotten to the core (whether con-sciously or unconsciously)."
- *Sexuality*: "Has difficulty directing both tender feelings and sexual feelings toward the same person (e.g., sees others as nurturing and virtuous or sexy and exciting, but not both)."

To what extent such processes could be captured by self-reports is un-known, but we suspect the fact that these processes are largely not available to introspection (i.e., they are implicit rather than explicit) and the fact that they generally have not been captured in over 60 years of objective testing may provide an indication. At the same time, it seems highly unlikely that the traits identified by trait theorists (particularly the Big Four psycho-pathology traits) that have proven so generative of research, replicable across samples and instruments, and useful for behavior genetic (and, increasingly, genetic and neuroimaging) research could be of little relevance from a clini-cal standpoint. One potential strategy for integrating traditional trait ap-proaches with more process- and function-oriented clinical language might be to correlate the 200 items of the SWAP with measures of the Big Four or Big Five. Thus, one might begin to translate the empirical lexicon of the FFM or Big Four psychopathology traits into a more clinically rich lan-guage.

In any case, it seems likely that the most important hurdle to be faced by trait researchers whose goal is to replace traditional personality disorder diagnoses with factor-analytically derived traits in DSM-V will be to dem-onstrate not their empirical strengths, which are considerable, but their clinical utility. The DSM is intended as a manual for clinicians as well as re-searchers. However, over the past 25 years, revisions have tended to focus on increasing its utility for research purposes (e.g., identifying diagnostic criteria that may be readily assessed by structured interview and hence use-ful in identifying "clean" diagnostic groups), with the assumption that such changes will "trickle down" to clinical practice in the form of better research evidence. As the manual has become more unmanageable, however, with its explosion of diagnostic categories and laundry-list criterion sets that lack any grounding in functional or causal relations that are helpful in human categorization (see Kim & Ahn, 2002; Westen & Bradley, 2005), it may have become less rather than more relevant to clinical practice. Thus, it seems likely that the revision process for DSM-V may take more seriously questions of clinical utility (First et al., 2004).[5]

Conclusions

We conclude with one final thought regarding the relation between personality and psychopathology. A prime characteristic of the approaches to personality that emerged from the clinic during the past century, beginning with the theories advanced by Freud to explain and guide clinical observation and intervention, was that they were personality *theories*, not just models (in the more narrow sense). Thus, not only did they describe domains on which individuals differed, but they also specified functional relations among mental processes and behavior and implicit and explicit rules that could guide interpretation and clinical understanding of a given patient.

Consider, for example, the case of a young woman interviewed by one of us at a clinical case conference some time ago (Westen, 1995). The patient had been orphaned until her 10th year and, like many such children, had grown up to have difficulty forming attachments as a young adult. She spoke in clipped sentences, offering as few words as possible. Indeed, this had made her a very frustrating patient on the inpatient unit where she was being briefly treated. About 10 minutes into the interview, the interviewer asked her if she also spoke to *herself* in clipped sentences—that is, in her own mind. The patient was initially startled by the question, having never thought about her own mental processes this way. After some reflection, she acknowledged that this was indeed the case and became engaged in the first genuine dialogue in which she engaged during her hospitalization. What became clear to her over the next few minutes was how she used this strategy to avoid painful thoughts, particularly about herself. If she avoided reflection, she avoided the object of reflection.

The interviewer had never asked a patient this question before. So, what suggested that this might be a fruitful line of inquiry? What guided the interviewer was a dynamic theory of affect regulation, which suggested that the patient's clipped way of speaking could be a way of protecting herself interpersonally, protecting herself intrapsychically, or both. By exploring the *meaning* to her of letting her thoughts flow without rigidly controlling them, he and the patient learned something very important that might not be readily captured by adjectival descriptions such as "introverted" or "taciturn" that are no doubt accurate descriptors of her behavior but do not offer enough help in understanding who she is—that is, her personality.

Our point is that a clinically useful theory of personality and psychopathology must lead both to accurate predictions *and* to interpretive understanding. In this respect, empiricist and hermeneutic philosophies of science are less contradictory than complementary, as each offers one way of using—and testing—a theory (Westen & Gabbard, 1999; Westen & Weinberger, in press). Although clinical observation is far less useful than more systematic empirical methods in deciding among competing hypotheses, an adequate theory of personality cannot choose between utility for prediction and utility for interpretive understanding. All of our strictures of empirical inquiry are essential in hypothesis testing and in model generation, but they do not guarantee that we test the right hypotheses or that the hypotheses we test are the ones most useful for clinical practice. As we move into an era in which personality once again assumes its place as central to the understanding of psychopathology, we may find that clinical approaches to personality are not only clinically useful but also theoretically indispensable.

NOTES

1. In keeping with psychoanalytic parlance, we use the terms personality, character, personality structure, character structure, and personality organization interchangeably to describe the patterned organization of personality processes.
2. Factor analysis of items (for simplicity, assuming the items assess the domains of personality relatively comprehensively) typically reveals trait dimensions that cut across domains rather than segregates them.
3. Kernberg tied this continuum to developmental fixations and regressions, which is probably not an optimal way of characterizing the relation between development and psychopathology. He also initially did not distinguish episodic psychosis (e.g., mania with psychosis in an otherwise relatively high-functioning personality) from chronic psychosis, although he has done so more recently (Kernberg, personal communication to DW, December 2003). Nevertheless, the basic framework he offered is extremely useful from a descriptive and dynamic point of view.
4. To what extent this problem is inherent in the use of factor analysis for taxonomic purposes is unclear. For example, in prior research, we a priori identified multiple clinically relevant subdomains of functioning involved in object relations, such as complexity of representations of people, affect tone of relationship paradigms (the extent to which the person tends to expect and experience relationships to be pleasurable or painful), capacity for emotional investment in relationships (ability to care about another person), self-esteem, and dominant interpersonal concerns (Westen, 1991b). Each of these dimensions, coded from narrative data using a five- or seven-point scale, is associated with predictable correlates. To see if we could reproduce something like this structure factor ana-

lytically, we developed a questionnaire that assessed the same domains of functioning by using many of the descriptors from the narrative coding manual as items. Instead of identifying domains of functioning, however, factor analysis grouped items by type of psychopathology, cutting across domains. For example, a borderline pattern emerged that included items suggesting a tendency toward black-and-white representations, malevolent affect tone, a self-serving approach to emotional investment, self-loathing, and interpersonal themes such as rejection or abandonment. We doubt that a factor analysis of statements from the coding manual of Loevinger's Sentence Completion Test (Loevinger & Wessler, 1970), which has generated hundreds of studies demonstrating impressive construct validity (Westenberg et al., 1998), would similarly reproduce her dimension of ego development.

5. Although some researchers may be concerned about "contaminating" the diagnostic manual with considerations of clinical utility, we would suggest that if clinicians do not find empirically derived models or diagnoses clinically useful, we should consider their response data and should try, in a nondefensive way, to understand that response. Practitioners in other areas of medicine tend to welcome discoveries from the laboratory, such as new treatments, whereas clinical psychologists and psychiatrists often find academic research academic. One hypothesis, of course, is that the minds of clinicians are simply filled with cognitive biases and "romantic" ideas of knowledge that cloud their thinking (Garb, 2005), and hence what is needed is psychoeducation (or more effective "dissemination," e.g., of knowledge about new treatments). An alternative (or complementary) hypothesis, however, is that the different observational vantage points of clinicians and researchers might mean that they have something to teach one another. In this respect, we might pause to wonder why clinicians hypothesized the importance of personality (or unconscious processes) in psychopathology for decades, while researchers were asserting, based on the best available empirical evidence, that they could study phenomena such as depression independent of the person who happens to be hosting the symptom. If clinical observation leads to the recognition of functional domains that are inadequately addressed by models of personality structure derived from self-reports, we should welcome their observations and bring them into the research process. Our own view is that experienced clinical observers provide a vast untapped resource for research if we simply quantify their observations using the same psychometric procedures applied for decades to patient self-reports (Westen & Weinberger, 2004, in press).

REFERENCES

Ackerman, S. J., Clemence, A. J., Weatherill, R., & Hilsenroth, M. J. (1999). Use of the TAT in the assessment of DSM-IV Cluster B personality disorders. *Journal of Personality Assessment, 73*, 422–442.

Adams, H. E., Wright, L. W., & Lohr, B. A. (1996). Is homophobia associated with homosexual arousal? *Journal of Abnormal Psychology, 105*, 440–445.

Agrawal, H. R., Gunderson, J., Holmes, B. M., & Lyons-Ruth, K. (2004). Attachment studies with borderline patients: A review. *Harvard Review of Psychiatry, 12*, 94–104.

American Psychiatric Association. (1952). *Diagnostic and statistical manual of mental disorders* (1st ed.). Washington, DC: Author.

American Psychiatric Association. (1968). *Diagnostic and statistical manual of mental disorders* (2nd ed.). Washington, DC: Author.

American Psychiatric Association. (1980). *Diagnostic and statistical manual of mental disorders* (3rd ed.). Washington, DC: Author.

Anderson, S. W., Bechara, A., Damasio, H., Tranel, D., & Damasio, A. R. (1999). Impairment of social and moral behavior related to early damage in human prefrontal cortex. *Nature Neuroscience, 2*, 1032–1037.

Aron, L. (1996). *A meeting of minds: Mutuality in psychoanalysis* (Vol. 4). New York: The Analytic Press.

Aron, L., & Harris, A. (2005). *Relational psychoanalysis: Innovation and expansion* (Vol. 2). New York: Analytic Press.

Baker, L., Silk, K. R., Westen, D., Nigg, J. T., & Lohr, N. E. (1992). Malevolence, splitting, and parental ratings by borderlines. *The Journal of Nervous and Mental Disease, 180*, 258–264.

Baldwin, M. W., Fehr, B., Keedian, E., Seidel, M., & Thomson, D. W. (1993). An exploration of the relational schemata underlying attachment styles: Self-report and lexical decision approaches. *Personality and Social Psychology Bulletin, 19*, 746–754.

Barratt, E. S. (1993). Impulsivity: Integrating cognitive, behavioral, biological, and environmental data. In W. G. McCown & J. L. Johnson (Eds.), *The impulsive client: Theory, research, and treatment* (pp. 39–56). Washington, DC: American Psychological Association.

Bateman, A. W., & Fonagy, P. (2003). The development of an attachment-based treatment program for borderline personality disorder. *Bulletin of the Menninger Clinic, 67*, 187–211.

Bateman, A. W., & Fonagy, P. (2004). Mentalization-based treatment of BPD. *Journal of Personality Disorders, 18*, 36–51.

Baumeister, R. F., Dale, K., & Sommer, K. L. (1998). Freudian defense mechanisms and empirical findings in modern social psychology: Reaction formation, projection, displacement, undoing, isolation, sublimation, and denial. *Journal of Personality, 66*, 1081–1124.

Bayer, R., & Spitzer, R. L. (1985). Neurosis, psychodynamics, and DSM-III: A history of the controversy. *Archives of General Psychiatry, 42*, 187–196.

Beck, A., Freeman, A., & Davis, D. (2004). *Cognitive therapy of personality disorders* (2nd ed.). New York: Guilford Press.

Bellak, L., Chassan, J. B., Gediman, H. K., & Hurvich, M. (1973). Ego function assessment of analytic psychotherapy combined with drug therapy. *Journal of Nervous and Mental Disease, 157*, 465–469.

Benjamin, L. S. (1996a). *Interpersonal diagnosis and treatment of personality disorders* (2nd ed.). New York: Guilford Press.

Benjamin, L. S. (1996b). An interpersonal theory of personality disorders. In J. F. Clarkin & M. F. Lenzenweger (Eds.), *Major theories of personality disorder* (pp. 141–220). New York: Guilford Press.

Bettelheim, B. (1983). *Freud and man's soul*. New York: Knopf.

Bieling, P. J., Beck, A. T., & Brown, G. K. (2004). Stability and change of sociotropy and autonomy subscales in cognitive therapy of depression. *Journal of Cognitive Psychotherapy, 18,* 135–148.

Blais, M. A., Hilsenroth, M. J., Fowler, J., & Conboy, C. A. (1999). A Rorschach exploration of the DSM-IV borderline personality disorder. *Journal of Clinical Psychology, 55,* 563–572.

Blanck, G., & Blanck, R. (1974). *Ego psychology: Theory and practice.* Oxford, UK: Columbia University Press.

Blanck, G., & Blanck, R. (1979). *Ego psychology II: Theory and practice.* New York: Columbia University Press.

Blatt, S., & Zuroff, D. (1992). Interpersonal relatedness and self-definition: Two prototypes for depression. *Clinical Psychology Review, 12,* 527–562.

Blatt, S. J. (1974). Levels of object representation in anaclitic and introjective depression. *Psychoanalytic Study of the Child, 29,* 7–57.

Blatt, S. J. (2004). Anaclitic and introjective depression in clinical and nonclinical settings. In *Experiences of depression: Theoretical, clinical, and research perspectives* (pp. 153–186). Washington, DC: American Psychological Association.

Blatt, S. J., & Lerner, H. D. (1983). The psychological assessment of object representation. *Journal of Personality Assessment, 47,* 7–28.

Blatt, S. J., Quinlan, D. M., Chevron, E. S., McDonald, C., & Zuroff, D. (1982). Dependency and self-criticism: Psychological dimensions of depression. *Journal of Consulting and Clinical Psychology, 50,* 113–124.

Block, J. (1971). *Lives through time.* Berkeley, CA: Bancroft.

Borkovec, T. D., Shadick, R. N., & Hopkins, M. (1991). The nature of normal and pathological worry. In R. M. Rapee & D. H. Barlow (Eds.), *Chronic anxiety: Generalized anxiety disorder and mixed anxiety-depression* (pp. 29–51). New York: Guilford Press.

Borkovec, T. D., & Sharpless, B. (2004). Generalized anxiety disorder: Bringing cognitive-behavioral therapy into the valued present. In S. C. Hayes, V. M. Follette & M. M. Linehan (Eds.), *Mindfulness and acceptance: Expanding the cognitive-behavioral tradition* (pp. 209–242). New York: Guilford Press.

Brennan, K. A., & Shaver, P. R. (1998). Attachment styles and personality disorders: Their connections to each other and to parental divorce, parental death, and perceptions of parental caregiving. *Journal of Personality, 66,* 835–878.

Brenner, C. (1982). *The mind in conflict.* New York: International Universities Press.

Brenner, C. (1994). The mind as conflict and compromise formation. *Journal of Clinical Psychoanalysis, 3,* 473–488.

Brown, T. A., Chorpita, B. F., & Barlow, D. H. (1998). Structural relationships among dimensions of the DSM-IV anxiety and mood disorders and dimensions of negative affect, positive affect, and autonomic arousal. *Journal of Abnormal Psychology, 107,* 179–192.

Carlson, E. A. (1998). A prospective longitudinal study of attachment disorganization/disorientation. *Child Development, 69,* 1107–1128.

Carver, C. S. (2001). Affect and the functional bases of behavior: On the dimensional structure of affective experience. *Personality and Social Psychology Review, 5,* 345–356.

Cassidy, J., & Mohr, J. J. (2001). Unsolvable fear, trauma, and psychopathology: Theory, research, and clinical considerations related to disorganized attachment across the life span. *Clinical Psychology: Science and Practice, 8*, 275–298.

Cicchetti, D., Rogosch, F. A., Maughan, A., Toth, S. L., & Bruce, J. (2003). False belief understanding in maltreated children. *Development and Psychopathology, 15*, 1067–1091.

Cicchetti, D., & Toth, S. L. (2003). Child maltreatment: Past, present, and future perspectives. In R. P. Weissberg & H. J. Walberg (Eds.), *Long-term trends in the well-being of children and youth: Issues in children's and families lives* (pp. 181–205). Washington, DC: Child Welfare League of America.

Cloninger, R. C., & Svrakic, D. (1994). Differentiating normal and deviant personality by the seven-factor personality model. In S. Strack & M. Lorr (Eds.), *Differentiating normal and abnormal personality* (pp. 40–64). New York: Springer.

Cohn, L. D., & Westenberg, P. (2004). Intelligence and maturity: Meta-analytic evidence for the incremental and discriminant validity of Loevinger's measure of ego development. *Journal of Personality and Social Psychology, 86*, 760–722.

Coleman, M. J., Levy, D. L., Lenzenweger, M. F., & Holzman, P. S. (1996). Thought disorder, perceptual aberrations, and schizotypy. *Journal of Abnormal Psychology, 105*(3), 469–473.

Crowell, J. A., Treboux, D., & Waters, E. (2002). Stability of attachment representations: The transition to marriage. *Developmental Psychology, 38*, 467–479.

Daley, S. E., Burge, D., & Hammen, C. (2000). Borderline personality disorder symptoms as predictors of 4-year romantic relationship dysfunction in young women: Addressing issues of specificity. *Journal of Abnormal Psychology, 109*, 451–460.

Daley, S. E., Hammen, C., Burge, D., Davila, J., Paley, B., Lindberg, N., et al. (1999). Depression and Axis II symptomatology in an adolescent community sample: Concurrent and longitudinal associations. *Journal of Personality Disorders, 13*, 47–59.

Davidson, R. J., Jackson, D. C., & Kalin, N. H. (2000). Emotion, plasticity, context, and regulation: Perspectives from affective neuroscience. *Psychological Bulletin, 126*, 890–909.

Endicott, J., Spitzer, R. L., Fleiss, J. L., & Cohen, J. (1976). The Global Assessment Scale: A procedure for measuring overall severity of psychiatric disturbance. *Archives of General Psychiatry, 33*, 766–771.

Erikson, E. (1986). *Childhood and society.* New York: Norton.

First, M. B., Pincus, H. A., Levine, J. B., Williams, J. B. W., Ustun, B., & Peele, R. (2004). Clinical utility as a criterion for revising psychiatric diagnoses. *American Journal of Psychiatry, 161*, 946–954.

First, M. B., & Spitzer, R. L. (2005). *User acceptability of five dimensional systems for personality diagnosis: A pilot study.* Unpublished manuscript, Columbia University.

First, M. B., Spitzer, R. L., Gibbon, M., & Williams, J. B. W. (1997). *Structured Clinical Interview for DSM-IV Personality Disorders (SCID-II).* Washington, DC: American Psychiatric Press.

Fisher, S., & Greenberg, R. P. (1996). *Freud scientifically reappraised: Testing the theories and therapy.* Oxford, UK: Wiley.

Fonagy, P. (2002). Understanding of mental states, mother–infant interaction, and the development of the self. In J. M. Maldonado-Duran (Ed.), *Infant and toddler mental health: Models of clinical intervention with infants and their families* (pp. 57–74). Washington, DC: American Psychiatric Publishing.

Fonagy, P., Steele, H., & Steele, M. (1991). Maternal representations of attachment during pregnancy predict the organization of infant–mother attachment at one year of age. *Child Development, 62*, 891–905.

Fonagy, P., & Target, M. (1997). Attachment and reflective function: Their role in self-organization. *Development and Psychopathology, 9*(4), 679–700.

Fonagy, P., Target, M., Gergely, G., Allen, J. G., & Bateman, A. (2003). The developmental roots of borderline personality disorder in early attachment relationships: A theory and some evidence. *Psychoanalytic Inquiry, 23*, 412–459.

Freud, A. (1936). *The ego and the mechanisms of defense.* New York: International Universities Press.

Freud, S. (1908). Character and anal erotism. *Standard Edition of the Complete Works of Sigmund Freud, 9*, 169–175.

Freud, S., & Breuer, J. (1957). *Studies on hysteria.* New York: Basic Books. (Original work published 1895)

Gabbard, G. O. (1998). Vertigo: Female objectification, male desire, and object loss. *Psychoanalytic Inquiry, 18*, 161–167.

Gabbard, G. O. (2005). *Psychodynamic psychiatry in clinical practice* (4th ed.). Washington, DC: American Psychiatric Publishing.

Garb, H. N. (2005). Clinical judgment and decision making. *Annual Review of Clinical Psychology, 1*, 67–89.

Gardner, H. (1999). *Intelligence reframed: Multiple intelligences for the 21st century.* New York: Basic Books.

Gilbert, D. T. (1998). Ordinary personology. In D. T. Gilbert, S. T. Fiske, & G. Lindzey (Eds.), *Handbook of social psychology* (4th ed.; Vol. 2, pp. 89–150). New York: McGraw-Hill.

Goldberg, T. E., Egan, M. F., Gscheidle, T., Coppola, R., Weickert, T., Kolachana, B. S., et al. (2003). Executive subprocesses in working memory: Relationship to catechol-O-methyltransferase Val158Met genotype and schizophrenia. *Archives of General Psychiatry, 60*, 889–896.

Gray, J. A. (1990). Brain systems that mediate both emotion and cognition. *Cognition and Emotion, 4*, 269–288.

Greenberg, J. R., & Mitchell, S. (1983). *Object relations in psychoanalytic theory.* Cambridge, MA: Harvard University Press.

Gross, J. J. (1998). Sharpening the focus: Emotion regulation, arousal, and social competence. *Psychological Inquiry, 9*, 287–290.

Gunderson, J. G. (2001). *Borderline personality disorder: A clinical guide.* Washington, DC: American Psychiatric Publishing.

Gunderson, J. G., Shea, T., Skodol, A. E., McGlashan, T. H., Morey, L. C., Stout, R. L., et al. (2000). The Collaborative Longitudinal Personality Disorders Study: Development, aims, design, and sample characteristics. *Journal of Personality Disorders, 14*, 300–315.

Haan, N. (1977). *Coping and defending.* New York: Academic Press.

Harter, S. (1999). *The construction of the self: A developmental perspective.* New York: Guilford Press.

Hartmann, H. (1958). *Ego psychology and the problem of adaptation.* Oxford, UK: International Universities Press. (Original work published 1939)

Hartmann, H., Kris, E., & Loewenstein, R. M. (1946). Comments on the formation of psychic structure. *Psychoanalytic Study of the Child, 2,* 11–38.

Heim, A., & Westen, D. (2005). Theories of personality and personality disorders. In J. Oldham, A. Skodol, & D. Bender (Eds.), *Textbook of personality disorders.* Washington, DC: American Psychiatric Press.

Heim, A., Thomas, C., & Westen, D. (unpublished data).

Higgins, E. T. (1990). Personality, social psychology, and person–situation relations: Standards and knowledge activation as a common language. In L. Pervin (Ed.), *Handbook of personality: Theory and research* (pp. 301–338). New York: Guilford Press.

Hilsenroth, M. J., Ackerman, S. J., Blagys, M. D., Baumann, B. D., Baity, M. R., Smith, S. R., et al. (2000). Reliability and validity of DSM-IV axis V. *American Journal of Psychiatry, 157*(11), 1858–1863.

Horowitz, M. (1999). Modes of conscious representation and their exploration through psychotherapy. In J. A. Singer & P. Salovey (Eds.), *At play in the fields of consciousness: Essays in honor of Jerome L. Singer.* Mahwah, NJ: Erlbaum.

Huprich, S. K., & Greenberg, R. P. (2003). Advances in the assessment of object relations in the 1990s. *Clinical Psychology Review, 23,* 665–698.

Ishikawa, S. S., & Raine, A. (2003). Prefrontal deficits and antisocial behavior: A causal model. In B. B. Lahey, T. Moffitt & A. Caspi (Eds.), *Causes of conduct disorder and juvenile delinquency* (pp. 277–304). New York: Guilford Press.

Johnston, M. H., & Holzman, P. S. (1979). *Assessing schizophrenic thinking.* San Francisco: Jossey-Bass.

Kernberg, O. (1967). Borderline personality organization. *Journal of the American Psychoanalytic Association, 15,* 641–685.

Kernberg, O. (1975). *Borderline conditions and pathological narcissism.* Northvale, NJ: Aronson.

Kernberg, O. (1983). Object relations theory and character analysis. *Journal of the American Psychoanalytic Association, 31,* 247–272.

Kernberg, O. (1996). A psychoanalytic theory of personality disorders. In J. Clarkin & M. Lenzenweger (Eds.), *Major theories of personality disorder* (pp. 106–140). New York: Guilford Press.

Kernberg, O. F. (1984). The couch at sea: Psychoanalytic studies of group and organizational leadership. *International Journal of Group Psychotherapy, 34,* 5–23.

Kim, N. S., & Ahn, W. (2002). Clinical psychologists' theory-based representations of mental disorders predict their diagnostic reasoning and memory. *Journal of Experimental Psychology, 131*(4), 451–476.

Klohnen, E. C., & Bera, S. (1998). Behavioral and experiential patterns of avoidantly and securely attached women across adulthood: A 31-year longitudinal perspective. *Journal of Personality and Social Psychology, 74,* 211–223.

Koenigsberg, H. W., Harvey, P. D., Mitropoulou, V., Schmeidler, J., New, A. S., Goodman, M., et al. (2002). Characterizing affective instability in borderline personality disorder. *American Journal of Psychiatry, 159,* 784–788.

Koos, O., & Gergely, G. (2001). A contingency-based approach to the etiology of "disorganized" attachment: The "flickering switch" hypothesis. *Bulletin of the Menninger Clinic, 65,* 397–410.

Krueger, R. F. (1999). The structure of common mental disorders. *Archives of General Psychiatry, 56,* 921–926.

Krueger, R. F., Hicks, B. M., Patrick, C. J., Carlson, S. R., Iacono, W. G., & McGue, M. (2002). Etiologic connections among substance dependence, antisocial behavior, and personality: Modeling the externalizing spectrum. *Journal of Abnormal Psychology, 111*(3), 411–424.

Krueger, R. F., Markon, K. M., Patrick, C. P., & Iacono, W. (in press). Externalizing psychopathology in adulthood: A dimensional-spectrum conceptualization and its implications for DSM-V. *Journal of Abnormal Psychology.*

Krueger, R. F., & Piasecki, T. M. (2002). Toward a dimensional and psychometrically-informed approach to conceptualizing psychopathology. *Behaviour Research and Therapy, 40,* 485–499.

Lancelot, C., & Nowicki, S., Jr. (1997). The association between receptive nonverbal processing abilities and internalizing/externalizing problems in girls and boys. *Journal of Genetic Psychology, 158,* 297–302.

Larsen, R. J., Billings, D. W., & Cutler, S. E. (1996). Affect intensity and individual differences in informational style. *Journal of Personality, 64,* 185–207.

Larstone, R. M., Jang, K. L., Livesley, W., Vernon, P. A., & Wolf, H. (2002). The relationship between Eysenck's P-E-N model of personality, the five-factor model of personality, and traits delineating personality dysfunction. *Personality and Individual Differences, 33,* 25–37.

Linehan, M. M. (1993). *Cognitive-behavioral treatment of borderline personality disorder.* New York: Guilford Press.

Loevinger, J. (1979). Construct validity of the Sentence Completion Test of Ego Development. *Applied Psychological Measurement, 3,* 281–311.

Loevinger, J., & Wessler, R. (1970). *Measuring ego development: Construction and use of a Sentence Completion Test* (Vol. 1). San Francisco: Jossey-Bass.

Luborsky, L., & Crits-Christoph, P. (1990). *Understanding transference: The core conflictual relationship theme method.* New York: Basic Books.

Lyons-Ruth, K., & Jacobvitz, D. (1999). Attachment disorganization: Unresolved loss, relational violence, and lapses in behavioral and attentional strategies. In J. Cassidy & P. R. Shaver (Eds.), *Handbook of attachment: Theory, research and clinical applications* (pp. 550–554). New York: Guilford Press.

Lyons-Ruth, K., Melnick, S., Bronfman, E., Sherry, S., & Llanas, L. (2004). Hostile–helpless relational models and disorganized attachment patterns between parents and their young children: Review of research and implications for clinical work. In L. Atkinson & S. Goldberg (Eds.), *Attachment issues in psychopathology and intervention* (pp. 65–94). Mahwah, NJ: Erlbaum.

Macklin, M. L., Metzger, L. J., Litz, B. T., McNally, R. J., Lasko, N. B., Orr, S. P., et al. (1998). Lower precombat intelligence is a risk factor for posttraumatic stress disorder. *Journal of Consulting and Clinical Psychology, 66,* 323–326.

Main, M., Kaplan, N., & Cassidy, J. (1985). Security in infancy, childhood, and adulthood: A move to the level of representation. *Monographs of the Society for Research in Child Development, 50*(1–2), 66–104.

Markon, K. E., Krueger, R. F., & Watson, D. (2005). Delineating the structure of normal and abnormal personality: An integrative hierarchical approach. *Journal of Personality and Social Psychology, 88*, 139–157.

Masterson, J. (1976). *Psychotherapy of the borderline adult: A developmental approach.* New York: Brunner/Mazel.

McClelland, D. C., Koestner, R., & Weinberger, J. (1989). How do self-attributed and implicit motives differ? *Psychological Review, 96*, 690–702.

McClure, E. B., & Nowicki, S., Jr. (2001). Associations between social anxiety and nonverbal processing skill in preadolescent boys and girls. *Journal of Nonverbal Behavior, 25*, 3–19.

McNally, R. J., & Shin, L. M. (1995). Association of intelligence with severity of posttraumatic stress disorder symptoms in Vietnam combat veterans. *American Journal of Psychiatry, 152*, 936–938.

McWilliams, N. (1994). *Psychoanalytic diagnosis.* New York: Guilford Press.

McWilliams, N. (1998). Relationship, subjectivity, and inference in diagnosis. In J. W. Barron (Ed.), *Making diagnosis meaningful: Enhancing evaluation and treatment of psychological disorders* (pp. 197–226). Washington, DC: American Psychological Association.

McWilliams, N. (1999). *Psychoanalytic case formulation.* New York: Guilford Press.

Menninger, K. A., Mayman, M., & Pruyser, P. W. (1962). *A manual for psychiatric case study* (2nd ed.). Oxford, UK: Grune & Stratton.

Mischel, W. (1968). *Personality and assessment.* New York: Wiley.

Mischel, W., & Shoda, Y. (1995). A cognitive–affective system theory of personality: Reconceptualizing situations, dispositions, dynamics, and invariance in personality structure. *Psychological Review, 102*(2), 246–268.

Mitchell, S. A. (1988). *Relational concepts in psychoanalysis: An integration.* Cambridge, MA: Harvard University Press.

Mitchell, S. A., & Aron, L. (Eds.). (1999). *Relational psychoanalysis: The emergence of a tradition* (Vol. 14). Hillsdale, NJ: Analytic Press.

Mitropoulou, H. C., New, A. S., Koenigsberg, H. W., Silverman, J., & Siever, L. J. (2001). Affective instability and impulsivity in borderline personality and bipolar II disorders: Similarities and differences. *Journal of Psychiatric Research, 35*, 307–312.

Newman, L. S., Duff, K., Schnopp-Wyatt, N., Brock, B., & Hoffman, Y. (1997). Reactions to the O. J. Simpson verdict: "Mindless tribalism" or motivated inference processes? *Journal of Social Issues, 53*(3), 547–562.

Nigg, J. T., Lohr, N. E., Westen, D., Gold, L. J., & Silk, K. R. (1992). Malevolent object representations in borderline personality disorder and major depression. *Journal of Abnormal Psychology, 101*, 61–67.

Nigg, J. T., Silk, K. R., Westen, D., Lohr, N. E., Gold, L. J., Goodrich, S., et al. (1991). Object representations in the early memories of sexually abused borderline patients. *American Journal of Psychiatry, 148*(7), 864–869.

Nowicki, S., Jr., & Duke, M. (2002). *Will I ever fit in?: The breakthrough program for conquering adult dyssemia.* New York: Free Press.

Pennebaker, J. (1997). Writing about emotional experiences as a therapeutic process. *Psychological Science, 8*, 162–166.

Perry, W., Minassian, A., Cadenhead, K., Sprock, J., & Braff, D. (2003). The use of the

Ego Impairment Index across the schizophrenia spectrum. *Journal of Personality Assessment, 80,* 50–57.

Plutchik, R. (1980). *Emotions: A psychoevolutionary synthesis.* New York: Harper & Row.

Rapaport, D., Gill, M., & Schafer, R. (1945). *Diagnostic psychological testing: The theory, statistical evaluation, and diagnostic application of a battery of tests: Vol. I.* Oxford, UK: Year Book Publishers.

Redl, F., & Wineman, D. (1951). *Children who hate: The disorganization and breakdown of behavior controls.* Glencoe, IL: Free Press.

Reich, W. (1931). The characterological mastery of the Oedipus complex. *International Journal of Psycho-Analysis, 12,* 452–467.

Scharff, J. S. (2004). The British object relations theorists: Fairbairn, Winnicott, Balint, Guntrip, Sutherland, and Bowlby. In M. S. Bergmann (Ed.), *Understanding dissidence and controversy in the history of psychoanalysis* (pp. 175–200). New York: Other Press.

Schimmack, U., & Diener, E. (1997). Affect intensity: Separating intensity and frequency in repeatedly measured affect. *Journal of Personality and Social Psychology, 73,* 1313–1329.

Shapiro, D. (1965). *Neurotic styles.* New York: Basic Books.

Shaver, P. R., & Mikulincer, M. (2005). Attachment theory and research: Resurrection of the psychodynamic approach to personality. *Journal of Research in Personality, 39,* 22–45.

Shedler, J., Mayman, M., & Manis, M. (1993). The illusion of mental health. *American Psychology, 48,* 1117–1131.

Shedler, J., & Westen, D. (2004a). Dimensions of personality pathology: An alternative to the Five Factor Model. *American Journal of Psychiatry, 161,* 1743–1754.

Shedler, J., & Westen, D. (2004b). Refining personality disorder diagnoses: Integrating science and practice. *American Journal of Psychiatry, 161,* 1350–1365.

Spitzer, R. L., Endicott, J., & Robins, E. (1978). Research diagnostic criteria: Rationale and reliability. *Archives of General Psychiatry, 35,* 773–782.

Strauman, T. J. (1992). Self, social cognition, and psychodynamics: Caveats and challenges for integration. *Psychological Inquiry, 3,* 67–71.

Strauman, T. J., & Higgins, E. (1993). The self construct in social cognition: Past, present, and future. In Z. V. Segal & S. J. Blatt (Eds.), *The self in emotional distress: Cognitive and psychodynamic perspectives* (pp. 3–40). New York: Guilford Press.

Stricker, G., & Healey, B. J. (1990). Projective assessment of object relations: A review of the empirical literature. *Psychological Assessment, 2,* 219–230.

Tangney, J. P. (1994). The mixed legacy of the superego: Adaptive and maladaptive aspects of shame and guilt. In J. M. Masling & R. F. Bornstein (Eds.), *Empirical perspectives on object relations theory: Empirical studies of psychoanalytic theories* (Vol. 5, pp. 1–28). Washington, DC: American Psychological Association.

Thompson-Brenner, H., & Westen, D. (2005). Personality subtypes in eating disorders: Validation of a classification in a naturalistic sample. *British Journal of Psychiatry, 186,* 516–524.

Tolpin, L. H., Gunthert, K. C., Cohen, L. H., & O'Neill, S. C. (2004). Borderline personality features and instability of daily negative affect and self-esteem. *Journal of Personality, 72,* 111–137.

Toth, S. L., Cicchetti, D., & Kim, J. (2002). Relations among children's perceptions of maternal behavior, attributional styles, and behavioral symptomatology in maltreated children. *Journal of Abnormal Child Psychology, 30,* 487–501.

Toth, S. L., Cicchetti, D., Macfie, J., Maughan, A., & Vanmeenen, K. (2000). Narrative representations of caregivers and self in maltreated pre-schoolers. *Attachment and Human Development, 2,* 271–305.

Trull, T., & Durrett, C. (2005). Categorical and dimensional models of personality disorder. *Annual Review of Clinical Psychology, 1,* 355–380.

Vaillant, G. (Ed.). (1992). *Ego mechanisms of defense: A guide for clinicians and researchers.* Washington, DC: American Psychiatric Press.

Vaillant, G. E. (1977). *Adaptation to life.* Boston: Little Brown.

Vaillant, G. E., & McCullough, L. (1998). The role of ego mechanisms of defense in the diagnosis of personality disorders. In J. W. Barron (Ed.), *Making diagnosis meaningful: Enhancing evaluation and treatment of psychological disorders* (pp. 139–158). Washington, DC: American Psychological Association.

Vasquez, K., Durik, A. M., & Hyde, J. S. (2002). Family and work: Implications of adult attachment styles. *Personality and Social Psychology Bulletin, 28,* 874–886.

Walker, E. F., & Gale, S. (1995). Neurodevelopmental processes in schizophrenia and schizotypal personality disorder. In A. Raine, T. Lencz, & S. A. Mednick (Eds.), *Schizotypal personality* (pp. 56–75). New York: Cambridge University Press.

Walker, E. F., Logan, C. B., & Walder, D. (1999). Indicators of neurodevelopmental abnormality in schizotypal personality disorder. *Psychiatric Annals, 29,* 132–136.

Wang, W., Du, W., Wang, Y., Livesley, W., & Jang, K. L. (2004). The relationship between the Zuckerman–Kuhlman Personality Questionnaire and traits delineating personality pathology. *Personality and Individual Differences, 36,* 155–162.

Ward, M. J., Lee, S. S., & Lipper, E. G. (2000). Failure-to-thrive is associated with disorganized infant–mother attachment and unresolved maternal attachment. *Infant Mental Health Journal, 21,* 428–442.

Watson, D., & Clark, L. A. (1984). Negative affectivity: The disposition to experience aversive emotional states. *Psychological Bulletin, 96*(3), 465–490.

Watson, D., & Clark, L. A. (1992). Affects separable and inseparable: On the hierarchical arrangement of the negative affects. *Journal of Personality and Social Psychology, 62,* 489–505.

Watson, D., & Tellegen, A. (1985). Toward a consensual structure of mood. *Psychological Bulletin, 98,* 219–235.

Weber, M. (1949). *The methodology of the social sciences.* Glencoe, IL: Free Press.

Webster, C. D., & Jackson, M. A. (Eds.). (1997). *Impulsivity: Theory, assessment, and treatment.* New York: Guilford Press.

Wegner, D. M., & Bargh, J. A. (1998). Control and automaticity in social life. In D. T. Gilbert & S. T. Fiske (Eds.), *The handbook of social psychology* (4th ed., Vol. 2, pp. 446–496). New York: McGraw-Hill.

Westen, D. (1985). *Self and society: Narcissism, collectivism, and the development of morals*. New York: Cambridge University Press.

Westen, D. (1990a). The relations among narcissism, egocentrism, self-concept, and self-esteem: Experimental, clinical and theoretical considerations. *Psychoanalysis and Contemporary Thought, 13*, 183–239.

Westen, D. (1990b). Towards a revised theory of borderline object relations: Contributions of empirical research. *International Journal of Psycho-Analysis, 71*, 661–693.

Westen, D. (1991a). Cognitive-behavioral interventions in the psychoanalytic psychotherapy of borderline personality disorders. *Clinical Psychology Review, 11*, 211–230.

Westen, D. (1991b). Social cognition and object relations. *Psychological Bulletin, 109*, 429–455.

Westen, D. (1992). The cognitive self and the psychoanalytic self: Can we put our selves together? *Psychological Inquiry, 3*(1), 1–13.

Westen, D. (1994). Toward an integrative model of affect regulation: Applications to social–psychological research. *Journal of Personality, 62*, 641–667.

Westen, D. (1995). A clinical-empirical model of personality: Life after the Mischelian ice age and the NEO-lithic era. *Journal of Personality, 63*, 495–524.

Westen, D. (1996). A model and a method for uncovering the nomothetic from the idiographic: An alternative to the five-factor model? *Journal of Research in Personality, 30*, 400–413.

Westen, D. (1997). Towards a clinically and empirically sound theory of motivation. *International Journal of Psycho-Analysis, 78*, 521–548.

Westen, D. (1998a). Case formulation and personality diagnosis: Two processes or one? In J. Barron (Ed.), *Making diagnosis meaningful* (pp. 111–138). Washington, DC: American Psychological Association Press.

Westen, D. (1998b). The scientific legacy of Sigmund Freud: Toward a psychodynamically informed psychological science. *Psychological Bulletin, 124*, 333–371.

Westen, D. (1999a). Psychodynamic theory and technique in relation to research on cognition and emotion: Mutual implications. In T. Dalgleish & M. Power (Eds.), *Handbook of cognition and emotion* (pp. 727–746). New York: Wiley.

Westen, D. (1999b). The scientific status of unconscious processes: Is Freud really dead? *Journal of the American Psychoanalytic Association, 47*, 1061–1106.

Westen, D. (2000). Integrative psychotherapy: Integrating psychodynamic and cognitive-behavioral theory and technique. In C. R. Snyder & R. Ingram (Eds.), *Handbook of psychological change: Psychotherapy processes and practices for the 21st century* (pp. 217–242). New York: Wiley.

Westen, D. (in press). Drizzling on the 5 plus or minus 3 factor parade: A response to Trull. In T. Widiger & E. Simonsen (Eds.), *Research agenda for DSM-V: Dimensional classification of personality disorder*. Washington, DC: American Psychiatric Press.

Westen, D., & Arkowitz-Westen, L. (1998). Limitations of Axis II in diagnosing personality pathology in clinical practice. *American Journal of Psychiatry, 155*, 1767–1771.

Westen, D., Blagov, P., Feit, A., Arkowitz, J., & Thagard, P. (2005). *When reason and passion collide: Cognitive and emotional constraint satisfaction in high-stakes political decision making.* Unpublished manuscript, Emory University.

Westen, D., & Bradley, R. (2005). Prototype diagnosis of personality. In S. Strack (Ed.), *Handbook of personology and psychopathology* (pp. 238–256). New York: Wiley.

Westen, D., Dutra, L., & Shedler, J. (2005). Assessing adolescent personality pathology: Quantifying clinical judgment. *British Journal of Psychiatry, 186,* 227–238.

Westen, D., & Gabbard, G. O. (1999). Psychoanalytic approaches to personality. In L. Pervin & O. John (Eds.), *Handbook of personality: Theory and research* (2nd ed., pp. 57–101). New York: Guilford Press.

Westen, D., & Gabbard, G. O. (2002). Developments in cognitive neuroscience: I. Conflict, compromise, and connectionism. *Journal of the American Psychoanalytic Association, 50,* 53–98.

Westen, D., & Harnden-Fischer, J. (2001). Personality profiles in eating disorders: Rethinking the distinction between Axis I and Axis II. *American Journal of Psychiatry, 165,* 547–562.

Westen, D., Huebner, D., Lifton, N., Silverman, M., & Boekamp, J. (1991). Assessing complexity of representations of people and understanding social causality: A comparison of natural science and clinical psychology graduate students. *Journal of Social and Clinical Psychology, 10*(4), 448–456.

Westen, D., Jenei, J., Walsh, K., & Bradley, R. (2005). *The trait structure of the DSM-IV personality disorders.* Unpublished manuscript, Emory University.

Westen, D., Klepser, J., Silverman, M., Ruffins, S. A., Lifton, N., & Boekamp, J. (1991). Object relations in childhood and adolescence: The development of working representations. *Journal of Consulting and Clinical Psychology, 59*(3), 400–409.

Westen, D., Lohr, N., Silk, K. R., Gold, L., & Kerber, K. (1990). Object relations and social cognition in borderlines, major depressives, and normals: A thematic apperception test analysis. *Psychological Assessment: A Journal of Consulting and Clinical Psychology, 2,* 355–364.

Westen, D., Ludolph, P., Lerner, H., Ruffins, S., & Wiss, F. C. (1990). Object relations in borderline adolescents. *Journal of the American Academy of Child and Adolescent Psychiatry, 29*(3), 338–348.

Westen, D., Ludolph, P., Silk, K., Kellam, A., Gold, L., & Lohr, N. (1990). Object relations in borderline adolescents and adults: Developmental differences. *Adolescent Psychiatry, 17,* 360–384.

Westen, D., & Muderrisoglu, S. (2003). Reliability and validity of personality disorder assessment using a systematic clinical interview: Evaluating an alternative to structured interviews. *Journal of Personality Disorders, 17,* 350–368.

Westen, D., & Muderrisoglu, S. (in press). Reliability of assessment of personality traits using the SWAP-200 Q-sort. *American Journal of Psychiatry.*

Westen, D., Muderrisoglu, S., Fowler, C., Shedler, J., & Koren, D. (1997). Affect regulation and affective experience: Individual differences, group differences, and measurement using a Q-sort procedure. *Journal of Consulting and Clinical Psychology, 65,* 429–439.

Westen, D., Novotny, C. M., & Thompson-Brenner, H. (2004). The empirical status of empirically supported psychotherapies: Assumptions, findings, and reporting in controlled clinical trials. *Psychological Bulletin, 130,* 631–663.

Westen, D., & Shedler, J. (1999a). Revising and assessing Axis II: Part 1. Developing a clinically and empirically valid assessment method. *American Journal of Psychiatry, 156,* 258–272.

Westen, D., & Shedler, J. (1999b). Revising and assessing Axis II, Part 2: Toward an empirically based and clinically useful classification of personality disorders. *American Journal of Psychiatry, 156,* 273–285.

Westen, D., & Weinberger, J. (2004). When clinical description becomes statistical prediction. *American Psychologist, 59,* 595–613.

Westen, D., & Weinberger, J. (in press). In praise of clinical judgment: Meehl's forgotten legacy. *Journal of Clinical Psychology.*

Westen, D., Weinberger, J., & Bradley, R. (in press). Motivation, decision making, and consciousness: From psychodynamics to subliminal priming and emotional constraint satisfaction. In M. Moscovitch & P. D. Zelazo (Eds.), *Cambridge handbook of consciousness.* Cambridge, UK: Cambridge University Press.

Westenberg, P., Jonckheer, J., Treffers, P. D. A., & Drewes, M. J. (1998). Ego development in children and adolescents: Another side of the impulsive, self-protective, and conformist ego levels. In P. Westenberg, A. Blasi, & L. D. Cohn (Eds.), *Personality development: Theoretical, empirical, and clinical investigations of Loevinger's conception of ego development* (pp. 89–112). Mahwah, NJ: Erlbaum.

Whisman, M. A. (1993). Mediators and moderators of change in cognitive therapy of depression. *Psychological Bulletin, 114,* 248–265.

Whitesell, N. R., & Harter, S. (1989). Children's reports of conflict between simultaneous opposite-valence emotions. *Child Development, 60,* 673–682.

Widiger, T., & Simonsen, E. (in press). Alternative dimensional models of personality disorder. In T. Widiger & E. Simonsen (Eds.), *Research agenda for DSM-V: Dimensional classification of personality disorder.* Washington, DC: American Psychiatric Press.

Widiger, T. A. (1993). The DSM-III—R categorical personality disorder diagnoses: A critique and an alternative. *Psychological Inquiry, 4*(2), 75–90.

Yeomans, F. E., Clarkin, J. F., & Kernberg, O. F. (2002). *A primer of transference-focused psychotherapy for the borderline patient.* Northvale, NJ: Aronson.

Young, J. (1990). *Cognitive therapy for personality disorders: A schema-focused approach.* Sarasota, FL: Professional Resource Exchange.

Zetzel, E. (1968). The so-called good hysteric. *International Journal of Psycho-Analysis, 49,* 256–260.

Index

Abuse
developing treatments and, 269–272
gene–environment interaction and, 161–162
relational self and, 307–308
Acquired sociopathy, 189
Activation theory of emotion, 176
Active genotype–environment correlation, 160
Actor–critic model, 185
Acute treatment, 282
Adaptive functioning
functional assessment and, 349–351
integration of with other personality components, 358–364, 363f
overview, 371n–372n
Addiction
dopamine system and, 185
individual differences in the regulation of emotions and, 198–199
Adversity, early
developing treatments and, 269–272
mentalization deficits and, 345
relational self and, 307–308
Affect regulation, 369
Affect systems
relational self and, 313–314
relations among, 195–199
transference and, 299
Affective basis of temperamental traits, 11–12, 12t

Affective regulation, 186–190, 190–199
Affiliation, 216–226, 219f. see also Agreeableness
Affiliative reward, 221–225
Age of onset
conduct problems and, 114–115
stability over time and, 74–75
Agency, 216–226, 219f
Agentic extraversion, 243
Aggression, 137
Agitated depression, 182. see also Depression
Agoraphobia
Extraversion/Positive Emotionality (E/PE) and, 20–21
Structured Clinical Interview for DSM-IV (SCID), 25
Agreeableness
dependent personality traits and, 59–60
five-factored model (FFM) and, 8, 43, 45t
neurobehavior model and, 216–226, 219f
personality disorders and, 54t, 213
prosociality and, 117
Alcohol consumptions
gene–environment interaction and, 161, 162–164
mu opiate receptors and, 226
Alcohol dependence, 162–164
Altruism, 126

Alzheimer's disease
   personality changes prior to, 155
   scar model of etiology and, 170
Amygdala
   anxiety and, 230–234, 231*f*
   defensive motivational systems and,
     179–182
   startle reflex and, 230
Anal phase of development, 340–341
Anger
   five-factored model (FFM) and, 46–
     47
   individual differences in the
     regulation of emotions and,
     199
Angry hostility, 46–47
Anhedonia, 20
Antagonism, 45*t*, 46–47
Anterior cingulate cortex
   emotional processing and, 190
   individual differences in the
     regulation of emotions and,
     196–197
Antisocial behavior
   behavior genetic approaches to, 129
   developmental model of, 3
   dispositions and, 119–123
   genetic factors and, 138, 161–163
Antisocial personality disorder
   alcohol consumption and, 162
   emotional responsiveness and, 272–
     273
   five-factored model (FFM) and, 53,
     54*t*, 55–56
   MAPP self-report scales and, 79–80
   Peer Nomination Study and, 102–
     104, 103*t*
   posttraumatic stress disorder and,
     158
Antisocial propensity. *see also* Conduct
     problems
   components of, 115–119
   overview, 113–114
Anxiety
   attachment system and, 310
   avoidant personality disorder and,
     266
   Big Two dimensions of temperament
     and, 26–31, 31*t*

   comorbidity and, 153
   ego psychology and, 342
   individual differences in the
     regulation of emotions and,
     192–193
   Mood and Anxiety Symptom
     Questionnaire (MASQ) and,
     22–23
   multidimensional model and, 247,
     247*f*
   neurobehavior model and, 227–229
   neurobiology of, 229–241, 231*f*,
     233*f*, 234*f*, 237*f*, 239*f*
   Peer Nomination Study and, 83–84,
     83*t*
   relational self and, 309–311
   transference and, 5
Anxiety disorders
   behavioral inhibition and, 118
   cognitive approaches to treatment
     of, 274–275
   differential relations within, 14–15
   heterogeneity of symptoms and, 15–
     16
   neuroticism/negative emotionality
     (N/NE) and, 13–14
   overview, 113
Anxiety sensitivity, 27
Anxiety Sensitivity Index (ASI), 27, 30
Anxious–Misery factor, 17
Anxious–preoccupied attachment, 270
Appetitive motivational systems
   neurobehavior model and, 224
   overview, 176–186
Approach–avoidance motivation, 302
Arousal, 177–178
Assessment, functional, 346–347, 348*t*,
     349–353
Assessment procedures
   functional assessment, 346–347,
     348*t*, 349–353
   in the Peer Nomination Study, 76–
     82, 78*t*, 80*t*, 81*t*
   role of in a managed care system,
     281
Attachment disturbances, 269–270
Attachment system
   anxiety and hostility and, 309–311
   functional assessment and, 353

level of pathology and, 355
relational self and, 293–294
self-regulation and, 303
social causality and, 352
Attachment theory
early adversity and, 269–272
mentalization deficits and, 345
Attention-deficit/hyperactivity disorder (ADHD)
genetic factors and, 138
overview, 113
spectrum model of etiology and, 169
Auditory-induced startle paradigm, 229–230
Automatic activation of mental processes, 298–299
Autonomy, 314
Avoidant attachment
level of pathology and, 355
suppression of hostility in, 310–311
Avoidant personality disorder
attachment disturbances and, 270
emotional responsiveness and, 273
five-factored model (FFM) and, 58, 266
Structured Interview for DSM-IV Personality (SIDP-IV) and, 81
Axis I personality pathology
conceptual models of, 263–264
developing treatments for, 262–263
negative cognition and emotion in, 272–275
Axis II personality pathology
conceptual models of, 263–264
developing treatments for, 262–263
facilitating engagement with valued life tasks and, 276–277
negative cognition and emotion in, 272–275
overview, 356

B

Beck Anxiety Inventory, 76, 82
Beck Depression Inventory, 76, 82
Bed nucleus of the stria terminalis (BNST), 180–182

Behavior genetic approaches. see also Genetic factors
conduct disorder and, 128–130
developmental propensity model and, 123–125, 126f
dispositional dimensions and, 125–128
mediational models of causes of CD symptoms and, 130–137, 131f, 133f, 136f
overview, 155–157
personality-as-risk model and, 157–165
role of personality and, 170–171
spectrum model of etiology and, 166–169, 167f, 168f
Behavioral activation system, 177, 266–267
Behavioral confirmation, 300–301
Behavioral disinhibition, 165
Behavioral inhibition
anxiety and, 228–229
compared to daring, 118
individual differences in the regulation of emotions and, 197
startle reflex and, 230
Behavioral inhibition system
neuroticism and, 266
overview, 177
Beliefs, negative, 272–275
Beliefs towards the self, 369
Biases
pathology and, 3
transference and, 297–299
Big Five Inventory (BFI), 11
Big Five model. see Five-factor model (FFM)
Big Four model, 365
Big Three structure
Mood and Anxiety Symptom Questionnaire (MASQ) and, 22–23, 24t
overview, 8–9
prosociality and, 125
Big Two dimensions of temperament
clinical traits and, 26–31, 31t
N/NE and E/PE dimensions of, 10–12, 12t

Big Two dimensions of temperament
    (*continued*)
    overview, 2, 9, 31–32
    psychopathology and, 12–22, 18*t*
Binge eating, 342
Biological vulnerabilities, 265–267
Bipolar affective disorder, 211
Borderline personality disorder
    attachment disturbances and, 270
    early adversity and, 269
    emotional responsiveness and, 272
    five-factored model (FFM) and, 54*t*,
        58, 60
    functioning and, 372*n*
    level of pathology and, 354, 355–356
    managed care and, 282
    mentalization deficits and, 345
    negative beliefs and, 273
    overlap of with other pathologies,
        263–264
    Peer Nomination Study and, 95,
        102–104, 103*t*
Brief acute treatment, 282
Bulimia nervosa, 342

C

California Q-set (CQS), 56
Center for the Study of Emotion and
    Attention (CSEA), 177
Character neurosis, 338–346
Child and Adolescent Dispositions
    Scale (CADS), 115–116
Cholesky decomposition model, 134–
    137, 136*f*, 139, 140
Cloninger's model of personality, 121
Cloninger's Tridimensional Personality
    Questionnaire, 162
Closedness to experience, 45*t*
Cocaine use
    incentive motivation and, 221–222
    mu opiate receptors and, 226
Coercive parenting, 161–162
Cognition, negative
    depression and, 311–312
    developing treatments and, 272–275
Cognitive abilities
    conduct problems and, 118–119
    prefrontal cortex and, 187–188

Cognitive style, 369
Cognitive theory, 311–312
Cognitive treatment approaches, 274–
    275, 279
Cognitive triad, 321
Collaborative Longitudinal Study of
    Personality Disorders (CLPS),
    57–58
Common cause model of etiology, 13
Common factor model, 278–280
Common pathways model, 166, 167*f*
Comorbidity
    behavior genetic approaches and,
        155–157
    five-factored model (FFM) and, 3
    integrating perspectives on
        personality structure and, 368
    overview, 335–336
    personality and psychopathology,
        153–154
    spectrum model of etiology and,
        167–169
Compensatory self-enhancement, 303
Complication model of etiology. *see
    also* Scar model of etiology
    overview, 13, 265
    relations between N/NE and
        psychopathology and, 19
Compulsivity, 265
Conduct disorders
    alcohol consumption and, 163
    behavior genetic approaches to, 128–130
    dispositions and, 119–123
    mediation of genetics and
        environmental influences on,
        137–140
    mediational models of, 130–137,
        131*f*, 133*f*, 136*f*
    neuroticism/negative emotionality
        (N/NE) and, 13–14
    overview, 112–113
    posttraumatic stress disorder and, 158
Conduct problems, 113–119
Conscientiousness. *see also* Constraint;
    Impulsiveness
    five-factored model (FFM) and, 8,
        43, 45*t*
    obsessive–compulsive traits and, 59–60
    personality disorders and, 54*t*, 213

Constraint. *see also* Conscientiousness; Impulsiveness
  five-factored model (FFM) and, 47–48
  interactive nature of, 243–246, 244*f*, 246*f*
  neurobehavior model and, 216
  neurobiology of, 236–231, 237*f*, 239*f*
  overview, 9
Constructs transcending approach, 5
Consummatory behavioral patterns
  motivational systems and, 220
  reward system and, 222
Contemporary factor analysis model, 166, 167*f*
Continuous treatment, 281–282
Convergent validity, 44, 45*t*, 46–48
Corticotropin-releasing hormone (CRH)
  anxiety and, 232–236, 233*f*
  overview, 181
Covariation relationship, 155–157
Criterion overlap problem, 154
Cross-cultural replication, 50–52
Culture, 8, 50–52

D

Daring
  behavior genetic approaches to, 127
  Cholesky decomposition model and, 136–137, 136*f*
  conduct problems and, 120
  dispositions and, 117–118
  mediation of genetics and environmental influences and, 137–140
  mediational models of causes of CD symptoms and, 131–132, 131*f*
Defenses
  ego psychology and, 341–343
  personality organization and, 357
  psychoanalytic theory and, 339
Defensive motivational systems, 176–186
Delinquency, 137
Dependency, 27
Dependent personality disorder, 213

Dependent personality traits
  agreeableness and, 59–60
  attachment disturbances and, 270
Depression
  Big Two dimensions of temperament and, 26–31, 31*t*
  cognitive approaches to treatment of, 274–275
  comorbidity and, 153
  diagnosis of, 154
  dopamine system and, 211
  ego psychology and, 342, 343
  Extraversion/Positive Emotionality (E/PE) and, 19–20, 21–22
  fear response system and, 182
  individual differences in the regulation of emotions and, 193
  Mood and Anxiety Symptom Questionnaire (MASQ) and, 22–23
  negative cognition and emotion and, 273–274
  object relations theory and, 344
  overlap of with other pathologies, 263–264
  overview, 113
  Peer Nomination Study and, 83–84, 83*t*
  relational self and, 311–320, 322–323
Depressive Experiences Questionnaire (DEQ), 27–28, 29, 30
Detachment, 24
Development, language
  conduct problems and, 118–119
  lexical foundation of, 40–41
Developmental model
  conduct problems and, 121–122
  overview, 3, 112–113
Developmental processes
  conduct problems and, 114–115
  developing treatments and, 276–277
Developmental propensity model of conduct problems
  antisocial propensity and, 119–123
  overview, 113–119

Diagnosis. *see also* DSM
  applying to clinical practice, 367,
    369–370
  comorbidity and, 153–154
  developing treatments and, 262–263
  DSM and, 335
  five-factored model (FFM) and, 58–
    59, 61–62
  integration of personality
    components, 358–364, 363*f*
  in the Peer Nomination Study,
    106*n*–107*n*
  personality organization and, 356–
    357
  problem of modeling personality
    disorders and, 213–215
  relations between N/NE and
    psychopathology and, 19
  role of in a managed care system,
    281
  validity analyses and, 25–26
Dialectical behavior therapy, 282
Direction of causation model, 131*f*,
    132–134, 132*f*
Discriminant validity, of the five-
    factored model (FFM), 44, 45*t*,
    46–48
Disinhibition
  five-factored model (FFM) and, 47–
    48
  individual differences in the
    regulation of emotions and,
    197–198
  overview, 9
Disinhibition versus Constraint (DvC),
    9
Dismissive–avoidant attachment,
    270
Disposition
  antisocial propensity and, 115–
    118
  behavior genetic approaches to,
    123–125, 125–128, 126*f*
  conduct disorder and, 119–123
  mediation of genetics and
    environmental influences and,
    137–140
Dissocial behavior, 265
Dissociation, 342

Distress
  neuroticism/negative emotionality
    (N/NE) and, 14–15, 16–17
  pathology and, 3
  Peer Nomination Study and, 82–86,
    83*t*, 84*t*
Dopamine projection system
  affiliate reward and, 221–225
  compared to mu opiate receptors,
    225–226
Dopamine system
  addictions and, 198–199
  appetitive motivational system and,
    182–186
  conduct disorder and, 138
  defensive and appetitive
    motivational systems and, 178
  motivational systems and, 210–211
DSM. *see also* Diagnosis; *entries for
    specific editions of the DSM*
  applying to clinical practice, 367–
    368, 369–370
  heritability of personality traits and,
    49
  neuroticism/negative emotionality
    (N/NE) and, 16–18, 18*t*
  overview, 174–175, 335
  personality organization and, 357–
    358
  validity analyses and, 25–26
DSM-I, 358
DSM-II, 357–358
DSM-III
  five-factored model (FFM) and, 53
  personality organization and, 357–
    358
DSM-III-R
  cross-cultural research and, 50–51
  five-factored model (FFM) and, 55
DSM-IV
  cross-cultural research and, 50
  five-factored model (FFM) and, 53,
    55, 56, 58–59, 61
  level of pathology and, 354, 355
  personality organization and, 358
  Shedler–Westen Assessment
    Procedure—200 (SWAP-200)
    and, 365
DSM-IV-TR, 40

Dual processing theory, 271
Dysphoria, 314–317
Dysregulation, 265

E

Eating disorders, 13–14
Ego, 337
Ego psychology
  functional assessment and, 347
  overview, 341–343
Emic studies, 50. *see also* Cross-
    cultural replication
Emotion
  affective regulation and control,
    186–190
  developing treatments and, 272–275
  functional assessment and, 350
  incentive motivation and, 221–222
  interactive nature of emotional traits
    and constraint, 243–246, 244*f*,
    246*f*
  primary motivational systems and,
    176–186
  regulation of, 190–199, 273–274,
    342–343, 350–351, 365
Emotional learning systems, 231
Emotional numbing, 307–308
Emotional regulation
  developing treatments and, 273–274
  ego psychology and, 342–343
  functional assessment and, 350–351
  individual differences in, 190–199
  Shedler–Westen Assessment
    Procedure—200 (SWAP-200)
    and, 365
Emotional stability, 45*t*
Emotional suffering, 304–311
Emotionality instability, 43
Emotionality, negative. *see* Negative
    emotionality
Emotionality, positive. *see* Positive
    emotionality
Empathy
  conduct problems and, 119
  prosociality and, 126
Endogenous endorphins, 222–225
Endophenotypes, 2
Engagement, 276–277

Environmental influences
  behavior genetic approaches and,
    123–125, 126*f*, 155–157
  conduct disorder and, 128–130
  developmental propensity model
    and, 122–123
  dispositional dimensions and, 137–
    140
  mediational models of causes of CD
    symptoms and, 131–132, 131*f*
  overview, 4
  personality-as-risk model and, 157–
    165
Erratic parenting, 161–162
Error-related negativity (ERN)
    response, 196–197
Etic studies, 50
Etiology
  Big Two dimensions of temperament
    and, 12–13
  common cause model of, 13
  pathoplasty model of, 12–13, 19,
    265
  of the relations between E/PE and
    psychopathology, 21–22
  of the relations between N/NE and
    psychopathology, 18–19
  scar model of, 13, 19, 155, 169–
    170, 265
  spectrum model of, 13, 155, 165–
    169, 167*f*, 168*f*, 265
  vulnerability model of, 12–13, 19,
    264–265
Evaluative trait
  developing treatments and, 273
  five-factored model (FFM) and, 42
  interpersonal perception and, 72–73
  transference and, 299
Evidence-based treatment, 278
Exacerbation model, 265. *see also*
    Pathoplasty model
Executive functioning, 118–119
Expanded Form of the Positive and
    Negative Affect Schedule
    (PANAS-X), 11–12, 12*t*
Expectancies
  behavioral confirmation of, 300–301
  role violations and, 305–306
  transference and, 300

Exposure-based treatments, 270–271
Extended amygdala, 230
Externalizing problems
  behavior genetic approaches to,
    128–130
  behavioral inhibition and, 118
  DSM and, 174–175
  emotionality and, 120
  individual differences in the
    regulation of emotions and,
    195–199
  negative emotionality and, 116–117
  spectrum model of etiology and,
    168–169
Extraversion
  affective basis of temperamental
    traits and, 11
  alcohol consumption and, 162
  dopamine system and, 210–211
  five-factored model (FFM) and, 8,
    43, 45t, 47–48
  impulsivity and, 236–238, 237f
  individual differences in, 243–246,
    244f, 246f
  neurobehavior model and, 215–216
  personality disorders and, 54t, 213
  positive emotionality and, 11–12
  in the two-factor model of
    personality, 9
Extraversion/Positive Emotionality (E/
    PE)
  clinical traits and, 29–31
  overview, 8–9, 31–32
  psychopathology and, 18t, 19–22
  temperamental basis of, 12t

F

Factor analysis, 371n–372n
Family members, in the Peer
    Nomination Study, 96–97
Family, perception of, 163
Fear
  individual differences in the
    regulation of emotions and,
    192–193, 199
  neurobehavior model and, 227–229
  neurobiology of, 229–241, 231f,
    233f, 234f, 237f, 239f

Fear dimension, 17
Fear response, 180
Fearful–avoidant attachment, 270
Fight-or-flight system, 116
Filipino culture, five-factored model
    (FFM) and, 51
Five-factor model (FFM)
  affective basis of temperamental
    traits and, 11–12, 12t
  applying to clinical practice, 367–
    368
  construct validity of, 44, 45t, 46–52
  lexical foundation of, 40–44
  overview, 2–3, 8, 265–266
  personality disorders and, 53, 54t,
    55–62
  problem of modeling personality
    disorders and, 213
  prosociality and, 125
  Shedler–Westen Assessment
    Procedure—200 (SWAP-200)
    and, 365
Frost Multidimensional Perfectionism
    Scale (FMPS), 28, 29
Functional assessment, 346–347, 348t,
    349–353
Functioning, adaptive
  functional assessment and, 349–351
  integration of with other personality
    components, 358–364, 363f
  overview, 371n–372n
Functioning, executive, 118–119
Functioning, psychological
  neuroticism/negative emotionality
    (N/NE) and, 13–14
  Structured Clinical Interview for
    DSM-IV (SCID), 25

G

Gene–environment correlation, 159–
    160
Gene–environment interaction, 161–
    165
Generalized anxiety disorders
  Extraversion/Positive Emotionality
    (E/PE) and, 20–21
  neuroticism/negative emotionality
    (N/NE) and, 14–15

Genetic factors. *see also* Behavior genetic approaches
  behavior genetic approaches and, 123–125, 126*f*, 155–157
  developing treatments and, 265–267
  developmental propensity model and, 122, 122–123
  dispositional dimensions and, 137–140
  five-factored model (FFM) and, 49–50
  mediational models of causes of CD symptoms and, 130–137, 131*f*, 133*f*, 136*f*
  N/NE and E/PE dimensions and, 10
  overview, 3–4
  personality-as-risk model and, 157–165
Global Assessment of Functioning (GAF)
  level of pathology and, 353–354, 355–356
  neuroticism/negative emotionality (N/NE) and, 14
Global positive affect, 309–310
Goals, personal, 306
Goals, treatment, 281

H

Health–sickness continuum, 353–354
Heritability of personality traits, 49–50. *see also* Genetic factors
Heritability of temperamental traits. *see also* Genetic factors
  N/NE and E/PE dimensions and, 10
  personality-as-risk model and, 157–165
Heterogeneity of symptoms, 15–16
Hierarchical structure of personality
  overview, 7–8, 31–32
  superfactor models of personality and, 8–9
Hippocampus
  emotional processing and, 190
  individual differences in the regulation of emotions and, 197

Histrionic personality disorder
  attachment disturbances and, 270
  personality organization and, 357
  problem of modeling personality disorders and, 213
  social functioning and, 85
Honesty–humility trait, 42
Hopelessness, 318–320
Hostility
  five-factored model (FFM) and, 46–47
  relational self and, 309–311
Hysterical personality style, 357

I

Id, 337
Imagination, 8
Impulse regulation, 351
Impulsiveness. *see also* Conscientiousness; Constraint
  five-factored model (FFM) and, 47–48
  individual differences in the regulation of emotions and, 196, 198
  interactive nature of, 243–246, 244*f*, 246*f*
  neurobehavior model and, 216
  neurobiology of, 236–241, 237*f*, 239*f*
Incentive motivation
  impulsivity and, 236
  multidimensional model and, 247, 247*f*
  neurobehavior model and, 221–225
Incentive salience model, 184–185
Independent pathways model, 166–167, 168*f*
Inferences, transference and, 297–299
Inhibitedness, 265
Inhibition, behavioral
  anxiety and, 228–229
  compared to daring, 118
  individual differences in the regulation of emotions and, 197
  startle reflex and, 230
Insight-oriented treatments, 270–271

Instability, behavioral, 243–246, 246*f*
Integrated treatment
   cognitive approaches to treatment
      and, 275
   for complex patients, 277–278
   early adversity and, 271
   overview, 283
Intellect
   conduct problems and, 118–119
   five-factored model (FFM) and, 8, 44
Internal working models
   anxiety and hostility and, 309
   early adversity and, 270
Internality, 9
Internalizing problems
   DSM and, 174–175
   fear response system and, 182
   individual differences in the
      regulation of emotions and,
      191–195
   negative emotionality and, 116–117
   overview, 16–17
   spectrum model of etiology and,
      167–169
International Affective Picture System
      (IAPS), 177
International Pilot Study of Personality
      Disorders (WHO, 1992), 50–51
Interoceptive stimuli, 218
Interpersonal behavior, 343
Interpersonal functioning
   functional assessment and, 349–353
   relational self and, 294
   transference and, 293
Interpersonal models, 312–314
Interpersonal perception, 72–73, 104–
      106. *see also* Peer Nomination
      Study
Interpersonal problems, 84–86
Interpersonal script, 295–296
Interpersonal treatment, 279
Introversion, 45*t*
Inventory of Interpersonal Problems
      (IIP), 85–86
   in the Peer Nomination Study, 106*n*

J

Judgmental evaluations, 42

L

Language development
   conduct problems and, 118–119
   lexical foundation of, 40–41
Lateral/basolateral complex, 179–180
Learned helplessness, depression and,
      318
Learning systems, 231
Life tasks, 276–277

M

Major depression. *see also* Depression
   comorbidity and, 153
   heterogeneity of symptoms and, 15–
      16
   individual differences in the
      regulation of emotions and,
      193
   neuroticism/negative emotionality
      (N/NE) and, 14–15
   overlap of with other pathologies,
      263–264
Maltreatment
   developing treatments and, 269–272
   gene–environment interaction and,
      161–162
   heritability of antisocial behavior
      and, 140
   mentalization deficits and, 345
   relational self and, 307–308
Managed care, 280–283
Mania, 211
Marriage, alcohol consumption and,
      161
Mediational models
   conduct disorder and, 130–137,
      131*f*, 133*f*, 136*f*
   developmental propensity model
      and, 121
   dispositional dimensions and, 137–
      140
Memory
   early adversity and, 271
   ego psychology and, 342
   expectancies and, 300
   mediational models of causes of CD
      symptoms and, 131–132, 131*f*
   prefrontal cortex and, 187–188

psychoanalytic theory and, 339
relational self and, 294, 295, 301
transference and, 297–298
Mental representations
attachment system and, 309–311
depression and, 311–312, 321–322
integrating perspectives on
personality structure and, 369
object relations theory and, 344–345
relational self and, 294, 305–307
relationships and, 292
Mentalization deficits, 344–345
Metaperception, 93–94
Mindfulness, 275
Monoamine oxidase A gene (MAOA),
162
Mood and Anxiety Symptom
Questionnaire (MASQ), 22–23,
24t
Mood disorders
differential relations within, 14–15
heterogeneity of symptoms and, 15–
16
neuroticism/negative emotionality
(N/NE) and, 13–14
Mood, transference and, 305–307
Morphine
affiliate reward and, 222–225
mu opiate receptors and, 226
Motivation, incentive
impulsivity and, 236
multidimensional model and, 247,
247f
neurobehavior model and, 221–225
Motivational interviewing technique,
279
Motivational systems
affective regulation and control,
186–190
approach–avoidant, 302
defensive and appetitive, 178–186
dopamine system and, 210–211
functional assessment and, 349
individual differences in, 190–199
multidimensional model and, 247,
247f
neurobehavior model and, 217–226,
219f
overview, 176–178, 199–200

Mu opiate receptors
affiliate reward and, 222–225
compared to dopamine projection
system, 225–226
Multi-source Assessment of Personality
Pathology (MAPP)
compared to peer data, 86–93, 87t,
88t, 91t
compared to the SNAP scales, 81t
metaperception and, 93–94
overview, 107n
in the Peer Nomination Study, 76–
78, 97
self-report section, 78–80, 80t
validity of, 98–101, 99t
Multidimensional model, 246–249,
247f
Multidimensional Personality
Questionnaire, 196
Multivariate behavior genetic models
conduct disorder and, 130
spectrum model of etiology and, 169

N

N–methyl-D-aspartate (NMDA), 180
Naloxone, 222, 224–225
Naltrexone, 222, 224–225
Narcissistic personality disorder
Multi-source Assessment of
Personality Pathology (MAPP)
and, 77
personality organization and, 356
semistructured diagnostic interviews
and, 98
National Institute of Mental Health
(NIMH)
translational research and, 39–40
Treatment of Depression
Collaborative Research
Program, 264
Negative cognition
depression and, 311–312
developing treatments and, 272–
275
Negative emotionality. see also
Neuroticism
behavior genetic approaches to,
127–128

Negative emotionality (*continued*)
  Cholesky decomposition model and,
    136–137, 136*f*
  clinical traits and, 29–31
  conduct problems and, 120
  dispositions and, 116–117
  individual differences in the
    regulation of emotions and,
    192
  mediation of genetics and
    environmental influences and,
    137–140
  mediational models of causes of CD
    symptoms and, 131–132, 131*f*
  motivational systems and, 177–178
  neuroticism and, 11
  overview, 8–9, 31–32
  psychopathology and, 12–22, 18*t*
  Shedler–Westen Assessment
    Procedure—200 (SWAP-200)
    and, 365
  temperamental basis of, 10–12, 12*t*
Negative temperament, 9
Neglect, 269–272
NEO Five-Factor Inventory
  gene–environment correlation and,
    160
  overview, 11
NEO Personality Inventory—Revised
    (NEO PI-R)
  five-factored model (FFM) and, 56
  overview, 44, 45*t*, 46–52
  problem of modeling personality
    disorders and, 214
Neurobehavioral model
  anxiety and, 229–241, 231*f*, 233*f*,
    234*f*, 237*f*, 239*f*
  higher-order personality traits and,
    215–229, 219*f*
  individual differences in personality
    traits and, 241–242, 242*f*
  interactive nature of emotional traits
    and constraint, 243–246, 244*f*,
    246*f*
  overview, 4–5, 210–212
  personality disturbances and, 246–
    249, 247*f*
  problem of modeling personality
    disorders and, 212–215

Neurobiological influences
  defensive and appetitive
    motivational systems and, 178–
    186
  overview, 4–5
Neuroticism. *see also* Negative
    emotionality
  affective basis of temperamental
    traits and, 11
  alcohol consumption and, 162
  avoidant personality disorder and,
    266
  behavioral inhibition system and,
    266
  clinical traits and, 29–31
  comorbidity and, 153
  five-factored model (FFM) and, 8,
    45*t*
  negative emotionality and, 11
  neurobehavior model and, 215–216,
    227–229
  overview, 8–9, 31–32
  personality disorders and, 54*t*
  posttraumatic stress disorder and,
    159
  predisposition to, 265
  problem of modeling personality
    disorders and, 213
  psychopathology and, 12–22, 18*t*
  Shedler–Westen Assessment
    Procedure—200 (SWAP-200)
    and, 365
  temperamental basis of, 10–12, 12*t*
  in the two-factor model of
    personality, 9
Neuroticism Extraversion Openness
    Personality Inventory (NEO-PI-
    R), 154
Neuroticism/negative emotionality (N/
    NE)
  clinical traits and, 29–31
  overview, 8–9, 31–32
  psychopathology and, 12–22, 18*t*
  temperamental basis of, 10–12, 12*t*
Neurotransmitters, 138–139
Nonaffective constraint, 240–241
Nonshared Environment in Adolescent
    Development (NEAD) project,
    170

Noradrenergic function, 138
Novelty seeking, 47–48
Nucleus reticularis pontis caudalis
    (nRPC), 181
Numbing
    early adversity and, 307–308
    ego psychology and, 342

O

Object relations theory
    functional assessment and, 347,
        351–352
    overview, 343–346
Obsessive–compulsive disorder
    Extraversion/Positive Emotionality
        (E/PE) and, 20–21
    five-factored model (FFM) and, 53,
        54t, 55
    heterogeneity of symptoms and, 15–
        16
    level of pathology and, 355
    overlap of with other pathologies,
        263–264
    Peer Nomination Study and, 102–
        104, 103t
    psychoanalytic theory and, 339–
        340
Obsessive–compulsive traits, 59–60
Openness to experience
    Big Three structure and, 9
    five-factored model (FFM) and, 8,
        44, 45t
    personality disorders and, 54t, 213
    schizotypal traits and, 59–60
Opiate antagonists, 222, 224–225
Oppositional defiant disorder (ODD)
    behavior genetic approaches to,
        128–129
    overview, 113
Other-protective self-regulation, 304
Overlap between personality
    pathologies, 263–264
Oxytocin antagonists, 224

P

Panic, 20–21
Panic disorder, 182
Paragiganticocellularis (PGi), 234–235

Paranoid personality disorder
    ego psychology and, 341
    level of pathology and, 355
    MAPP self-report scales and, 79–80
    neurobehavior model and, 214
    Peer Nomination Study, 95
Parenting
    early adversity and, 269–270
    gene–environment interaction and,
        161–162
Passive genotype–environment
    correlation, 160
Pathology, levels of
    integration of with other personality
        components, 358–364, 363f
    overview, 353–356
Pathoplasty model of etiology
    overview, 12–13, 265
    relations between N/NE and
        psychopathology and, 19
Pavlovian associative learning, 220–
    221, 226
Peer groups, 96–97
Peer Nomination Inventory. see Multi-
    source Assessment of
    Personality Pathology (MAPP)
Peer Nomination Study
    assessment procedures, 76–82, 78t,
        80t, 81t
    comparison of self-report and peer
        data in, 86–93, 87t, 88t, 91t
    distress and social impairment, 82–
        86, 83t, 84t
    informants and, 94–97
    metaperception and, 93–94
    overview, 104–106
    participants in, 73–76
    predictive validity of peer
        nominations and, 101–104,
        103t, 104t
    validity of semistructured diagnostic
        interviews and, 98–101, 99t
Perceiver effects, 72
Perception of self, 71
Perceptions of family, 163
Perfectionism, 28
Personality
    Cloninger's model of, 121
    function of, 154–155

Personality-as-risk model, 157–165
Personality Disorder Interview-IV
 (PDI-IV), 80
Personality Disorder Questionnaire
 (PDQ-IV), 107n
Personality disorders
 five-factored model (FFM) and, 2–3,
  53, 54t, 55–62
 forms of, 356–358
 level of pathology and, 354
 neuroticism/negative emotionality
  (N/NE) and, 13–14
 overview, 106n–107n
 personality-as-risk model and, 157–
  165
 problem of modeling, 212–215
 spectrum model of etiology of, 165–
  169, 167f, 168f
Personality disturbances
 model of, 246–249, 247f
 rather than the terminology of
  "personality disorders", 214–
  215
Personality organization, 356–358
Personality structure
 clinical conceptualizations of, 346–
  347, 348t, 349–364, 363f
 integrating perspectives on, 364–
  365, 366t, 367–371
 overview, 337–338
Personality traits. see also Big Two
  dimensions of temperament;
  Five-factor model (FFM); Two-
  factor model
 applying to clinical practice, 367–
  370
 forms of, 356–358
 individual differences in, 241–242,
  242f
 integration of with other personality
  components, 358–364, 363f
 interactive nature of, 243–246, 244f,
  246f
 neurobehavioral systems and, 215–
  229, 219f
 psychoanalytic theory and, 340–341
Physical attractiveness, 42
Pleasantness, 177
Pleasurable emotion, 194–195

Positive emotionality
 motivational systems and, 177–178
 overview, 9
Positive incentive motivation, 218
Posttraumatic stress disorder (PTSD)
 cognitive processes and, 273
 ego psychology and, 342
 fear response system and, 182
 heterogeneity of symptoms and, 15–16
 individual differences in the
  regulation of emotions and, 194
 overlap of with other pathologies,
  263–264
 personality-as-risk model and, 157–
  160
Potentiated startle paradigm, 181
Predicting psychopathology, 13–14
Prediction error, 183
Predisposition/vulnerability model,
  264–265. see also Vulnerability
  model
Prefrontal cortex
 emotional processing and, 186–190
 individual differences in the
  regulation of emotions and,
  196–197
Preoccupied attachment, 310
Prevention focus, 303
Primary care models, 282
Primary motivational systems. see also
  Motivational systems
 affective regulation and control,
  186–190
 defensive and appetitive, 178–186
 dopamine system and, 210–211
 individual differences in, 190–199
 overview, 176–178, 199–200
Promotion focus, 303
Prosociality
 behavior genetic approaches to,
  125–127
 Cholesky decomposition model and,
  136–137, 136f
 dispositions and, 117, 119–120
 mediation of genetics and
  environmental influences and,
  137–140
 mediational models of causes of CD
  symptoms and, 131–132, 131f

Proximal exteroceptive stimuli, 218
Psychoanalytic ego psychology, 341–343
Psychoanalytical theory
    functional assessment and, 347
    level of pathology and, 353–356
    overview, 336–337
    from symptom to character in, 338–346
    transference and, 294–295
Psychodynamic perspective, 5–6, 346–347, 348t, 349–364, 363f
Psychopathology
    behavior genetic approaches to, 123–125, 126f
    Big Two dimensions of temperament and, 12–22, 18t
    dispositions and, 115–116
Psychoticism
    Constraint and, 9
    level of pathology and, 354
Punitive parenting, 161–162

Q

Q-factor analysis, 358
Q-sort methodology, 90–91, 91t

R

Reactive genotype–environment correlation, 160
Reactivity, 272–275
Regulatory focus theory, 303
Relatedness, 43
Relational schema model, 295–296
Relational self
    depression and, 311–320
    evidence that supports, 296–311
    limitations of the research on, 320–322
    overview, 292–293, 293–296, 322–323
Relationships. see also Relational self
    affiliative reward and, 220
    object relations theory and, 343–346
    overview, 72
Religiosity
    alcohol consumption and, 164–165
    five-factored model (FFM) and, 42

Representation of others. see also Transference
    attachment system and, 309
    functional assessment and, 351–352
    overview, 245–246
    relational self and, 304
Representation of self, 351–352
Response Style Questionnaire (RSQ), 27, 29, 30
Responsiveness, emotional, 272–275
Revised Eysenck Personality Questionnaire (EPQ-R)
    alcohol consumption and, 162
    gene–environment correlation and, 160
Reward behavior, 182–186
Reward-learning model, 184–185
Reward system
    interactive nature of emotional traits and constraint and, 244–245
    multidimensional model and, 247, 247f
    neurobehavior model and, 217–226, 219f, 221–225
Rewarding goals, 217–218
Risk factors
    developing treatments and, 264–265
    personality as, 157–165
Risk model, 154–155
Role violation, 305–306
Ruminative response style
    Big Two dimensions of temperament and, 27
    depression and, 319–320

S

Scaffolding, 343
Scar model of etiology. see also Complication model
    overview, 13, 155, 169–170, 265
    relations between N/NE and psychopathology and, 19
Schedule for Nonadaptive and Adaptive Personality. see SNAP scales
Schema, self
    depression and, 311–312, 317–320
    overview, 295–296

Schizoid personality disorder
  five-factored model (FFM) and, 53
  MAPP self-report scales and, 79–80
  personality organization and, 356–357
  Structured Interview for DSM-IV Personality (SIDP-IV) and, 81–82
Schizophrenia
  cross-cultural research and, 51
  Extraversion/Positive Emotionality (E/PE) and, 21–22
  neurobehavior model and, 214
  neuroticism/negative emotionality (N/NE) and, 13–14
  relation with psychopathology, 20
  spectrum model of etiology and, 165
Schizotaxia, 165
Schizotypal personality disorder
  case example of, 359–364, 363f
  five-factored model (FFM) and, 57
  integrating perspectives on personality structure and, 365, 366t, 367
  neurobehavior model and, 214
  Structured Interview for DSM-IV Personality (SIDP-IV) and, 81–82
Schizotypical traits, 59–60
Secure attachment, 270
Self-consciousness, 266
Self-criticism, 27
Self-discrepancy theory
  agitation-related affect and, 314
  depression and, 313
Self-enhancement, 303
Self-fulfilling prophecy, 301. see also Behavioral confirmation
Self-harm
  Structured Clinical Interview for DSM-IV (SCID), 24
  validity analyses and, 25
Self-insight, 3
Self–other agreement, 86–93, 87t, 88t, 91t
Self-perception. see Perception of self
Self psychology, 347
Self-Realization, 9
Self-reflection, 369

Self-regulation, 302–303, 305
Self-report measures
  compared to peer data, 86–93, 87t, 88t, 91t, 94
  integrating perspectives on personality structure and, 369
  in the Peer Nomination Study, 78–80, 80t, 85
  semistructured diagnostic interviews and, 98–101, 99t
Self-schema, 295–296
Semistructured diagnostic interviews
  in the Peer Nomination Study, 80–82, 82t
  validity of, 98–101, 99t
Sensation seeking. see also Impulsiveness
  association of with being a victim of rape, 159
  five-factored model (FFM) and, 47–48
  neurobiology of, 236–241, 237f, 239f
Serotonin receptors
  conduct disorder and, 138–139
  interactive nature of emotional traits and constraint and, 244–246, 246f
  nonaffective constraint and, 240–241
Seven-factor model, 367
Sexuality, 369
Shedler–Westen Assessment Procedure—200 (SWAP-200)
  case example of, 359–364, 363f
  integrating perspectives on personality structure and, 364–365, 366t, 367–371, 368–369
  personality organization and, 358
Situationally accessible memory, 271
SNAP scales
  clinical traits and, 30
  compared to the MAPP, 79–80, 81t
  five-factored model (FFM) and, 46–47
  Mood and Anxiety Symptom Questionnaire (MASQ) and, 22
  overview, 32
  in the Peer Nomination Study, 76, 92–93, 102–103, 103t, 106n
  validity analyses and, 25–26

Sociability
  behavior genetic approaches to,
    125–126
  Extraversion/Positive Emotionality
    (E/PE) and, 21–22
  prosociality and, 119
Social Adjustment Scale (SAS-SR), 83,
    84–85, 106n
Social anxiety
  Extraversion/Positive Emotionality
    (E/PE) and, 20, 21–22
  Structured Clinical Interview for
    DSM-IV (SCID), 24–25
Social causality, 351–352
Social closeness. see Agreeableness
Social functioning
  depression and, 315
  Peer Nomination Study and, 84–86
Social Functioning Questionnaire
    (SFQ), 83, 84
Social impairment, 82–86, 83t, 84t
Social learning approaches, 113
Social network techniques, 89
Social phobia
  cognitive processes and, 273
  Extraversion/Positive Emotionality
    (E/PE) and, 20
Social relations model, 72
Socialization, 303
Socioeconomic status, 118–119
Sociotropy, 314
Somatoform disorders, 13–14
Spectrum model of etiology, 13, 155,
    165–169, 167f, 168f, 265
Stability, behavioral, 244–246, 246f
Stability of traits
  five-factored model (FFM) and, 48
  N/NE and E/PE dimensions and, 10
  personality disorders and, 74–75
Standards of others, 312–313
Startle reflex
  amygdala and, 181
  neurobiology of, 229–232, 231f,
    233f
Stress response system, 235–236, 312
Structure, personality, 5–6
Structured Clinical Interview for DSM-
    IV (SCID)
  level of pathology and, 354–355

neuroticism/negative emotionality
    (N/NE) and, 15, 17
  validity analyses of, 24–25
Structured Interview for DSM-IV
    Personality (SIDP-IV), 76, 80–
    82, 82t, 100, 105–106
Substance use
  dopamine system and, 185
  incentive motivation and, 221–222
  individual differences in the
    regulation of emotions and,
    197–198
Substance use disorders
  neuroticism/negative emotionality
    (N/NE) and, 13–14
  overlap of with other pathologies,
    263–264
Superego, 337
Symptom-based analyses, 15
Symptom neurosis, 338–346
Symptom overlap, 212. see also
    Comorbidity
Symptoms, heterogeneity of, 15–16

T

Target effects, 72
Taxonomic classifications, 16–18, 18t
Temperament
  developing treatments and, 267–269
  dimensions of, 2, 7–9, 31–32. see
    also Extraversion/Positive
    Emotionality (E/PE);
    Neuroticism/negative
    emotionality (N/NE)
  dispositions and, 116
  N/NE and E/PE dimensions of, 10–
    12, 12t
Temperament-based models of
    personality, 7. see also
    Extraversion/Positive
    Emotionality (E/PE);
    Neuroticism/negative
    emotionality (N/NE)
Temporal stability of traits
  five-factored model (FFM) and, 48
  N/NE and E/PE dimensions and, 10
  personality disorders and, 74–75
Therapeutic alliance, 279–280

Thought disorder, 368
Thought processes, 350
Thought suppression, 275
Threshold response, 238–239, 239f
Tonic inhibitory influence, 240
Traits of personality, 26–31, 31t
Transference
    anxiety and, 5
    depression and, 311–320
    evidence that supports, 296–311
    limitations of the research on, 320–
        322
    overview, 293–296
Translational research, 39–40
Trauma
    early adversity and, 271
    personality-as-risk model and, 158–
        160
Treatment goals, 281
Treatment of Depression Collaborative
    Research Program, 264
Treatments, developing
    biological/genetic vulnerabilities and,
        265–267
    common factors and processes, 278–
        280
    for complex patients, 277–278
    facilitating engagement with valued
        life tasks and, 276–277
    integrated treatment and, 283
    managed care and, 280–283
    negative cognition and emotion and,
        272–275

overview, 262–263
risk and, 264–265
temperamental vulnerabilities and,
    267–269
Two-factor model. see Big Two
    dimensions of temperament

U

Unconventionality, 44
Undependability, 45t
Univariate behavior genetic models,
    130

V

Verbally accessible memory,
    271
Vigilance, 180
Vulnerability
    avoidant personality disorder and,
        266
    depression and, 311–320
Vulnerability model of etiology
    overview, 12–13, 264–265
    relations between N/NE and
        psychopathology and, 19

W

Working memory, 131–132, 131f
Working models, internal
    anxiety and hostility and, 309
    early adversity and, 270